*f*P

The TRIPLE WHAMMY CURE

THE BREAKTHROUGH WOMEN'S HEALTH PROGRAM FOR FEELING GOOD AGAIN IN 3 WEEKS

DAVID EDELBERG, M.D.

WITH HEIDI HOUGH

FREE PRESS
New York London Toronto Sydney

FREE PRESS
A Division of Simon & Schuster, Inc.
1230 Avenue of the Americas
New York, NY 10020

FREE PRESS and colophon are trademarks
of Simon & Schuster, Inc.

Designed by Kris Tobiassen

Manufactured in the United States of America

ISBN-13: 978-0-7432-6907-0
ISBN-10:   0-7432-6907-1

ACKNOWLEDGMENT

Some years ago, I was attending my first meeting of the American Holistic Medical Association. It was there I heard for the first time Christiane Northrup, M.D., and Caroline Myss. The audience, mainly physicians nervously crossing over into the realms of holistic and alternative medicine, was spellbound. By the time the afternoon was over, Chris had changed forever all I had previously learned about women's health and Caroline, describing chakras and energy systems, altered forever my understanding of the human body. A decade later, I offer this book with heartfelt thanks.

CONTENTS

III. Triple Whammy Cure Plus: Healing Paths for Triple Whammy Disorders

IV. Triple Whammy Resources

A NOTE TO YOU, THE READER:

WHY I WROTE THIS BOOK

My patients frequently tell me a lot about themselves as we jointly try to understand their health. And when they do, I feel blessed to be allowed this glimpse into the heart and mind of a fellow human being. Each tale is unique, and I'm perpetually astonished by the profound courage, pain, and endurance that my female patients display. One morning recently, it came to me that, on virtually every working day for the past thirty years, I've been taking care of people, listening as they revealed their lives and pains, their anxieties and fears. In fact it was my patients' stories that led me to write this book.

As a holistic doctor, I'm committed to treating whole people. I don't simply treat their diseases and believe that all people are pretty much interchangeable—that they have the same reactions to the causes of illness or to the illnesses themselves—the way I was taught in medical school. I listened as my patients told me the details of their lives, and I began to see patterns of poor health. So many women came to me to ask why they felt so unwell even after endlessly hearing doctors tell them that all their tests were normal and nothing was really wrong.

Does any part of this sound like your own story? You've been feeling just plain crummy for too long. In fact, you're beginning to have some difficulty remembering when you last felt "just fine."

Quite reasonably, you want an explanation for your chronic ill health. You don't want to be told you look fine and that your test results are normal. You're getting weary of seeing doctors, getting referrals, and taking medicines that don't help. You want a way out of this mess. You want your health back.

Let's clear the air right away: your symptoms are valid and you do feel awful. You are not a hypochrondriac. "So," you say, "if my tests are normal, and my doctor says I don't have a disease, what exactly do I have?"

Follow this carefully: what you're experiencing is not a disease, as doctors think of disease, but rather the consequences of a susceptibility you have as a woman on three separate fronts. Your symptoms are the result of a three-pronged assault—a "triple whammy" so to speak—consisting of:

- stress

- a shortage of a chemical in your brain called serotonin

- your ever-shifting female hormones

You can't get a gene transplant hoping to erase your factory-installed genetic susceptibility to low serotonin. But there are definite steps you can take to prevent this susceptibility from manifesting itself—steps that are simple and effective.

And that's why I wrote this book. I decided that the five finest words any doctor can ever hear are "I think I'm feeling better," and my patients tell me they do feel better when they follow the Triple Whammy Cure. In fact, some of them say they feel like they got their lives back.

Up to now, you've probably been losing against the Triple Whammy assault. Some women have come to believe that feeling crummy is unavoidable, but it's not. Your situation is far from hopeless. In fact, with a few lifestyle changes, nutritional supplements, and some safe, gentle alternative therapies, women with the Triple Whammy can get their lives back. So it's time to turn things around. It's time to:

- develop healthy strategies to deal with stress

- increase your serotonin levels

- balance your hormones

This book will show you how.

PART I

UNDERSTANDING THE TRIPLE WHAMMY

1.

WHAT IS THE TRIPLE WHAMMY?

Believe me, I tried to think of a more scientific name for what's going on here. But really, what would *you* call a health problem that affects tens of millions of women, and is caused by three separate but tightly connected factors that work together? Furthermore, it's a health problem that's not a disease but that does underlie women's most common medical conditions. Doctors certainly agree that any of the three components of the Triple Whammy taken separately can cause all sorts of unpleasant symptoms. But they'll also tell you things like, "You have to learn to live with it" or "There's not a lot that can be done."

What makes up the Triple Whammy? It's a devilish interaction among three factors: non-stop stress, low levels of stress-buffering serotonin (a brain chemical that is behind good moods), and imbalances in your female hormones. That's right. The situation that's making so many women feel anywhere from the euphemistic "less-than-well" all the way to the "utterly crummy" consists of stress, serotonin, and hormones. Here's why:

– **WOMEN ARE POORLY PROTECTED AGAINST THE RAVAGES OF STRESS** on their bodies because they have less available serotonin, which acts as a buffer to damp down the physical effects of chronic stress.

- **WOMEN ARE GENETICALLY PREDISPOSED TO LOW SEROTONIN,** one of the feel-good neurotransmitters in our brains. Women actually have more serotonin than men, but it doesn't work as efficiently.

- **WOMEN HAVE SHIFTING TIDES OF HORMONES**—which themselves control serotonin levels and function—monthly and throughout life.

And the result? These three factors conspire to make millions of women feel miserable, living their lives with Triple Whammy symptoms that often progress to one or more Triple Whammy disorders.

TRIPLE WHAMMY SYMPTOMS

Produced by the tangled influence of chronic stress, low levels of serotonin, and fluctuating hormones, Triple Whammy symptoms include feeling "beaten up"—tired, achy, anxious, depressed, forgetful, headachy, and lacking energy and focus. Forgetfulness and sleep problems are common, as is a bloated feeling, with constipation or diarrhea. Craving carbohydrates (a cry for the body to produce more serotonin) is another symptom. Women with these symptoms chug through life feeling less than well most of the time. When things get really bad, women with Triple Whammy symptoms go to their doctor and hear the discouraging refrain "all your tests are normal."

Here's something I want to repeat, because it's hopeful: your Triple Whammy is not a disease. But if you don't resolve its symptoms, one or more of the Triple Whammy disorders listed on page 24 usually develops. Each disorder involves a low level of serotonin aggravated by stress and is made worse by shifts in your female hormones, estrogen and progesterone.

To complicate matters, low-serotonin disorders run through families like fault lines in California. While all women have less serotonin than men, some women also carry the "depression gene," making them even more vulnerable to Triple Whammy disorders.

HOW YOU CAN FEEL WELL AGAIN

Repeat after me: "Simple, fixable, not a disease. I can feel well again." Notice that I didn't lighten up the Triple Whammy by calling it "just an imbalance." Girl, this is an imbalance from hell.

In this book, I offer you some powerful ways to quell the effects of the Triple Whammy. The Triple Whammy Three-Week Cure is all-natural, easy to follow, and inexpensive. It produces results very quickly, clearing the vast array of symptoms you've been experiencing and restoring the good health that seems like a remote memory. So it's time to turn things around. Time to get your life back. So, now you can turn to Chapter 4 and begin the Three-Week Cure, or stay with me here while we look at the Whammies, so you can learn why the cure works.

THE WHAMMIES, EXPLAINED

WHAMMY #1: THE CHEMISTRY OF STRESS

What exactly is stress and why does it affect us so badly? Here's one definition: stress is any situation in which you've unwillingly relinquished the ability to control your life. The controlling force can be a person (a dictator of a country, a boss, a boyfriend) or something inanimate (a deadline, a tax audit, the "dark"). Adapting to stress in a positive way can lead to good things, like ambition, accomplishment, courage, and creativity. But stress can also be destructive.

When faced with stress of any kind, our bodies are hardwired to respond in a series of ways that are designed to protect us. This series of events, called the stress response, allows us to either fend off stress (fight) or escape it (flight), leading to its common name, the fight-or-flight response. The system is triggered when the adrenal glands, a pair of walnut-sized glands sitting one each atop your kidneys, receive distress messages from your brain. The adrenals then release the hormone adrenalin, which in the right situation—such as escaping a mugger—can be lifesaving.

As these hormones pour into your system, they kick up your heartbeat, raise your blood pressure, churn your intestines, increase your blood sugar, tighten your muscles, and rechannel the blood flow in your body so that you're primed to respond physically, either with a swift kick to the crotch or the fastest hundred yard dash imaginable. Fleeing (or fighting off) the mugger is followed by panting relief, shakiness as your body processes the wash of hormones, and ultimate recovery. But let's say the person you thought was a mugger turns out to be a friend. You didn't have to fight or flee, it turns out, but your body, in preparation, would have undergone the stress response anyway, and now you feel utterly drained. Even though you "did" nothing—your body simply got you ready to do something—you're exhausted. Remember this "exhausted" part, because it becomes very important later on.

Our truly elegant, primitive response to an actual threat was designed to be turned on and off. It was not built to accommodate chronic stress. Our bodies simply can't cope with the jolts of one stress response after another. Repeated bursts of adrenalin tighten muscles painfully ("I carry my stress in my neck"), change the way blood circulates in your body ("my hands and feet are always cold"), and throw digestion out of whack ("I get diarrhea whenever I'm nervous"). When stress shifts from being an occasional isolated event into a way of life, additional symptoms begin to appear. Chronic stress makes you feel anxious, depressed, and tired all the time, interferes with sleep, causes you to eat carbohydrates to generate stress-buffering serotonin, and bollixes up concentration and short-term memory.

But in modern life, chronic stress does enter our lives. And let's face facts. During the past fifty years, the day-to-day stresses faced by women have multiplied exponentially. As the many women I treat tell me, they are stretched so thin that they feel as if they're always avoiding the spinning blades of a Cuisinart. Contemporary women are, in the vast majority of families, responsible for meeting the needs of partners, children, and aging parents while maintaining the house, paying the bills, and organizing their own and their family's life. Many also hold a paying job. And single women have a different range of stressors that are just as valid.

Of course, each of these factors in itself is no mugger with a gun, but taken together they're extraordinarily stressful. With constant stress, though, you don't have a rush of adrenalin alone. Unrelenting stress stimulates a different system in your body—your endocrine glands. Constant stress will turn some of these glands to "high," ultimately exhausting them, while deliberately suppressing your ovaries (also endocrine glands), which interferes with sex drive, ovulation, and the timing of your periods. This shows the body's common sense: it's not a good idea to get pregnant when the world is sending a constant stream of stressful messages. What happens next is that chronic stress sends alarm signals to a small section of your brain called the hypothalamus, which in turn relays volleys of stress information on to your pituitary gland. A cherry-sized little thing, the pituitary is the "master" gland in your body, tucked safely out of harm's way on the underside of your brain, resting royally in a curve of bone whose Latin name translates to "Turkish saddle." (Try to imagine your master-gland pituitary sitting there, piloting you around like a Boeing 747.)

The back end of the pituitary releases a single hormone, vasopressin, which jacks up your blood pressure and speeds up your heart. The front end controls your other endocrine glands: the thyroid (essentially your body's gas pedal); a portion of your adrenal glands (called the *adrenal cortex*), which release the hormone cortisol; and your ovaries (which produce sex hormones).

ENDOCRINE ACTIVATION AND CHRONIC STRESS

In the chronic stress of your harried life, it will be endocrine activation that dominates your stress response. Your adrenaline fight-or-flight response never gets turned off during chronic stress, however. Rather, during a particularly bad week it will pepper your constant-stress endocrine response with adrenalin bursts during especially stressful moments. As each of your glands gears up in response to chronic stress, you may feel any of the following sensations, each of which represents *a physical change in your body trying to resist the stressor:*

- **THYROID:** nervousness, excessive sweating, tremulousness. Obviously this is very similar to an adrenalin rush but slower, and more prolonged.

- **ADRENAL CORTEX (THE OUTSIDE PART OF THE ADRENAL GLANDS):** elevated blood sugar, fuzzy thinking, rise in blood pressure, fall in awareness of pain (the hormone cortisol acts as an antiinflammatory, similar to aspirin or ibuprofen), gas and bloating, constipation and diarrhea.

- **OVARIES:** diminished sex drive, change in menstrual cycle.

Again, your body wasn't meant to be hit with a bevy of stressors without some downtime in between. As it tries to cope with the various stressors of your day, your body turns your endocrine gland system to high—and holds it there. You don't have to know much about cars to realize that if you put the gears in neutral and keep the gas pedal pressed to the floor, you'll burn out your motor before too long. And if your stressors continue unchecked, that's precisely what will happen to you.

Both stress responses, acute and chronic, are meant to be temporary, the acute for a few minutes (the mugger); the chronic for a few hours or days (final exam week, finishing a board report). Each of these responses is meant to come to an end. The human body simply cannot tolerate a nonstop stress response of any kind.

SEROTONIN IS YOUR FACTORY-INSTALLED BUFFER
AGAINST STRESS—YOUR RESISTANCE

This is a good time for me to introduce serotonin briefly, although I discuss it in more detail on page 12. Serotonin is a brain chemical called a neurotransmitter,

WHAT ABOUT MEN AND LOW SEROTONIN?

Men are susceptible to all Triple Whammy disorders except the obvious, like PMS and postpartum depression. But recently, during a conference on antidepressants, I learned something that seemed almost like that last piece in a jigsaw puzzle.

Some background: when reviewing the life stories of women with Triple Whammy disorders, I'd heard frequently how Dad "may have been depressed, but his real problem was anger," or "we always walked on eggshells around Dad," or "an alcoholic, a mean drunk." And, sadly, almost a fifth of fibromyalgia patients report physical and/or sexual abuse, usually from a male relative, often Dad.

So, at the meeting, I asked about this.

The psychiatrist answered, "In men, we now know that low serotonin disorders often manifest as impulse control disorders and anger disorders. In fact, chronic sexual offenders, who are almost always male, obviously have a real impulse control issue. And yes, they're treated with SSRI antidepressants to control their otherwise uncontrollable behavior."

and for the time being, consider it your factory-installed buffer against stress—your resistance. The more you have, the better you're able to tolerate stress, both sudden and chronic. But women have less available serotonin than men, so you're poorly protected, and your susceptibility to stress is much greater. To give you a sampling of serotonin's effect, consider what many people say when, by means natural or pharmaceutical, their serotonin levels rise. They'll say "What used to really stress me out doesn't anymore" or "I simply don't feel as anxious as I once did." On the surface, it may sound as if they've been handed a tranquilizer. But serotonin isn't a tranquilizer; it's simply a chemical already present in your brain that increases your resistance to stress. And if you follow the steps in this book to increase your serotonin, within no time it will soar. As it does, your mood, energy, and sex drive will improve, your cravings for junk carbs and sugar will disappear, and you'll feel like a new woman.

EXHAUSTION LEADS TO TRIPLE WHAMMY DISORDERS

Let's talk about the exhaustion of chronic stress. As your body becomes overwhelmed by the relentless task of resisting multiple constant stressors, your protective mechanisms start to fail. Understanding how the stress response goes awry and wreaks its destructive effects on the body is key to understanding the

Triple Whammy. The whole array of Triple Whammy symptoms and disorders is triggered by unrelenting stress that is able to attack your body freely because you're unprotected by adequate serotonin and buffeted by shifts in your hormones. But let me quickly add that, if you're going through any of this, you can get out of it and have your health restored to normal.

Emotionally, as your systems crash under constant stress, you may get tired, moody, irritable, and withdrawn and ultimately develop depression. Your level of anxiety about relatively minor stressors may increase so much that you're not even sure what's making you anxious anymore. You just feel anxious all the time, and may even experience surges of panic. Some women might fall back to an old abnormal behavior pattern or develop a new one. If you had an eating disorder as a teen, it may resurface. You may find yourself repeatedly checking the locks on your doors or whether you turned off the stove, working over and over in your mind the same negative thoughts, first signs of what may be later diagnosed as obsessive-compulsive disorder.

Moving on to physical symptoms, your muscles may remain so constantly tight that you can no longer relax them. Certain spots within your muscles become so tender that a massage therapist can feel hard, painful knots. If the muscle pain persists, you may go on to develop fibromyalgia (which means simply "muscle pain"). This is not a disease, but rather a reaction of your muscles having become "stuck" trying to resist chronic stress.

Your internal organs will suffer from stress, too. The intestinal churning from stress may proceed to the cramping, bloating, pain, nausea, and diarrhea/constipation that defines irritable bowel syndrome. Surges of hormones—adrenalin from your adrenal gland and vasopressin from your pituitary—contract blood vessels throughout your body and may affect an especially vulnerable blood vessel in your brain. As it pulsates, you feel the throbbing of a migraine approaching.

Always tense and irritable, you may clamp your jaw tight, and if it fails to relax, you're stuck with chronic pain in your temporomandibular joint (TMJ). Part of the stress response includes racing thoughts, triggered by the cortisol that's secreted by your adrenal gland. Over a period of time, this cortisol washing through your body actually blocks short-term memory and your ability to focus on details or fully concentrate fades. Hormones from your stress-driven pituitary cause a shift in your sex hormones that can change your periods, impair your fertility, or trigger symptoms of premenstrual syndrome (PMS).

Finally (and, fortunately, only rarely), overwhelmed with unchecked stress, you may collapse into an exhausted heap, first for days, then for weeks or even months, staggering into your doctor's office, to learn that you have all the signs of chronic fatigue syndrome (CFS), again not a disease, but one of the most dramatic outcomes of stress.

HOW THE TRIPLE WHAMMY IS A REFLECTION OF THE STRESS RESPONSE

Triple Whammy symptoms and Triple Whammy disorders are actually intense exaggerations of all the body changes that occur during the stress response. Please read that sentence again. The stress response is central to all these Triple Whammy problems. But stress plays a commanding role in the onset of many diseases. For instance, researchers recently discovered the so-called depression gene and found that people born with it are more likely to develop depression after exposure to stress.

FATIGUE AND EXHAUSTION OF THE THYROID, ADRENAL GLANDS, AND OVARIES

All doctors don't agree, but I'm convinced that the demands of chronic stress on these three endocrine glands impairs their function—first overstimulating them and then exhausting them. In fact, some Triple Whammy symptoms may well be caused by this glandular fatigue. Your thyroid, adrenals, or ovaries aren't "diseased" in any way, but with exhaustion (depletion) simply produce less of their hormones.

Symptoms of stress-related thyroid fatigue and exhaustion include fatigue, dry skin, intolerance to cold, mild constipation, and fuzzy thinking. These are the very same symptoms caused by an underactive thyroid due to thyroid disease, and if you tell your doctor you have these symptoms she'll probably (and possibly correctly) diagnose you as having an underactive thyroid. To verify, she may do a test to check your levels of thyroid-stimulating hormone (TSH), which, if high, indicates an underactive thyroid gland. (As an aside, TSH does not come from the thyroid gland, but rather is a stimulant sent from your pituitary gland to get your thyroid to produce more hormone. A high level of TSH indicates a low level of thyroid function, a fact that endlessly confuses medical students, because the pituitary keeps sending out TSH in an effort to get the thyroid to function properly.)

If your test results come back showing normal levels of TSH, both you and your doctor may be surprised, given your symptoms. But these normal test results do not (repeat, *do not!*) necessarily indicate that your thyroid is functioning normally. There are two reasons for this:

- The so-called normal range for TSH is currently questioned by leading endocrinologists. Now it seems that many people who'd been told in past years that their thyroid was normal may need treatment. For years, any TSH above 5.0 was interpreted to mean the person had an underactive thyroid. Now an increasing number of physicians will begin treating those with a TSH of 3.5 or higher if they show other signs of underactive thyroid.

- Some doctors (myself included) are beginning to question altogether the value of a normal TSH. We're asking "What happens to our patients who have all the symptoms of an underactive thyroid (hypothyroidism) but a completely normal TSH test result?"

What I do is this: if your TSH test results are normal but you have the symptoms (fatigue, dry skin, cold intolerance, mild constipation, muddled thinking), we recheck your thyroid gland using an old-fashioned screening test that measures basal body temperature (p. 75) for several days. If temperatures average 97.6 or lower after testing for a number of days, I prescribe a small dose of thyroid replacement hormone, usually 30 mg (one half grain). This basal temperature diagnostic test was used by conventional doctors for more than fifty years and is extremely accurate.

Interestingly, stress-related thyroid exhaustion can reverse itself after stress is addressed, your serotonin is increased, and your body starts functioning smoothly again—unlike other forms of thyroid underactivity. For this reason, taking thyroid replacement hormone for stress-induced thyroid fatigue/exhaustion is rarely a lifetime commitment, as it is when you have actual thyroid disease. In other words, you likely won't have to stay on the small hormone dose forever.

Symptoms of stress-related adrenal fatigue or exhaustion include fatigue, low blood pressure, and feeling especially lightheaded when you rise suddenly from a stooped position. And just as the symptoms of stress-related thyroid problems are the same as low thyroid caused by a thyroid disease, adrenal fatigue symptoms are the same as an uncommon adrenal gland disorder called Addison's disease. As you might suspect, the treatment for Addison's disease is to take adrenal hormones.

To diagnose adrenal fatigue/exhaustion, doctors measure levels of cortisol (an adrenal hormone) and DHEA (a building block of adrenal hormones), collected via blood or saliva during one twelve-hour period. If you have adrenal fatigue or exhaustion, you may need to take a short course of adrenal gland hormones along with nutritional supplements to restore proper function to your adrenal gland.

Therapies I use, and which you can request from your doctor, include 5 mg of hydrocortisone (cortisol) once or twice a day, 10–25 mg daily of DHEA, and other nutritional supplements combined and sold as adrenal support products. Again, these are not permanent therapies and usually you can discontinue them in fewer than four months, once you get a handle on your stress and take steps to improve your serotonin levels.

Symptoms of stress-related ovarian fatigue include changes in your menstrual cycle and PMS, which is triggered by an imbalance between estrogen and progesterone, and almost always worsens during periods of stress. The interplay of pituitary hormones affects the maturation of an egg and its release for fertilization, as well as the amount of estrogen and progesterone produced by your ovaries. In addition, the adrenal gland is a secondary source of sex hormones, DHEA being a building block of progesterone.

The effects of chronic stress on your ovaries may also contribute to infertility. Doctors are beginning to appreciate that infertility caused by the ominous-sounding "ovarian failure" may have a lot to do with the effect of unchecked stress on ovulation. It is possible that women could avoid the need for many extraordinarily stressful (and expensive) infertility treatments if they reduced their stress.

WHAMMY #2: SEROTONIN, POWERFUL STRESS BUFFER

Serotonin is needed in the brain to allow nerve cells to communicate with each other. Without neurotransmitters, the billions of nerve cells that make up your brain would sit idle and you'd be unable to think or even move. Depression is perhaps the best-known low-serotonin disorder, but serotonin is also intimately involved in the action of your intestines, blood vessels, and blood clotting. That's a pretty broad role for a single molecule, so you can see why serotonin might be involved in such seemingly unrelated Triple Whammy conditions as depression, migraines, and irritable bowel syndrome.

A genuinely annoying fact about serotonin is that it is unfairly distributed between the sexes. Women actually have more serotonin in their brains than men, but it simply doesn't work as well. Men's levels of serotonin operate much (much!) more efficiently than women's. And because women's brains are deprived of adequate serotonin, they're poorly equipped to handle stress. To make matters more complex, serotonin levels are influenced by your hormones.

To understand how neurotransmitters like serotonin work, consider this sequence of events: you remember you need to add milk to your grocery list, see the list on the fridge, grab a pen, and write down the word "milk." Sounds simple enough, but your family dog will never master this. Fetching the pen and writing the word gives the illusion that there's a single thread-like nerve traveling from your brain to your fingertips. But this isn't the case. Picture instead that your brain consists of billions of nerve cells, each separated from hundreds of its neighbors by extremely tiny gaps, called synapses. When information—an electrical impulse, actually—in one brain cell needs to get to the next cell, the particle of information needs to jump the gap. I use the phrase "one brain cell" only to describe the mechanics of the process, because just to think of the word "milk" and then picture the container, you're actually activating millions of brain cells.

NEUROTRANSMITTERS AND RECYCLING?

Here's how jumping the synapse gap works. When information reaches the transmitting end of one nerve cell, it's carried by neurotransmitter molecules across the gap to the receiving end of the next nerve cell, where it locks onto a receptor site and transmits the information. The neurotransmitter molecule is then recycled back into the first nerve cell for reuse. (Remember this recycling process because it's very important when we talk about how antidepressants work.)

Every thought you have, every emotion, perception (like hearing, seeing, or feeling), and movement—whether voluntary, like reaching for the pen, or involuntary (your beating heart)—involves your nervous system and requires neurotransmitters. Without them every aspect of your existence would come to a screeching halt.

Researchers have identified several different neurotransmitters working inside the brain, each involved in different activities. Serotonin is predominant; others are norepinephrine, acetylcholine, and dopamine. Part of serotonin's predominance comes from the idea that it seems to control the release of other neurotransmitters, and can attach itself to a greater variety of nerve cell receptor sites than the others. Large amounts of serotonin are also located elsewhere in your body, including your gastrointestinal system, blood vessels, and platelets (small particles in your blood needed for clotting).

The other neurotransmitters play significant roles, too. Norepinephrine is involved with focus and concentration (the treatment of attention deficit disorder includes increasing the levels of norepinephrine). Acetylcholine is linked to memory, and the new drugs for slowing Alzheimer's disease increase its levels. Dopamine is involved in movement, and is the mainstay of Parkinson's disease treatment.

WOMEN, EVOLUTION, AND SEROTONIN

Doctors know that the rates of depression, anxiety and panic disorder, obsessive-compulsive disorder, eating disorders, fibromyalgia with chronic fatigue, irritable bowel syndrome, and migraines are always higher among women than men. They knew this even before they knew the chemistry behind these disorders. When doctors discovered the relationship between low serotonin and emotional disorders, they started comparing the serotonin levels between sexes and found that women simply were not making enough and that it can be plentiful in certain parts of your female brain, but not in others—at least not enough to protect you against stress.

But nobody is exactly positive why this is. One guess—and it's only a guess—shifts us back to our prehistoric days, when men were hunter-gatherers and women stayed back at the cave or camp and took care of the kids. Out in the woods, their lives perpetually at risk, men needed to develop some adjustment in their brain chemistry to avoid having a panic attack when they heard something crunching the twigs behind them. Hence, they evolved an increased amount of serotonin, a stress buffer. Women, on the other hand, didn't need this same protection until relatively recently, during the past several generations, when the playing field for women changed considerably, and their lives underwent tremendous transformation. Even though you face more stress than ever, more than your ancestors, today's women rely on a serotonin buffer little changed from tens of thousands of years ago.

Some years ago, doctors first began to note a link between low levels of serotonin and depression when studies showed that reserpine (a drug for high blood pressure no longer used) could trigger depression to the extent that suicide was actually a possibility among users. Then it was discovered that reserpine depleted serotonin inside the brain, so researchers began measuring serotonin in the spinal fluid of previously depressed patients. They found that serotonin levels were consistently low and that serotonin levels could be increased using medication. This eventually led to serotonin's nickname as the "feel-good" neurotransmitter.

Discovering this biochemical cause for disorders like depression and anxiety is indeed one of the miracles of twentieth-century medical research. As recently as fifty years ago, a woman with severe depression might have found herself committed to a state mental hospital, often for years. Some of my interest in women's health came about when I gained access to the medical records of my grandmother, years after she'd died in one of these hospitals. Because of the stigma associated with mental illness, I'd been told she had died as a young woman, when in fact she'd spent virtually her entire adult life institutionalized. I had not even known she was alive when I was young. Years later, as I looked through her doctor's notes, I realized sadly that she could have lived a real life if only antidepressants had been invented a few decades earlier.

HOW SEROTONIN BUFFERS STRESS AND WHAT OCCURS IF YOU DON'T HAVE ENOUGH

Research during the past few years has taught us a lot about serotonin and other neurotransmitters. For example, a combination of serotonin and norepinephrine (which helps us focus and concentrate) regulates how well we react in response to both positive and negative stress. A soldier preparing to defend her comrades or a high school senior taking her SATs becomes more focused, even hyperalert, as levels of norepinephrine rise, helping her concentration and attention in the face of an impending task. But both women also need adequate levels of serotonin to prevent—buffer, actually—their hyperalert state from intensifying into a panic attack or despair. For both soldier and student, stress can escalate even further in one of two ways:

- In the first case, stress escalates because the stress itself actually increases. In other words, the actual event triggering the stress can get more intense: a bombing begins or the test booklet is opened.

- In the second case, the stressor itself is unchanged, but without an adequate serotonin stress buffer, the perception of stress escalates.

In both situations—actual stress or stress perceived—*the result can be the same.* With escalating stress of either type, the brain sends a distress signal to the adrenal glands to release additional stress hormones: epinephrine and, to a lesser extent, cortisol. These hormones flood into the soldier and the student, putting their bodies into overdrive, speeding up their hearts, tensing their muscles, racing their thoughts. Obviously, the stress response is a two-edged sword, helpful for the soldier if the bombing is actually under way, but definitely the wrong re-

A URINE TEST THAT
MEASURES YOUR SEROTONIN

Until recently, it's been costly and time consuming to determine levels of serotonin and other neurotransmitters (like epinephrine, dopamine, and norepinephrine) in the human body. Recently, however, researchers have developed techniques to measure neurotransmitters in a urine sample. Several labs now offer this, but I've mainly been using NeuroScience (www.neurorelief.com), which offers its services only through your health care provider. The test comes in a convenient kit; you collect a small urine sample and mail it directly to the lab. Your doctor can obtain levels of both neurotransmitters and sex hormones in this way. Since these are FDA-approved tests and really not alternative medicine, many insurance companies will reimburse without batting an eyelash. You just need to be nice to your doctor because many physicians are still resistant to this kind of evidence and aren't familiar with the research. If your doctor is hesitant, contact the lab above for a list of doctors in your area who will provide you with a prescription for the test during an appointment. I've ordered dozens of these tests and the most common pattern I see in my Triple Whammy patients is low serotonin and low epinephrine (adrenalin). This combination shows me their predisposition to stress susceptibility (low serotonin) and the effect of unrelenting stress on the internal portion of the adrenal gland (the medulla), which depletes its supply of epinephrine. I also test the outside portion of the adrenal gland (the cortex) using samples of saliva to measure the levels of cortisol and the "prehormone" building block DHEA (dehydroepiandrosterone). Low levels of cortisol and DHEA mean the adrenal gland has been dealing with unrelenting stress but still trying to keep the body running as smoothly as possible. It's important to understand that the adrenal gland is not diseased, but rather exhausted (see p.11). By lowering stress, increasing your stress buffer serotonin, and taking personal time for self healing you can return the numbers to the normal range. To me, the most important aspect of the test results is how a patient can see for herself that her symptoms are real—that she isn't "just a little depressed," as her doctor may have said. And although her doctor may have also told her "all your tests are normal," it may be that the doctor has simply been ordering the wrong tests.

action for the student to feel ten minutes (or ten hours) before the exam even starts—or after it's over.

When faced with a stressful situation, whether actual and dangerous or created by unrealistic worry, if you don't have enough serotonin, two things can happen: your mood may plummet and you'll become apathetic or you'll become anxious in the extreme, sometimes to the point of panic.

Although you need the hyperalert state of norepinephrine and the stress response of epinephrine, you also need serotonin to act as a buffer against those situations. Triple Whammy disorders are not diseases as we usually define disease, but rather the emotional and physical symptoms of stress unchecked by sufficient amounts of serotonin.

SEROTONIN'S ROLE IN PLEASURE AND PAIN

Serotonin is also involved with our appetites. Our enjoyment of the scents and flavors of food correlates to levels of serotonin. For depressed people, for example, food often loses its taste and scent and instead they may crave substances that either mimic neurotransmitters (like alcohol, tobacco, or caffeine) or change the levels of neurotransmitters in the brain (like sugar, carbohydrates, and other comfort foods).

People with low levels of serotonin also perceive pain more strongly than those with normal levels because they have an increased sensitivity to a chemical called Substance P (for Pain). People with chronic pain disorders have reduced levels of serotonin and are more susceptible to depression. Serotonin also causes the smooth muscles of your intestines to contract, and increasing serotonin levels alleviates the symptoms of irritable bowel syndrome (p. 103). Likewise, changes in serotonin levels affect our susceptibility to migraine headaches (p. 136), triggered by stressful spasms of blood vessels.

SEROTONIN AND ESTROGEN: THE ROLLER-COASTER EFFECT

The relationship between serotonin activity and your sex hormones is complex. Estrogen increases the amount of all neurotransmitters, including serotonin, and also increases the number of receptor sites for them. With more receptor sites, you can make more connections in your brain. To put it simply, with higher levels of neurotransmitters and more receptor sites for them, you're smarter, and can think faster and more creatively.

The relationship between estrogen and feel-good serotonin is so sensitive that I think of it as a two-car roller coaster, with estrogen the front car, pulling serotonin behind. When estrogen is high, as it is during pregnancy or during the two weeks after your period, most women feel pretty good because their estrogen and serotonin levels are both moving upward. The drop in estrogen during PMS days can make you cry at a Hallmark commercial or bite the head off your partner. That same estrogen-serotonin drop is also responsible for the misery of postpartum depression and the increased frequency of mild depression in women going through the menopause transition.

This relationship between serotonin and estrogen is fundamental to how you'll be treating Triple Whammy symptoms and disorders. The mild depression of perimenopause can respond quite well to the natural serotonin-boosters in the Three-Week Cure; sometimes you'll also need small doses of either bioidentical hormone replacement, serotonin-boosting herbs, or prescription serotonin-raising antidepressants. Likewise, you can resolve any moodiness you feel during PMS days by following the serotonin-boosting steps in the Three-Week Cure, taking herbs that increase serotonin, antidepressants, or (sometimes) birth control pills.

Here's another statistic to consider: it's estimated that some 40 percent of the population has a genetic susceptibility to serotonin-related disorders and that a majority are female. This means almost half of us have been born with a trait that prevents us from having enough serotonin when the situation calls for it— on top of the fact that all women have less available serotonin. This is why you need to know how to make more for yourself.

HOW TO MAKE SEROTONIN WITHOUT TAKING A PILL

Since serotonin is so thoroughly useful, it would be handy if we could just "take some" to build up our stress barrier, ease pain, and get quick relief from Triple Whammy disorders. Currently, we just can't do this. Serotonin is a delicate molecule and would be destroyed by your stomach acid before it could be absorbed. And even if you could get serotonin into your bloodstream, it wouldn't be able to cross the internal shield known as the blood-brain barrier, a specialized system of cells designed to keep any but the most essential nutrients away from your vulnerable brain. Even though serotonin is necessary to the brain, the molecule itself is too large and too complex to pass through this guardian barrier.

You might be asking yourself, "But what about antidepressants—don't they contain serotonin?" We're coming to that, but first let me say that it's not particularly difficult to increase the serotonin in your brain without drugs. And since we can always use some extra protection from the stress in our lives, having above-average serotonin levels is almost always a good idea. There are three immediate steps you can take to help your brain make more serotonin and they're outlined in the Three-Week Cure: sunlight, exercise, and carbohydrate timing. There are also two bonus serotonin boosters: laughter and kindness. Learn jokes, visit comedy clubs, rent only comedies from your video store. And perform acts of kindness. People who regularly volunteer to help others have measurably higher levels of serotonin.

HOW SSRI ANTIDEPRESSANTS INCREASE SEROTONIN

With the help of your doctor and her prescription pad, you can increase serotonin by taking prescription antidepressants. They work by increasing the levels of serotonin (and other neurotransmitters) in the synapse gap between two nerve cells—specifically by blocking your brain's neurotransmitter recycling system. Remember on page 13 we discussed that neurotransmitters jump the synapse gap between nerve cells to move information from one brain nerve cell to another, and are then recycled back into the first nerve cell for reuse. This recycling is how today's antidepressants work. Older antidepressants, like amitriptyline, simply made more serotonin. These are still in use, but side effects like drowsiness and dry mouth have made them less popular. The newer antidepressants—Prozac, Paxil, Lexapro, and others—are called selective serotonin reuptake inhibitors, SSRIs for short. These drugs block the reentry (reuptake) of released serotonin. SSRIs keep the serotonin from getting back inside the original brain cell, leaving serotonin in the gap, where it accumulates, causing levels in the gap itself to rise and work their magic.

The process of recycling released serotonin by blocking reentry takes from two to six weeks. It takes that long for enough serotonin to build up in the gap to make a noticeable difference.

Other antidepressants, like Effexor and Wellbutrin, work with other neurotransmitters and thus are not SSRIs.

There's a difference between the sexes when using antidepressants. For many women, a tiny dose—as little as one-fourth the dose used for men—works nicely. Pharmacologists believe that women in general are more drug-sensitive than men, again possibly because of low serotonin levels. It's best for women to start with a small dose and work slowly upward to avoid side effects. Everyone, but especially women, must be cautious when stopping antidepressants. Your brain has grown accustomed to the added neurotransmitters and doesn't want the boat rocked. Unless you gradually taper off your dose (your doctor can tell you the best way), you can experience headaches, dizziness, problems walking, and a return of your depression and anxiety. These effects almost never occur when your dose is reduced gradually.

NUTRITIONAL SUPPLEMENTS THAT INCREASE SEROTONIN

Now that you understand the two ways of increasing serotonin—making more on your own and recycling it using antidepressants—you'll see how nutritional supplements can be helpful. Because nutritional supplements are generally safe and simple to take, I often recommend that my patients first try the make-your-own-serotonin steps and these supplements before turning to an antidepressant.

- **ST. JOHN'S WORT** This herb crosses the blood-brain barrier and acts in the brain like a mild version of an SSRI antidepressant, allowing serotonin to accumulate slowly in the synapse gap. Because it works like an antidepressant, you shouldn't take both St. John's wort and a prescription antidepressant simultaneously. Doing so can make you feel nervous, "wired," and can interrupt your sleep. A February 2005 study in the *British Medical Journal* finally put to rest the effectiveness of St. John's wort as an antidepressant for people with moderate to severe depression. Half the study's partcipants took the antidepressant Paxil (paroxetine); the other half took a minimum 900 mg daily of St. John's wort. After six weeks on these regimens, one third of those taking the Paxil felt less depressed; but one half of those taking St. John's wort were less depressed. The well-designed study also showed that St. John's wort caused fewer side effects than Paxil.

- **5HTP** Along with St. John's wort, to increase serotonin further you can add the amino acid 5HTP (5-hydroxytryptophan). Although serotonin can't pass the blood-brain barrier, 5HTP can, and once it's in the brain it converts to serotonin, making 5HTP a building block for new serotonin.

- **B VITAMINS AND FISH OIL** These are needed to grease the wheels for smooth serotonin production, which is why they're an integral part of the Three-Week Cure.

WHAMMY #3: THE BIOLOGY OF HORMONES

Women can only guess how mysterious they are to men. I was highly impressed when I learned that menstrual cycles and moon cycles were the same length. And women's bonding impresses men, too. Men have buddies and pals, but generally we tackle life alone, rarely experiencing the degree of intimacy women share with friends, endlessly supportive. Sisterhood implies a man-free barrier, the "we'll talk about it later" look that passes between women when a man enters the room. The menstrual cycles of women living together start synchronizing, so it could be said that women are not only connected by emotional and spiritual bonds, but their bodies are magically linked together as well. Very, very impressive.

Hormonally speaking, every day something different is happening within you. With periods, PMS, pregnancy, and the menopause transition, there's a lot

Q & A: MENOPAUSE

Q. I've had a little forgetfulness and minor depression during menopause, plus some annoying hot flashes. Is there a connection between this and the Triple Whammy?

A. Yes. At menopause (and before, during perimenopause), estrogen and progesterone levels decline. As these hormones drop, so do your levels of serotonin—the feel-good neurotransmitter. The result is that some women feel more depressed or anxious and may have problems with concentration and memory.

To fix this: first, follow the Triple Whammy Three-Week Cure to shore up your serotonin, balance hormones, and, of course, reduce stress. If brain fog and poor focus continue to be an issue, read and follow the Memory Loss and Brain Fog healing path on page 111.

Here's an interesting fact that shows you how closely hormones and neurotransmitters like serotonin work together: a study published a year and a half ago proved that stubborn hot flashes can be dramatically relieved by taking very small doses of the antidepressant Effexor or Prozac. If after following the Three-Week Cure for a couple of months you don't see improvement in your mild depression and hot flashes, ask your doctor about taking a minidose of Effexor XR. The smallest capsule is 37.5 mg, but you can open it and shake out about half the granules inside to take a small dose.

If depression or anxiety predominates, ask about the antidepressant Lexapro. The standard starting dose of Lexapro is 10 mg but my patients often start with a minidose of as little as 2.5 mg or 5 mg to minimize the drug's side effects.

going on. Your body produces three sex hormones. Most familiar are your female hormones, estrogen and progesterone, mainly made in the ovaries. The third is the male hormone testosterone, a small amount of which is secreted from your ovaries and adrenal glands. Levels of estrogen and progesterone are controlled by your pituitary gland, the body's master gland, which controls your ovaries, thyroid, and adrenals. The pituitary affects your ovaries by releasing two hormones—follicle-stimulating hormone (FSH) and luteinizing hormone (LH). How much of each is secreted depends on two separate factors:

- First, your pituitary "reads" the amount of estrogen and progesterone circulating in your blood at any given moment and then pumps up or turns down FSH and LH.

- Second, your pituitary responds to emotional information relayed from an area of your brain called the hypothalamus, a key command center for the interaction between your mind and body. The hypothalamus is very sensitive to stress. Most women have had their periods thrown off cycle by stress at one time or another.

Here's an example of how the control system works: during the menopause transition, when the amounts of estrogen and progesterone being produced by the ovaries are very low, your pituitary responds by pumping out large amounts of FSH and LH in an attempt to get the ovaries started up again. This is fruitless because your ovaries are pretty much done producing these hormones. (Women who want to confirm that they're in the menopause transition sometimes have their levels of FSH and LH tested, and very high readings confirm the diagnosis. The same holds true for women undergoing infertility testing; doctors measure FSH and LH levels to see if the ovaries are functioning. If they're not, FSH and LH levels will be high.)

Your hormones fluctuate day to day, month to month, and year to year in a cycling system that kicked in when you were about twelve. Your brain and pituitary gland are always working to control your cycle. This constant hormonal shifting gives you an idea why "measuring" your hormone levels on any given day, or even during a single month, may not be all that helpful. Smaller amounts of your hormones were around several years before puberty, making you decidedly different from your brother but not enough to get your period started. Most women have sufficient hormones to keep their periods going until their late forties or early fifties, when things change and your periods become irregular and scantier because levels of uterus-stimulating progesterone are in decline. Ultimately, your periods will stop altogether, although your ovaries will continue to produce some hormones for the next few years.

TWO HORMONE SHIFTS . . . AND POSSIBLE IMBALANCE

There are really two separate hormone shifts throughout the course of your life. You have your monthly rise and fall of estrogen and progesterone, as well as a lifetime s-l-o-w rise and fall of these hormones. The situation is not unlike how the earth itself cycles, rotating on its axis as it travels around the sun. Ideally, this lifetime of hormonal tides should proceed without any problems, uninterrupted except by pregnancy. What generally causes trouble—meaning uncomfortable symptoms rather than disease—are imbalances in the system.

Stress is a frequent source of this hormone imbalance. The entire hormonal system is highly sensitive, and when your pituitary gland receives stress-laden messages relayed from the hypothalamus, the changes in FSH and LH that follow can throw off your cycle or interfere with ovulation. Stress reduction becomes a key factor in getting your hormones back on track when dealing with PMS, the menopause transition, and even infertility. You might also be surprised by the extent that unhealthful food choices play in hormonal imbalances. Junky diets are a recipe for PMS. The Triple Whammy Food Plan is an easy eating program that can help bring everything back into alignment, sometimes without any other therapies at all.

You may unwittingly bring upon yourself one of the most common hormone problems. If you ever took birth control pills and simply couldn't stand how they made you feel, you were experiencing one of those imbalances: too much estrogen. Side effects were a real problem with the first generation of oral contraceptives because the estrogen content was so high. Now birth control pills contain synthetic estrogens in microgram-sized doses (that's one ten-thousandth of a gram), and side effects are less common. But despite these minuscule doses, many women continue to report nausea, breast swelling and tenderness, bloating, headaches, and vaginal yeast infections, all symptoms of excessive estrogen that stop abruptly when the pill is discontinued. On the other hand, many women report feeling much better when taking the pill. They simply do better when an outside influence runs their hormonal system, correcting any subtle imbalances.

If the symptoms of excessive estrogen sound suspiciously like another common hormone problem, premenstrual syndrome (PMS), you're absolutely right. During the second half of your cycle, after you ovulate, estrogen falls slowly as progesterone rises. In the days before your period, progesterone falls as well. But for many women, the estrogen does not fall quickly enough, bringing about estrogen-dominant (or progesterone-deficient) PMS, along with breast tenderness, bloating, and fluid retention. This can be easily treated (see PMS, p. 153) using the herb chasteberry, which acts on the pituitary and balances the two hormones. Or you can simply increase your progesterone levels by applying a progesterone-containing skin cream or taking capsules of progesterone itself.

To some degree, every woman experiences hormonal imbalance when she goes through menopause. Unlike PMS and its estrogen excess / progesterone deficiency, in menopause your body encounters an overall estrogen lack. Potential symptoms (not all women experience them) include hot flashes, night sweats, vaginal dryness, headaches, fatigue, and urinary incontinence. Virtually all can be eliminated in a few weeks with hormone replacement therapy. But I know you might not be thrilled with that idea. So in the Menopause Transition healing path (p. 120) we'll talk about alternative approaches to menopause, including easy changes in your eating habits, herbs like black cohosh, and bioidentical replacement hormones.

TRIPLE WHAMMY DISORDERS

As you read this list, remember that each condition involves a low level of the stress-protector serotonin that's further aggravated by chronic stress and made worse by shifting hormones, which themselves control serotonin levels. Triple Whammy disorders tend to appear and reappear throughout a susceptible woman's life. Most important, though, these disorders *can* be resolved by starting the Triple Whammy Three-Week Cure and following the appropriate healing path in Triple Whammy Cure Plus (p. 57).

- ANXIETY DISORDERS

- CHRONIC FATIGUE SYNDROME

- DEPRESSION

- FIBROMYALGIA

- IRRITABLE BOWEL SYNDROME (IBS)

- MENOPAUSE TRANSITION

- MEMORY LOSS AND BRAIN FOG

- MIGRAINE HEADACHES

- POSTPARTUM DEPRESSION

- PREMENSTRUAL SYNDROME (PMS)

- SEASONAL AFFECTIVE DISORDER (SAD) AND WINTERTIME BLUES

- SLEEP PROBLEMS

- SMOKING

- TEMPOROMANDIBULAR JOINT DISORDER (TMJ)

- WEIGHT LOSS AGONIES

TESTOSTERONE AND SEX DRIVE

Women joke that men, primed with testosterone, are capable of having sex with anything that moves. And indeed that's the purpose for the tiny amount of testosterone in your female body—to give you a sex drive. Doctors prescribe testosterone to men and women to enhance declining sexual energy and interest. But too much testosterone can make you one of the guys, giving you a masculine voice, more facial hair, even some acne. Obviously, a woman's dose needs to be an exceedingly small one. The ever-helpful pharmaceutical industry provides several forms of estrogen-testosterone products for menopausal women to boost libido.

THE ROLLER COASTER THAT IS SEROTONIN + HORMONES

Your hormones demand attention and respect. They are powerful, with a capital P. Many women are well aware of the mood-related hormone symptoms: mental fuzziness, poor focus and concentration, depression, anxiety, moodiness, irritability, panic attacks, anger, and flares of rage. Hormone imbalance can also occur during the vulnerable weeks after delivering a baby, when susceptible women can be plunged into deep depression or develop obsessive-compulsive tendencies.

All these symptoms are examples of the intimate relationship between Whammy #2, low serotonin, and Whammy #3, your hormones. As I will remind you throughout this book, estrogen and serotonin are intimately related. When estrogen rises, as it does in the two weeks after your period and also during pregnancy, up goes serotonin, and with it your mood. But when estrogen falls, as it does before your period and also during the menopause transition or after delivering a baby, so does your mood and life can get difficult.

Add to all this Whammy #1, stress. Remember that serotonin is not only a neurotransmitter allowing brain cells to talk to each other, but also a buffer against stress. When you realize that you as a woman have only a fraction of the amount of serotonin available for stress-buffering as men, stressful events can have life-shattering consequences. When a stressful event happens during PMS days or perimenopause, when serotonin is even lower, your Triple Whammy symptoms (p. 4) and disorders can get a lot worse.

THYROID FATIGUE AND EXHAUSTION

"Although Carla's thyroid gland was basically only doing its job,
it had almost been destroyed by her doctor for doing so."

Carla's story is important, because it shows what can go wrong when conventional doctors confuse the stress response with actual disease. It's now recognized, for example, that tens of thousands of people are inappropriately taking medicines for high blood pressure when they really don't have a blood pressure problem at all. They just get nervous in the doctor's office and their blood pressure goes up when they're being tested. Carla, on the other hand, came within days of permanently losing her thyroid gland.

A bright woman in her mid-thirties, Carla was seeing a supportive non-MD counselor for depression because she'd been going through the worst year of her life. After a long engagement, her relationship was ending. An only daughter, Carla had elderly parents who were heartbroken for her unhappiness, and because the likelihood of seeing a grandchild now seemed pretty remote. Carla knew she'd be relearning how to be single, and while the thought frightened her a bit, with her counselor's help she'd come to recognize that it was preferable to being in a bad marriage.

Carla's depression seemed to be worsening, so the therapist had referred her to a psychiatrist, who could prescribe antidepressants. When the psychiatrist asked Carla to tell her everything she was feeling, Carla described times when she felt anxious—even "wired"—and of not being able to sleep at night because of a racing heart. The psychiatrist diagnosed her with bipolar disorder and prescribed medication for it. After taking it for a few weeks, Carla told her therapist that the new medication allowed her to sleep at night, but that she was still depressed and very tired.

The therapist suggested Carla visit her internist for a checkup—that perhaps she was anemic or her thyroid was underactive. Now on a hunt to determine exactly what was wrong, Carla saw her internist, who phoned the following day to share news that had surprised the doctor too: tests showed Carla's thyroid to be overactive rather than underactive (which would be expected given her fatigue). Her blood test had shown an increased blood level of thyroxine, the hormone produced by the thyroid gland. The internist wanted Carla to see a thyroid specialist, and so she did.

The specialist looked at Carla's blood tests and immediately started her on a medication to turn off thyroid hormone production. Carla took the drugs faithfully, along with her medicine for bipolar disorder. In the meantime, her break-up had been messy and stressful. Her father, during all this, had a mild heart attack, and Carla somehow blamed herself for it.

As weeks turned to months, Carla continued to feel miserable. Concerned that her heart seemed to be beating too rapidly, her thyroid specialist added a second medicine, called a beta-blocker, to slow it down. This made Carla's fatigue and depression even worse. Finally the specialist suggested that "to solve this thyroid issue once and for all," she take radioactive iodine to permanently destroy her thyroid gland. This way, the doctor explained, Carla could control the amount of hormone in her body by taking one thyroid pill a day for the rest of her life.

FATE INTERVENES

But then things seemed to change Carla's life. Summer arrived. She landed a job she enjoyed, and with it she was able to afford a nice apartment. Although she wasn't really interested in dating yet, she received a dinner invitation during the first month on her new job and was pleased to discover there were nice men in the world who were neither ex-fiancés nor lawyers.

Now feeling pretty good, her energy returning, Carla actually felt happy for the first time in a year. But she was scheduled for thyroid destruction in three weeks. In preparation, her specialist had taken her off her medications the month before. She was reasonably anxious about the thought of having her thyroid destroyed forever but she was also feeling fine without all the drugs, so Carla scheduled an appointment with me to see if there was "anything alternative" she could do instead.

Having taken no medicines to damp down her thyroid for weeks, Carla should have shown some signs of thyroid overactivity when I saw her, but there was none. Carla with no thyroid medicine at all looked healthy, almost vibrant. Her physical exam was normal, as were her thyroid blood tests.

What the psychiatrist had diagnosed as bipolar disorder and the thyroid specialist as an overactive thyroid were simply two manifestations of perfectly appropriate reactions to prolonged stress. Carla's stress glands—the adrenal glands and thyroid—had both been in overdrive, stimulated by her pituitary gland to help her withstand her tumultuous year.

Carla wasn't manic in the bipolar sense, or even wired. Her glands, faced with wave after wave of emotional or physical stress, simply pumped more and more thyroid and adrenal hormones into her bloodstream, speeding up her heart rate and occasionally interfering with sleep. Even her blood test had shown this increased hormone production, but her doctors had wrongly interpreted the effects of stress as disease.

Ironically, although her thyroid gland was basically only doing its job, it had almost been destroyed by her doctor for doing so. But Carla was healthy and didn't need a lot of medical care. I agreed to continue rechecking her thyroid as it recovered from being overworked, and recommended she stay with her therapist because she was still vulnerable to stress. Now was the time for her to get back to the gym, eat a healthful diet, and get into a stress-reducing yoga class. In short, she needed to follow the Triple Whammy Cure.

2.

TRIPLE WHAMMY QUESTIONNAIRE

This questionnaire is a simple way to discover if you're being affected by the Triple Whammy.

For each question you answer yes, circle the number. Then add the numbers to get a total for each of the three sections.

WHAMMY #1: STRESS   YES

Do you feel your overall level of stress has been higher during
the past year than it's been at other times during your life? 25

Do you feel on the verge of being overwhelmed by responsibilities? 25

Have you been in any especially difficult relationship during the
past year (this can include partner, boss, parents, children)? 15

Do you feel you've lost control of your life? 15

Do you spend little or no time taking care of yourself? 15

Do you feel everything in your life changed for the worse after
an especially traumatic event, such as an illness, surgery, injury,
death of a loved one, or physical, emotional, or sexual abuse? 10

STRESS TOTAL _____

WHAMMY #2: LOW SEROTONIN   YES

Throughout your life, have you ever had periods of significant depression, anxiety, panic, obsessive-compulsive disorder, an eating disorder, or social anxiety for which you considered or had professional counseling? 35

Have you ever taken antidepressant medication?..25

Did the antidepressant significantly help your symptoms? 10

Have you been diagnosed with any of the following: fibromyalgia, chronic fatigue syndrome, irritable bowel syndrome, migraine headaches?.................35

Were any of your blood relatives treated
for any of the disorders listed so far?..25

Do you feel a sense of depression when the days start
getting shorter or the sky is overcast for weeks at a time? 10

Are you especially sensitive or uncomfortable
when exposed to perfumes or chemical smells?...5

If you're given a prescription medication, do you frequently
have to stop taking it because of side effects? 5

Have you discovered that the smallest dose of a medicine (one
half or even one quarter of a tablet) is often adequate for you? 5

Do you crave carbohydrates, sugar, or chocolate,
especially during the days before your period? 10

LOW SEROTONIN TOTAL _____

WHAMMY #3: HORMONES   YES

Do any of the disorders listed so far get worse
during the week before your period? 25

Do you experience moodiness, irritability, breast tenderness,
or bloating during the days before your period?...15

Is the week after your period the week
when you feel best during a month? 10

If you've taken birth control pills, did
you get depressed while taking them?..10

If you've ever given birth, did you experience
depression after delivery?..10

Are you now in perimenopause or menopause and
experiencing any uncomfortable symptoms? 10

HORMONES TOTAL _____

TRIPLE WHAMMY SYMPTOMS

For each symptom, write the number that best describes how it applies to you.

0 = NEVER   3 = MILD   6 = FREQUENT   9 = SO SEVERE IT DISRUPTS EVERYDAY LIFE

Fatigue/lethargy

Poor memory

Can't concentrate

Insomnia

Unrefreshing sleep

Overwhelmed

Depressed

Anxious

Panic attacks

Tobacco addiction

Alcohol addiction

Regular recreational drug use (including alcohol), mainly to relieve symptoms
of stress and anxiety

Widespread muscle aches

"I carry stress in my neck"

Brain fog _____

Feeling drained _____

Constipation _____

Frequent loose bowel movements _____

Frequent abdominal cramping _____

Headaches (migraine, tension, or sinus) _____

Jaw grinding _____

Loss of sex energy _____

Excessive thirst _____

Binge eating _____

ADD NUMBERS TO GET SYMPTOMS TOTAL _____

SCORING THE TRIPLE WHAMMY QUESTIONNAIRE

Add your totals from the four sections (Stress, Serotonin, Hormones, and Symptoms) to get a total score. My total score is _____.

INTERPRETING YOUR RESULTS

The first part of the questionnaire is designed to help you see which of the three whammies might be causing you the most problems. Review your scores to see if a particular combination of whammies (such as hormones and stress, or low serotonin and hormones) requires your attention as you start the Three-Week Cure. Most women are affected by the interaction of all three whammies, scoring some points in each section. But some of my patients score higher in one or two areas. The Symptoms portion of the questionnaire can help steer you to further reading in Triple Whammy Cure Plus (p. 57).

IF YOUR TOTAL SCORE IS:

UNDER 50: You may have some symptoms of the Triple Whammy. Following the Three-Week Cure can help relieve them and will contribute to your overall good health.

50–100: Triple Whammy is very likely. Follow the Three-Week Cure to prevent your symptoms from progressing and to significantly improve the way you feel. In addition, review the subject areas in Triple Whammy Cure Plus (p. 57) and, if any stand out (PMS or migraine, for example), explore the appropriate healing path for more suggestions.

OVER 100: Triple Whammy is definitely present and in fact your doctor may already have diagnosed you as having one or more Triple Whammy disorders. Start by following the Three-Week Cure. Then read the healing path devoted to your disorder(s) in Triple Whammy Cure Plus. Obviously the content of the healing paths is not meant to replace the good services of your physician, but she may not be too offended if you copy some pages and subtly suggest she read them.

CHART YOUR HEALING PROGRESS

You can also use the Triple Whammy Questionnaire to chart your healing progress. Complete it using a pen or pencil of one color and write the date you answered the questions in that color as well. Then start following the Three-Week Cure and repeat the questionnaire using a different pen after three weeks and again after three months. If you follow all my suggestions, I think you'll be pleased with your progress.

3.

LOOKING FOR CLUES IN YOUR LIFE STORY

If you came to see me as a new patient whose symptoms suggested that you have the Triple Whammy, you might be surprised as we talked to see how early in your life these symptoms actually began. Many of my patients have told me it's a real eye-opener to recognize that other members of their family—usually female—have had Triple Whammy problems too. All of this emerges as we review your life story, which can help you see your symptoms in their clearest context—alongside the different stages of your life, the good times and the not so good—as well as a part of your biological inheritance.

As you consider your life and health history, look for clues that indicate patterns of events that were followed by symptoms or illnesses. Think of any relatives who may have felt the way you do.

You've probably had the experience of visiting a doctor for the first time and being handed a form that listed a vast array of diseases, many of which you'd never heard of, with instructions to mark the ones you've had. Your new doctor glanced over your check marks and made a decidedly brief inquiry about them. You might have responded with a variation of "I had that in college, but it hasn't been around for years." If whatever it was just cleared up on its own, both of you would just as soon forget about it.

This style of taking a medical history is the way doctors are taught in medical school. Most physicians still believe that the important information surfaces when you, the patient, describe what's called your "History of Present Illness," while the doctor interrupts your flow of thought every few seconds to ask for particulars. The flaw in this method is obvious: with your doctor clearly pressed for time, you relate the story of your illness starting when symptoms began to interfere with your life, but not *beforehand* when you weren't "ill" but might have had significant life challenges that contributed to your future illness.

To figure out Triple Whammy symptoms and disorders, we need to try a different form of history taking for two reasons:

– The symptoms and disorders usually surface after a period of significant stress.

– They've often been around for years, sometimes since childhood, just manifesting themselves in different forms and disguises. What may have been called "nervous stomach" during your childhood may later manifest as irritable bowel syndrome during finals week in college, premenstrual migraines during your twenties, food cravings in your thirties, and fibromyalgia in your forties.

You know you're more complicated than a hastily completed list of diseases or brief description to your doc of the symptoms you came to see her about. You, my friend, are in possession of a very complex life story. So, what we're going to do now is think about your health, illnesses, and symptoms in the context of that life story, complete with family background, upbringing, education, relationships, job history, joys, and disappointments. By examining your life story and the lives of your biological family, we can then appreciate the duration and intensity of what you're going through.

LET'S START WITH YOUR CHILDHOOD

Think back to your emotions as a child. Overall, was the predominant feeling one of happiness, or of sadness, anxiety, or loneliness? Maybe it was mixture. If you have negative memories, what was going on at home? What do you recall of the family dynamics? Was the blissful innocence of childhood disrupted by divorce or an alcoholic or abusive relative? How did you react to stressful events?

Childhood is also a good starting point to think about the health of your parents and siblings. Triple Whammy disorders are extremely common in families, especially among women. Some conditions like fibromyalgia and chronic fatigue went by other names years ago, so if you have a recollection that goes something like, "Mom always complained of hurting, but no one could ever find anything wrong," let's keep this in mind.

The emotional story of your life is very important, too. Even if a diagnosis of depression was never formally made (or treated) by a doctor, the sentence "I always thought my mother was depressed" strongly indicates that a susceptibility to Triple Whammy disorders runs in your family. In fact, the single most important Triple Whammy clue is some variation of "I (or my sister, aunt, or mother) once had some depression (or anxiety or panic) and when I (or my sister, aunt, or mother) started taking an antidepressant, it worked like a miracle." This is because serotonin, the stress buffer, is in shorter supply in people with depression, and antidepressants increase serotonin. So if an antidepressant worked well for you, everything else we uncover should be considered in the context that you are more biochemically susceptible to stress than others.

If this doesn't apply to you, however, you may *still* be vulnerable to the Triple Whammy. After all, antidepressants haven't been used for very many years and Triple Whammy disorders come in many forms.

Most of my Triple Whammy patients had childhood symptoms that ultimately became a Triple Whammy disorder later in life. Clues include phrases like, "I always had headaches as a child" or "I was kept out of school because of stomachaches, but they were never given a diagnosis." Common Triple Whammy symptoms that first surface during adolescence are headaches (tension/migraine-type headaches often misdiagnosed as sinus problems), irritable bowel syndrome, and PMS. Even fibromyalgia and chronic fatigue can appear during high school and college. My youngest fibro patient was eleven when her first symptoms appeared. I've lost track of the number of teens I've treated with chronic fatigue syndrome.

Psychiatrists now believe depression and anxiety disorders are common childhood problems, with treatment—counseling rather than medication—beginning for some as early as age eight.

Many women with the Triple Whammy feel physically well as teens, apart from what psychologists call age-appropriate anxieties regarding appearance and popularity. But it's important to remember if you had any depression, anxiety, panic disorder, eating disorders, or if you practiced any self-mutilation or obsessive habits.

LEAVING HOME

Let's imagine you're leaving home and off to college or your first job. College can be a mixed bag. For some, these years may be among their best: less depression, better energy, and relief from the aching of your undiagnosed fibromyalgia. For others, the stress of a new environment, homesickness, deadlines for school papers, final exams, poor food choices, and erratic sleeping hours are enough to trigger depression and anxiety, or flare-ups of IBS, TMJ, PMS, fibro, or severe fatigue.

Finally you enter what your parents called the real world. If you were already susceptible to stress—by virtue of your low serotonin—the next twenty or so years can be difficult indeed. Symptoms that were mild and intermittent during college become intense, constant, and sometimes disabling after a period of unchecked stress, especially when you don't know it's stress that's making you ill. Far too many women find "career" a euphemism for an unfulfilling, time-consuming, and stress-laden job. You may hate your job, but you've racked up some debts and the credit card bills hang heavily over you, creating monthly surges of stress as you open them. And you can't quit now because you need the health insurance.

What's your job history? Tell me about the first job that made you physically or emotionally sick. Did this ill health magically and dramatically improve when you quit? Or were you ever fired and then, a few days later, felt physically really well for the first time in months? Did your migraines or irritable bowel disappear when you went on vacation, away from the stress? This current job of yours, is it fulfilling or are you suffering through each day? You know you've landed in job hell when you start carrying your stress in your neck, are too tired each evening to mingle with friends or enjoy your family, awaken with your jaw clenched tightly, find yourself in the john with crampy diarrhea, or don't enjoy Sundays because of work the next day.

Of course, the stress of bad relationships can bring the same array of symptoms, especially if you're Triple Whammy–susceptible, so let's consider them too. Many women live good lives without being partnered, but others going it alone feel stressed, anxious, and depressed, worried that they'll spend their lives lonely and unloved. Being alone can look very good, however, if you find yourself in a rotten relationship. And then there's the stressful hell of a marriage going sour, the divorce proceedings, and relearning how to survive as a single woman or as a single mother.

HOW NOW REFLECTS THEN

By the time we get to the present moment, you probably have recognized some patterns in your life. Your irritable bowel or migraines may have first surfaced long ago, with the childhood tummyaches or headaches brought on by the stress of school, family alcoholism, or divorcing parents. We can link how you feel to your mother's "nervous migraines" or your sister's depression, because, remember, all Triple Whammy disorders involve some combination of stress, low serotonin (which often runs in families), and hormones. The phrase "it runs in the family" takes on new significance.

Maybe you felt fine during the summers or on vacation, away from the stress. Or maybe things have been going fairly well but now you're facing the pressure of your dad's illness and your mom needing more help. Has your PMS been raging out of control? Hormones ablaze, the third leg of the whammies.

Finally, consider the stressful background noise of simply being a woman. The "system" does not favor you. Please don't get me wrong. Most people who know me would call me a feminist. But women today can experience stress they don't even bother to think of as stress anymore—when you feel vulnerable and your guard is up, whether walking down a street or driving on a highway at night alone. Much in the male world is subtly threatening and adds further stress. You may be on your guard (in ways that I'm not) when you're alone in the house with a repairman or having your car fixed. Too many employers underpay you, overwork you, and don't accommodate the demands of raising a family. Even though you may not always be conscious of these tensions and worries because you've learned just to forge ahead and get on with it, they do take a toll on your mind and body.

You might ask "This is all stress?" The answer is no, not stress alone, but stress as a catalyst. It's a trifecta, really, the Triple Whammy: your low levels of stress-protecting serotonin, your fluctuating hormones, and the stress itself. If you're reading this section first, please read more about the Triple Whammy (p. 3), take the quiz that starts on page 28, begin the Three-Week Cure, and then do me a favor. Revisit this section and go through it again once you understand more how the Triple Whammy elements work together.

So here you are, and I'm hoping you've seen maybe a glimmer of how the patterns in your life have affected you. Ultimately what I hope is that by making some simple changes to reduce the stress in your life (and yes, for some of you this can include quitting a job you detest and taking one for less pay), boosting your serotonin reserves, and balancing out your hormones you can start feeling good again. Good enough to start taking more of those art history courses you liked so much in college. Good enough to laugh with your kids. A big part of settling the Triple Whammy is being willing to prioritize what's important.

DO TRIPLE WHAMMY DISORDERS RUN IN YOUR FAMILY?

Make a list of your blood relatives: siblings, parents and grandparents, aunts, and uncles. Were (or are) any of them significantly depressed or treated for depression? Also consider other Triple Whammy disorders, including anxiety, panic attacks, obsessive-compulsive disorder, and addictions to alcohol, tobacco, or other drugs. Then think about migraines, irritable bowel syndrome, and PMS. Remember that doctors weren't really diagnosing conditions like fibromyalgia until the last ten years or so, so an aunt who "always complained of her arthritis, even when she was young" may have had fibromyalgia. If you see a pattern of these disorders, follow the Triple Whammy Three-Week Cure to limit your own vulnerability.

TIRED. ALL THE TIME.

"Doctors can never find anything wrong with me . . ."

On her first visit to my office, Melissa had written the words "Tired. All the time," and "Hormones??" across her Patient Information Form. This form helps me get to know what's on my patients' minds before we talk. Melissa was in her thirties, smart and articulate, and she'd made the appointment at the suggestion of her best friend, though she added that she'd already been to her internist and gynecologist, both of whom told her they couldn't find anything wrong. Her internist had suggested antidepressants.

I told Melissa it would help me to know more about her as a person and asked her to imagine her entire life on videotape and then to press the rewind button. She was to stop the tape at the time when her health was last perfect. Not just a good week or even a good month, but a time when she had no health issues whatsoever—when doctors were for other people.

And here's what Melissa saw on her tape:

"Honestly, I think I was about nine when I didn't feel good a lot. I started getting terrible stomachaches—I think I was anxious about school. My mom took me to several doctors, but they could never find anything wrong. I went on diets, took pills, had X-rays. Nothing. And that's the story of my life—doctors never find anything wrong with me!

"My parents got divorced when I was eleven and that's when everything sort of fell apart. I remember feeling really sad most of the time. We were always short of money and my mom got really depressed too. I had an eating disorder for a while—I thought I was fat, but when I look at my high school photos, I just see a skinny, sad girl. Things definitely improved when I went to college. Just being away from my mother and the rest of the family helped. I was really shy, but made some very good friends. The only real problem then was that my PMS started. At first, it only wrecked one week a month; now it's almost up to two weeks. My stomachaches came back, usually around finals, with constipation and then diarrhea."

I asked Melissa what happened after college.

"When I graduated, I traveled for two months on a train through Europe, and that's probably the best I ever felt in my entire life—my energy was great and I was really happy. I didn't have stomachaches, and honestly, I don't even remember any PMS. When I came home I got my first job, at an ad agency, and I've been in advertising ever since."

Melissa readily acknowledged that her job was stressful. Long hours, looming deadlines, and demanding clients left little time to care for herself. She told me she used to keep going with regular visits to the gym, always feeling better after a vigorous workout, but now she spent so much time at work and in airports that she'd lost her workout rhythm. Recently, Melissa had been working even longer hours, harder than ever, as her division tried to avoid layoffs. When traveling, she ate airport-hotel food. Lunch is what she calls marginal foods, usually at her desk between phone calls. By the time she gets home, it's usually too late to cook anything real for dinner. She falls asleep watching TV, wakes up at 1 a.m., and has trouble getting back to sleep, worrying about everything from her job to her weight, from the health of her father to the health of her cat.

The main symptom that Melissa has reported to her doctors is that she's tired all the time, even after managing a good night's sleep. She also feels achy all over, but especially in her neck and shoulders. She showed me how she's always massaging her neck to help the pain, and tells me aspirin doesn't really help. A good total body massage can really work wonders for a day or so, but she never has the time. Melissa thought her immune system was weak, because she got every illness that went through the office, and this worried her.

And everything ("everything!") gets worse before her period. As Melissa put it: "During the two days before my period, I just want to crawl into bed with a box of Godivas and pull the covers up." She told me the only time during the month when symptoms seem to let up is the week after her period ends.

"Still," she added at the end of all this, "this may sound ridiculous, but despite all these symptoms, I think my health is basically good. My doctor checked me over for different diseases and all my tests are normal. She says I'm probably depressed but I really don't want to start taking Prozac. But I begin to think I'm going crazy with these doctors telling me everything's fine when I feel so crummy. I'm not a doctor, but in my opinion everything's out of balance. I think if I could get my body back on track, I could feel better." This made good sense, and I stressed that it was important to recognize that her symptoms were genuine even though her tests were negative.

MELISSA'S CLASSIC TRIPLE WHAMMY

Melissa has classic symptoms of the Triple Whammy. First, each one of her physical and emotional issues, from her tummyaches at age nine, her adolescent eating disorder and depression, to her current chronic fatigue, muscle aches, and even her PMS, was either triggered or aggravated by stress. But let's face it, life is stressful for all of us. Why is stress so damaging to Melissa?

The answer is Whammy #2: a shortage of serotonin, the stress buffer. Lacking this firewall, stress "gets" to Melissa, with the result that throughout most of her life she's simply been buffeted by one symptom after another. Endlessly feeling crummy, any joy in life gets steadily chipped away. And the fact that doctors have found no cause for her symptoms has only increased Melissa's stress.

Now add to this mess Whammy #3. Each month her hormones shift, and during the two weeks before her period, her estrogen falls, taking with it her already precarious serotonin buffer (remember, when estrogen goes down, so does feel-good serotonin). Every symptom she experiences during the first half of the month gets worse before her period. What she's going through is unique to women. Even the most sensitive man can't fathom how utterly awful Melissa feels.

Although her physical and emotional symptoms began during childhood, if

Melissa drew her family tree, she'd probably discover she was earmarked for trouble when she was born. Susceptibility to serotonin disorders is highly genetic, and runs through the women of multiple generations. Her problems surfaced during childhood, when fears (which are one form of the stress response) about school manifested themselves as morning tummyaches, and went into high gear after the divorce of her parents. Further questioning about her childhood revealed Melissa as a sad girl who struggled with a lurking depression in her teens by trying to be "extra popular" in high school and active in sports. Interestingly, her involvement in sports probably helped keep her depression at bay by raising her serotonin levels.

What began as school anxiety when she was nine became a steady event in her life when hormonal tides initiated her first period.

When we turned to the question of her family's health, she told me that her mother had struggled with migraines until she went into menopause, that her father was an "on again, off again alcoholic," and that her younger sister had had postpartum depression after the birth of her first child. I explained that everything she was saying provided vital clues to understanding the way Triple Whammy disorders affected her and her female relatives. We discussed the low-serotonin/hormonal features of mother's migraines and sister's postpartum depression, and how her childhood tummyaches surfaced in her college years as diarrhea and constipation—what's called irritable bowel syndrome today—in response to the stress of exams.

After replaying her life story for me, Melissa quickly appreciated the close correlation between periods of stress and the decline in her physical health. She wondered aloud if it were even fair to expect to feel as good as she did on vacation during day-to-day life. I responded that feeling healthy on vacation and crummy at home is a pretty good indicator that the Triple Whammy was a factor, driven by uncontrolled stress, and that yes indeed, we could feel as well day to day as we could during vacations.

Melissa acknowledged that the last two or three years had been the most consistently stressful of her life, with her symptoms intensifying. There was little sense in my repeating any of the diagnostic tests performed by her other doctors, which hadn't revealed any medical problem. I wanted Melissa to feel better, and quickly. While I'm not opposed to antidepressants (though I rarely suggest them as a first treatment), Melissa herself was. We agreed that she could take charge of her health without them; she'd also probably learn something about herself that could help her for the rest of her life. Melissa was not ill, but she was feeling the consequences of unrelenting stress and her susceptibility to hormone and serotonin imbalances.

MAKING A PLAN

We put together this plan, based on the Triple Whammy Three-Week Cure:

- **TO BOOST MELISSA'S SEROTONIN (AND HER IMMUNE SYSTEM),** she would start walking to work every day. She lived downtown and the office was about ten blocks away. This would be a good start. A brisk walk in the sun, with no sunglasses, to work every day, plus more on her lunch hour—even fifteen minutes more if possible. She would start "timing" her carbohydrates to get her brain making serotonin, focusing on powerhouse carbs like whole grains, veggies, and nuts, taking some with every meal. We discussed the Triple Whammy food plan (no more vending machine snacks). One Godiva per day was fine, but not as a meal plan.

- **TO BALANCE HER HORMONES,** the food plan would be an ideal start, reducing processed foods, saturated fats, sugar, caffeine, soft drinks. Dairy products interfere with magnesium absorption, and low magnesium can worsen PMS. Melissa could find alternate sources of calcium in dark green leafy vegetables, supplements, and even chewing a couple of Tums. We discussed nutritious foods she could take to work and on business trips (veggies, fruit, nuts, peanut butter on whole wheat) to steer her away from the grim food choices she'd been making.

- **TO IDENTIFY STRESS POINTS,** Melissa agreed to start a stress journal, following the guidelines on page 198. She would look into the lunchtime massage being offered down the street and would start a weekend yoga class. We agreed that her lapsed gym membership could stay lapsed for a few weeks until she worked the other steps into her schedule. But within a month, I wanted her working out seriously at least three times a week.

- **MELISSA JOTTED DOWN THE NUTRITIONAL SUPPLEMENTS** I asked her to start: magnesium for PMS and muscle pain; B complex, fish oil, St. John's wort, and 5HTP (at bedtime) to raise her serotonin and help with sleep; and an herbal combination containing chasteberry, dong quai, and black cohosh to get her hormones back on track.

I emphasized that her commitment to all this was vital, and that as she improved, she might even consider some short-term counseling just to explore the "why" of her life choices. I asked Melissa to come back in three weeks, though it was more like six before she returned. When she did, I heard voices from the front of my office, "Melissa! You look terrific!" I saw from her big smile that she'd jumped into the Triple Whammy Cure with both feet. She'd lost some of the puffiness in her face, her color was better, and she moved with a grace that hadn't been present six weeks earlier. This was a woman who felt well.

I told her that when she hadn't returned after three weeks, I'd wondered if I'd given her too much to do. "Not at all," she replied, "It was my travel schedule, but even travel didn't stop me. No more between-flight Bloody Marys! Instead, I'm drinking water and walking the terminal to rev up my serotonin.

"Best of all, I've finished up some work projects and I'm starting to say no when they try to throw more travel my way. I can't believe how much has changed in six weeks. My energy is back, the achiness is way down—even my PMS wasn't too bad last week."

She paused, tears starting, and said "I never thought I'd ever be able to say I'm feeling good again in my life."

PART II

TRIPLE WHAMMY
THREE-WEEK CURE

4.

THE TRIPLE WHAMMY THREE-WEEK CURE

The Triple Whammy Three-Week Cure is easy to follow. It requires no drugs and no expensive therapies. You'll make a maximum of nine simple changes—three per week—designed to help you manage stress, boost your serotonin levels, and smooth out your hormonal roller-coaster ride. Even in this era of high-tech medicine and fancy pharmaceuticals, the vast majority of my patients are searching for an all-natural way to feel better. Though it costs just a few dollars and a modest amount of your time, this plan produces powerful results, resolving the overwhelming imbalances caused by the Triple Whammy and significantly helping the symptoms and disorders it produces. Some of my patients report feeling better after just seven days. A majority see dramatic results within three weeks.

As you start the Three-Week Cure, I encourage you to read "What Is the Triple Whammy?" (p. 3) to get an overall sense of how the three whammies work together to sabotage your good health.

If you happen to be among the fortunate who can say, "But I feel just fine," following the recommendations here will have tremendous health benefits in the years ahead. Stress is and will continue to be a major risk to your health. Why not examine your life now for potential stressors and initiate the simple few steps in this plan to avoid future trouble? Remember that life eventually throws everyone a few curve balls. Shoring up your stress-buffering reserves of serotonin will lessen your chances of developing any of the numerous stress-related illnesses out there, Triple Whammy disorders included.

THREE-WEEK CURE AT A GLANCE

WEEK ONE

- **STRESS:** start your stress journal
- **SEROTONIN:** walk (briskly!) in the light
- **HORMONES:** start the Triple Whammy Food Plan

WEEK TWO

- **STRESS:** work out stress and overcome worry
- **SEROTONIN:** add B vitamins and fish oil
- **HORMONES:** start chasteberry or black cohosh; St. John's wort and 5HTP if needed.

WEEK THREE

- **STRESS:** manage anger and cultivate a positive attitude
- **SEROTONIN:** learn carbohydrate timing
- **HORMONES:** consider progesterone cream, in the dosage recommended

WEEK ONE

REDUCING STRESS: KEEP A STRESS JOURNAL

Women are especially vulnerable to stress, because you work far too efficiently in many different roles: partner, mother, volunteer, homemaker, employee, caregiver to parents, doing too much in too little time, and often placing yourself last in line. Many women are so busy coping with the stressors in their lives that they become oblivious to the damaging effects of nonstop stress on their bodies and minds. Keeping a stress journal will help you recognize the sources and effects of stress so you can start managing it or banish it altogether. Don't believe anyone who says you can't get rid of stress. Maybe you can't quit your much-hated job right now for a position you enjoy. That's clearly not a financial option for everyone, but it's worth considering. So, find a spiral notebook, get a pen, turn to page 198, and I'll walk you through it. In a few short days, you'll see some patterns emerging.

Here's an example of how a stress journal can help: I have a patient who is primary caregiver for her ailing mother. The daughter's visits—once filled with affection and eagerness to help—started to cause her sleepless nights, anxiety, and resentment. After keeping her stress journal for a couple weeks, she saw with great clarity that on days when she shared lunch with a co-worker who was going through a similar challenge, her stress level dropped significantly and her ability to cope improved. Recognizing the importance of a support system is a single but compelling example of the patterns, both positive and negative, that can be revealed by keeping such a journal.

The connection between stress and symptoms became very apparent to one of my patients whose fibromyalgia had been under pretty good control until a change of surroundings triggered a flare-up. As a child, she had been sexually abused by her stepfather; by making her home in Chicago she avoided visiting her family in Seattle. Yet one holiday season, she felt determined to participate in a reunion. Driving westward, she felt her old fibro symptoms returning, with tight and painful spasms crisscrossing her neck and shoulders. By the time she pulled into her parents' driveway, she could barely get out of the car. Even though her stepfather was now a very old man, she felt her body tense up every time she was in the same room with him. Ultimately, she pleaded some excuse and left for home as quickly as possible. "It was amazing," she later told me. "I felt my muscles loosening the moment I started heading eastward. By the time I was driving through the Great Plains states, I was laughing and singing along with the country music on the radio. When I finally walked into my apartment, in the comfort and safety of my home, I was completely fine. Really an amazing experience."

RAISING SEROTONIN: WALK IN THE LIGHT

A daily twenty-minute brisk walk—outside during daylight hours—will increase your serotonin in two ways. First, exposure to light raises the amount of serotonin in your brain, although scientists are not exactly sure of the mechanism.

Second, the physical exertion of a simple twenty-minute brisk walk raises the level of a chemical in your brain called phenylethylamine, which in turn triggers the release of feel-good endorphins, including GABA, norepinephrine, dopamine, and the all-important serotonin. This is a mini version of a runner's high. (By the way, chocolate also raises phenylethylamine, so if you're like my many chocoholic patients, now you know the chemical behind the pleasure that is chocolate.)

There are two ways to increase serotonin: you can either make more serotonin or prevent the serotonin sitting in the gaps (the synapses) between your brain cells from being reabsorbed and recycled. Exposing yourself to light acts like an SSRI antidepressant by keeping serotonin in the synapse gaps where it works on your mood.

Please don't wear sunglasses during your walk. The light needs to reach your brain through the optic nerves in your eyes. By this I don't mean you should walk for twenty minutes daily while looking directly at the sun. This is not a good idea because it increases your risk of cataracts. However, walking outside without sunglasses when the sun is shining carries no appreciable health risks—only benefits. For many other easy ways to increase the amount of light—and thus serotonin—in your life, read the seasonal affective disorder (SAD) healing path on page 164.

I'd like you to consider your walk sacrosanct—nothing should get in the way of doing it. Make it brisk, make it twenty minutes minimum, and do it every day rain, shine, or cold (yes, even on overcast days you can get enough light to your brain to make your walk worthwhile). At first you might want to wear a watch, walking ten minutes in one direction and then returning. Soon you'll have a good idea of the various routes that satisfy the twenty-minute requirement. Many of my patients integrate the walk into the infrastructure of their commute, getting off the subway or bus twenty minutes away from work and walking the rest of the way in. Others walk to decompress at a certain point during their days, such as during the lunch hour or after work.

Consistency is important. I understand that you're pressed for time, but twenty minutes is truly a small piece of your day to devote to your health. The benefits in addition to serotonin-boosting are wide-ranging: kicking up your metabolism (even after you're done walking), increasing energy, balancing hormones, helping you sleep more soundly, and improving cardiovascular fitness.

BALANCING HORMONES: START THE TRIPLE WHAMMY FOOD PLAN

This week you'll start following the Triple Whammy Food Plan, starting on page 245. The food plan is simple. You'll increase the amount of nutrient-rich whole

Q & A: MACULAR DEGENERATION
AND WALKING IN THE LIGHT

Q. I'm seventy-five and have been diagnosed with macular degeneration. My doctor says I should wear sunglasses with at least 98 percent UV protection whenever I'm outside. Regarding serotonin production, I'm guessing the sunglasses will block the beneficial effects of walking in the light. Any suggestions?

A. Your doctor is correct that bright sunlight can worsen the progression of macular degeneration, so your sunglasses are important. But please don't stop your twenty-minute daily walk just because you're wearing sunglasses—the breathing and moving will raise serotonin and improve your general health. Work on brightening the light sources in your home and workplace, which will boost your serotonin production while being safe and efficient for your eyes. You can also rely more on other methods to raise your serotonin, including the fish oil and B complex supplements. Additionally, there are many lifestyle changes that can slow the degenerative process overall and in your eyes specifically: eat a healthful diet (p. 245) with plenty of fruits and dark green leafy vegetables, and reduce your saturated fat intake. If you're diabetic or have high blood pressure, keep these under good control. Take high-quality antioxidants (vitamin C, E, grapeseed extract, and zinc) and have a glass of red wine daily to get protective antioxidants.

foods you eat and reduce the less healthful choices. You'll eat well on the food plan, and you'll feel the results as your hormonal symptoms decline. Additional benefits include a stronger immune system, better digestion, and vibrant skin, hair, and nails (nutrients really work!). Most of my patients also happily report a real increase in energy after about a week of eating the Triple Whammy way and walking in the light.

You might wonder about the relationship between good nutrition and keeping your hormones balanced. Eating too much sugar and refined carbohydrates interferes with your body's absorption of magnesium, which is essential for hormone production. Too much salt causes fluid retention, swelling of your hands and feet, and abdominal bloating. Eating a lot of saturated fat throws off the delicate balance of prostaglandin production and in the process triggers the symptoms of PMS, while making you vulnerable to menstrual cramps. If you're going through the menopause transition, you want to maximize the effectiveness of your declining estrogen, and this food plan shows you how.

WEEK TWO

REDUCING STRESS: WORK OUT STRESS AND OVERCOME WORRY

This week you'll boost your ability to fend off the inevitable stresses in your life. Read "Using Your Body to Calm Down Your Mind" (p. 200) and begin doing one stress-reducing technique daily. I'll give you a bunch of options here, but I ask that you select one or more (feel free to rotate among them) and keep it in your schedule. This is the fun part! You'll review the Stress-Relief Menu and start doing something from the list every day. Ask a friend to join you in trying something new, like t'ai chi, or go get a massage. I'm prescribing it.

Your second project is learning how to overcome worry, a major source of stress. Turn to "Put Worry Behind You" (p. 200) and start viewing your worry realistically.

RAISING SEROTONIN: ADD B VITAMINS AND FISH OIL

Two inexpensive nutritional supplements—vitamin B complex and fish oil—will further increase your serotonin levels.

- **B VITAMINS, ESPECIALLY VITAMIN B_6 (PYRIDOXINE),** are necessary for the conversion in your body of tryptophan to serotonin (see Step Two: Boost Serotonin Naturally with Carbohydrate Timing, p. 263). In Week 1 we discussed how light and SSRI antidepressants increase serotonin in your brain by blocking the reabsorption and recycling of serotonin. Both the B vitamins and fish oil help the brain with the other mechanism—making more serotonin itself. In addition, some of the B vitamins assist your liver in flushing out stress hormones and help keep your nervous system on an even keel. Get some B complex-100 capsules (any brand) and start taking one a day, with food. The "100" designation refers to the number of milligrams of each B vitamin inside. Bottles of B complex-100 are available at any drugstore and typically contain 100 micrograms of B_{12} and biotin, and 100 milligrams of all the other B vitamins. B vitamins are water soluble, so even if you're already getting some B vitamins in your multiple vitamin, adding the B complex will only help, with any extra being flushed out of your body in urine.

- **FISH OIL** from cold-water fish offers high concentrations of polyunsaturated fats called omega-3 fatty acids, which your body can't produce on its own. Although the exact mechanism of production isn't known, the omega-3 DHA (docosahexaenoic acid) increases the amount of serotonin in your brain and enhances its efficiency. Take 1000 mg (1 gram) of fish oil twice a day, with meals. Fish oil is available at health-food stores and most drugstores. A newer source of fish oil—krill oil, extracted from the shrimp-like crustaceans that blue whales feed on—has two advantages over other sources. First, the component needed for brain health seems to enter the nervous system more readily than standard fish oil. Second, krill oil is an extremely powerful antioxidant. One study on krill oil showed a dramatic improvement of PMS symptoms in comparison to a placebo.

CONTAMINANTS AND FISH OIL

You've probably read about mercury and PCB contaminants in fish and you may be wondering about fish oil supplements. ConsumerLab.com, which evaluates supplements, tested more than forty brands of fish oil and found that none contained any mercury or PCBs. In February 2004, in response to a rising concern about the possibility of mercury and PCBs in fish, Canada TV hired two separate diagnostic laboratories to evaluate different brands of fish oil in both the US and Canada. No contamination was found, and some doctors remarked that it now appeared safer to take fish oil capsules than to eat actual fish.

BALANCING HORMONES: ADD CHASTEBERRY OR BLACK COHOSH; ST. JOHN'S WORT AND 5HTP IF NEEDED

Whether you're menstruating or in the menopause transition, the best choices for balancing your hormones are exercise and a healthful diet. This week's step, adding the herb chasteberry or black cohosh, is necessary only if you have symptoms related to PMS or menopause. Any discomforts that appear or escalate during the seven to ten days before your expected period are likely a variation of PMS. You'll definitely want to read the PMS healing path on page 153 in greater detail, but this week if you've got symptoms of PMS you'll start chasteberry. If you're having perimenopause/menopause symptoms, you'll start black cohosh, and also have a look at the Menopause Transition healing path (p. 120).

For menstruating women
One aspect of PMS is caused by a hormonal imbalance between estrogen and progesterone, while another involves serotonin. Hormonal symptoms include breast tenderness, bloating, headaches, and fluid retention; they're caused by a little too much estrogen in your system during the week before your period. Since you can't remove excess estrogen, the best treatment is to shore up progesterone. The herb chasteberry contains no hormones or hormone-like substances, but it brings hormones into balance by stimulating your pituitary gland to produce more luteiniz-

Q & A: IS A DOUBLE WHAMMY POSSIBLE?

Q. Two-thirds of the whammy material rings so true for me—stress and serotonin. I know that stress is a major factor in how I feel day to day, and I already feel better after three weeks of taking the fish oil and B complex, plus the walking. My hormones don't seem to be involved. Is it possible to have a double whammy?

A. Absolutely. In fact, the hormone cycle runs quite smoothly for many women, and if you're one of them the effect of your hormones on your serotonin levels may be quite mild. I'm delighted your daily walks and supplements are helping, but be aware that unchecked stress can trigger symptoms of hormonal imbalance and get you a ticket to Triple Whammy Land, so please be sure to read Chapter 20 and choose at least one stress reliever in addition to your walking to keep you balanced.

ing hormone and less prolactin. These changes then signal your ovaries to balance their hormones in favor of progesterone. In a study of women with PMS, 90 percent of those taking chasteberry reported a reduction in PMS symptoms and in one-third of them, symptoms disappeared altogether. That's a very high positive result.

Chasteberry, whose botanical name is *Vitex agnus-castus,* comes from the chaste tree, a small shrub that bears violet flowers and reddish-black berries. It's indigenous to the Mediterranean region, but is now grown in subtropical climates around the globe. In the fall, its ripe berries are dried and used medicinally. Chasteberry plays a vital role in balancing the hormone fluctuations of the Triple Whammy. Because chasteberry affects hormone levels, you shouldn't use it if you're taking prescription hormones like hormone replacement therapy or birth control pills (it can reduce their effectiveness), or if you're pregnant or nursing.

CHASTEBERRY DOSE: Take 175 to 225 mg of standardized extract (containing 0.5 percent agnuside, the active ingredient in chasteberry) once a day when not menstruating, before a meal to maximize absorption. Be aware that chasteberry can work rather slowly, so it may take two to four cycles before you can appreciate its effect. Please don't give up on it.

The second aspect of PMS is caused when your monthly premenstrual decline in estrogen drags down your stress-buffering, feel-good neurotransmitter serotonin. Symptoms include mood swings, irritability, anger, or crying. Here's the solution: try all the serotonin-boosting ideas in the Three-Week cure. They may provide just enough of a boost to eliminate your symptoms. After a couple of months, if you're still experiencing the snarky-sadness of PMS, you can kick up your serotonin even higher by using the amino acid 5HTP (p. 20) and the herb St. John's wort (p. 20). 5HTP is a building block of serotonin, whose man-ufacturing process is already being hastened along by the B vitamins and fish oil. St. John's wort acts like a gentle SSRI antidepressant, allowing serotonin to in-crease in the gap between brain cells. Be patient. It may take a couple of cycles be-fore these supplements erase your PMS mood miseries, but it will happen.

5HTP/ST. JOHN'S WORT DOSE: Take 100 mg of 5HTP at bedtime and 450 mg of St. John's wort twice a day on this schedule: start both about two calendar weeks before your period and stop when your period starts.

For women in the menopause transition
Shifting hormone levels in the years up to and after menopause can cause hot flashes, sweating, vaginal dryness, and mild depression. Here the problem is not excess estrogen, but a lack of estrogen. Black cohosh reduces your luteinizing hormone (LH) levels, which increases the amount of estrogen your ovaries pro-duce; it also contains phytoestrogens, plant compounds that have an estrogen-like effect (soy also has these effects).

Black cohosh (*Cimicifuga racemosa*) is an herb native to the east coast of America, a wildflower, really, related to the buttercup, and its medicinal proper-ties are in its black root. Generations of women have taken black cohosh: some Native American tribes used it for "female problems" like menstrual cramps and it was also an ingredient in Lydia Pinkham's Vegetable Compound for Women, one of the best selling patent medicines of all time.

BLACK COHOSH DOSE: Take 40 mg of black cohosh (available as Remifemin) twice a day, standardized to contain 2.5 percent of triterpenes, the active compo-nents of black cohosh.

WEEK THREE AND THEREAFTER

REDUCING STRESS: MANAGE ANGER
AND CULTIVATE A POSITIVE ATTITUDE

Anger and stress are inextricably linked, with chronically stressed people more prone to anger. If this sounds familiar, turn to page 202 for a quick course in anger management.

Cultivating a positive attitude will be an eye-opening assignment for you, I hope. In this exercise, described on page 202, you'll use the back portion of your stress journal to record a daily thought that brought you a sense of happiness, optimism, or even wonder. Once you start, you'll start seeing positive things everywhere. As a bonus, research shows that doing helpful things for others kicks up your serotonin. Aren't you lucky?

RAISING SEROTONIN: CARBOHYDRATE TIMING

To keep your body producing a steady supply of feel-good serotonin, each meal of your day (and especially breakfast) must contain some carbohydrates. This is carbo timing, and it's discussed more fully on page 263. High-quality carbs are the ones to eat, including vegetables, fruits, whole grain breads, and legumes such as kidney beans. Here's some quick background on how periodically eating carbohydrates helps make serotonin in your brain: the amino acid tryptophan, which comes from protein sources, ultimately converts to serotonin (the effect we're after), but in order for the tryptophan to reach your brain and convert, you need to eat carbohydrates. When you eat carbohydrates, they break down into sugar (glucose). Rising levels of glucose trigger your pancreas to release insulin. Insulin then carries the glucose into cells as an energy source, but also carries tryptophan to the brain for serotonin production. In other words, ultimately it's carbohydrates that determine how much serotonin reaches your brain. Carbs aren't called comfort foods for nothing.

BALANCING HORMONES: PROGESTERONE CREAM IF NEEDED

Our Week 2 hormone-balancing step included using chasteberry for PMS or black cohosh for the symptoms of menopause transition, and these are effective for most women. But for others with PMS, estrogen dominance is so strong that progesterone itself is needed to relieve symptoms caused by hormone shifts. These are the breast tenderness, bloating, back pain, and fluid retention symptoms of PMS, rather than the "mood" symptoms (irritability, crying easily). Generally I recommend you give chasteberry at least two or three cycles to work before moving to progesterone. If you've been using chasteberry and it hasn't helped, start using progesterone cream, purchased from your local health food store. The product must specifically contain progesterone and not just herbs or wild yam. Read the ingredient list carefully; if you don't see progesterone listed in a concentration of at least 400 mg per ounce, the cream won't work. Also, if the label lists only Mexican wild yam but no progesterone, the manufacturer is making the incorrect assumption that your body will convert the yam to progesterone. In fact, your body cannot make this conversion, and this cream won't be effective.

FOR PMS: Starting ten days before your period, apply a half teaspoonful twice a day to an area where your skin is naturally thinner, such as your inner thighs or forearms, tummy, or buttocks. Use the cream until your period starts, stopping use until ten days before your next period.

Women going through the menopause transition often find progesterone cream helps their symptoms too. Like black cohosh, progesterone suppresses the pituitary gland's production of luteinizing hormone (LH), increasing in turn the amount of estrogen your ovaries release. It's the combination of low estrogen and high LH that's thought to be a source of hot flashes and night sweat misery.

FOR MENOPAUSE TRANSITION SYMPTOMS: Using a calendar to keep track, apply one-quarter teaspoon of the cream twice a day on days 1 through 7. Increase your dose to one-half teaspoon, once or twice a day depending on symptoms, from day 8 through 21. Use no cream for the remainder of the month.

WAYS TO INCREASE SEROTONIN

EXERCISE Get out and about for your brisk twenty-minute walk every day. Physical exertion increases levels of all feel-good hormones (called endorphins), including serotonin. The more exercise you get, the more endorphins you generate, and the more serotonin you produce.

SUNLIGHT Expose your eyes to sunlight and your body will make more serotonin. No sunglasses please—the light needs to reach your brain through your eyes to create serotonin.

FISH OIL Take 2 grams (2000 mg) of fish oil every day. Fish oil from cold-water fish offers high concentrations of polyunsaturated fats called omega-3 fatty acids, which your body can't produce on its own. The omega-3 DHA (docosahexaenoic acid) increases the amount of serotonin in your brain and improves serotonin's operational efficiency. And, yes, these are the same omega-3s that help prevent heart attacks.

VITAMIN B COMPLEX Take vitamin B complex 100 (p. 50), one tablet daily. B vitamins, mainly B_6 (pyridoxine), are needed for your brain to convert tryptophan, found in protein, to serotonin.

CARBOHYDRATE TIMING (p. 263) Eat a small amount of high-quality carbohydrates with each meal and for snacks throughout your day. Via a series of reactions, the carbs help get more tryptophan into your brain for conversion to serotonin.

ST. JOHN'S WORT Extremely popular among Europeans for mild-to-moderate depression, this herb is very gentle, extremely safe, and acts like most antidepressants: it slowly raises your serotonin by preventing serotonin already sitting in the synapse gap between two brain cells from getting reabsorbed. Take 450 mg twice a day.

5HTP This amino acid, 5-hydroxytryptophan, is one of the building blocks of serotonin. The tryptophan molecule first changes to 5HTP as it converts to serotonin. 5HTP works nicely in combination with St. John's wort to increase your serotonin. Take 100 mg at bedtime.

SAMe (S-adenosyl methionine) This nutritional supplement is a slight alteration of the amino acid methionine and is very much needed in your brain's neurotransmitter-manufacturing process. SAMe was shown in clinical studies to be as effective as many prescription antidepressants. But you must take it on an empty stomach and at 400 mg a dose, twice a day.

PRESCRIPTION ANTIDEPRESSANTS The SSRI antidepressants (p. 19) don't actually contain serotonin. They work like this: when one brain cell transmits information to another brain cell, the two are separated by a small gap called a synapse. The sending cell releases serotonin to carry the information across the gap. Once the information is delivered, the used serotonin is reabsorbed and recycled. SSRIs block this reabsorption and, as a consequence, levels of serotonin in the synapse gap increase. Not all prescription antidepressants are SSRIs; some focus on the neurotransmitters dopamine and norepinephrine. Although all antidepressants of all classes work to some degree, some people actually seem to have a better response when these other neurotransmitters are increased.

COMBINING SEROTONIN BOOSTERS Now let's review how you can use these various serotonin boosters together. I recommend that you try to raise your serotonin with the minimum amount of pill taking. You'll make a lot of progress with mild Triple Whammy discomforts by walking briskly for twenty minutes every day, eating some nutritious carbs at regular intervals, getting into the sun, and taking B complex and fish oil every day.

After a couple of weeks, if you're not happy with your progress (you're still mildly depressed or anxious, PMS-y, or your energy isn't up to par), add the St. John's wort and 5HTP. Consider adding SAMe as well if depression is your predominant symptom. These will take at least three or four weeks for maximum effect.

Now obviously, if you feel you're slipping backwards—that is, you're constantly depressed, sleeping poorly, crying a lot, anxious, or even panicky—you should not be trying any do-it-yourself doctoring. Make an appointment with your physician for a serious discussion about antidepressant therapy. And remember, antidepressants work best when combined with talk therapy, so please ask your doctor for a referral for some counseling (p. 232).

You should not take 5HTP, St. John's wort, or SAMe while you're taking prescription antidepressants because you could get an overload of serotonin in your brain. I say this as a precautionary measure, although I've never seen it actually happen to anyone. This "serotonin syndrome," so named by doctors, usually occurs with high doses of multiple prescription antidepressants. If you do decide a prescription antidepressant is right for you, regular exercise, sunlight, and carb timing will only enhance the effect of the medication.

PART III

TRIPLE WHAMMY
CURE PLUS

Healing Paths for Triple Whammy Disorders

5.

ANXIETY DISORDERS

– GENERALIZED ANXIETY DISORDER (GAD)

– PANIC DISORDER

– PHOBIAS

– POSTTRAUMATIC STRESS DISORDER (PTSD)

– OBSESSIVE-COMPULSIVE DISORDER (OCD)

– BODY DYSMORPHIC DISORDER (BDD)

Anxiety disorders can be incapacitating. Don't try to handle these problems on your own. Get some professional help. Begin counseling (p. 232) with a non-physician psychotherapist, such as a clinical psychologist. The reason for this is that unless your anxiety disorder is especially serious, you stand a good chance of being successfully treated without medication by talking about your anxieties and learning some relaxation techniques. Too often an MD (your internist or a psychiatrist) will reach for her prescription pad before you've finished telling your story. Understand that sometimes medication is necessary, and when it works well it does so with jaw-dropping success. But the nonprescription nutritional supplements described on page 64 have helped many of my patients when combined with talk therapy. If you're able to manage without prescription drugs, so much the better. Most psychotherapists use a technique called cognitive-behavioral therapy, which will teach you to recognize the steps your mind went through before you got to the dreadful point of anxiety or panic. You'll learn to substitute positive thoughts for negative ones, master some coping skills, and use guided imagery (p. 214) to ease fears and anxiety.

VARIATIONS ON A THEME

Doctors now recognize that each of the anxiety disorders is a variation of generalized anxiety disorder. If it's of any comfort to you, both generalized anxiety disorder and panic disorder are extremely common. When I was a young doctor doing my tour of duty in emergency rooms, people with panic attacks convinced they were having heart attacks vastly outnumbered people with actual heart attacks. The emergency room was located at an expressway exit and, with great regularity, the emotions of people feeling trapped in rush hour traffic and having to be somewhere "important" would escalate from anxiety to panic to "I'm having a heart attack" in minutes.

- **GENERALIZED ANXIETY DISORDER (GAD)** Imagine walking around all day with all the worry, dread, and fear generated by your body's fight-or-flight stress response without any real reason to do so. This state of affairs is known as generalized anxiety disorder. GAD is a chronic condition, mening that it can last for weeks or months, and may be accompanied by physical symptoms like restlessness, insomnia, and low sex drive. For some people, GAD has become such a sustained part of life that they can no longer pinpoint any triggering event. It's as if their whole stress response system has been reprogrammed to be always hypersensitive, with almost any life event able to trigger some degree of anxiety.

- **PANIC DISORDER** The acute form of the stress response that occurs unpredictably, intensely, and without any true serious threat is the well-named panic disorder. It's almost as if someone turned up the heat under your anxiety symptoms. In less than ten minutes, worry thoughts spin out of control, your heart pounds, and you might feel nauseated, dizzy, or sweaty. You might have some chest pain or feel like you're choking, smothering, unable to take a deep breath. You feel like you can't control your mind, and think you might be going crazy. In fact, you think you just might die.

- **PHOBIA** With a phobia, you know exactly the triggering event for your anxiety or panic, but at the same time, on a rational level, you're aware of its harmlessness. You simply can't prevent the intense feeling of anxiety that occurs when the stage is set in a certain way. People are commonly phobic of certain insects, animals, or situations (spiders, heights, darkness, closed spaces). The newly named social anxiety disorder describes a phobia of social situations, such as giving a speech or attending a cocktail party where you don't know anyone. Although medications have a definite role in the treatment of both phobias and social anxiety disorder, talk therapy and learned relaxation techniques can be especially helpful.

- **POSTTRAUMATIC STRESS DISORDER (PTSD)** For a person with posttraumatic stress disorder, something associated with an emotionally charged event or period in the person's life triggers severe anxiety or even panic. It turns out there's a virtual epidemic of PTSD among women soldiers returning from their tour of duty in Iraq. Treating PTSD is very complex and talk therapy is vital. Many times the event occurred years previously—as far back as early childhood. One approach to PTSD is to reexamine the triggering event in a perspective that attempts to defuse the power it holds over a person's life and then inch forward, reframing life with this weakened (but not denied) event under control.

- **OBSESSIVE-COMPULSIVE DISORDER (OCD)** In OCD, the affected person may have seemingly endless repetitive thoughts (obsessions) on one topic that are not worries about real life problems, but rather inappropriate, intrusive, and, even to the person herself, irrational. An example is a straight-A student who obsesses endlessly about failure. She tries unsuccessfully to clear such thoughts from her mind but is unable to do so. In an attempt to clear obsessions, people with OCD may perform repetitive acts (compulsions) aimed at preventing some fear or dreaded event. A person with a germ phobia may obsess about disease and wash her hands repeatedly all day to keep herself germ free.

- **BODY DYSMORPHIC DISORDER (BDD)** In this condition, related to OCD, an affected person obsesses about an imagined defect in appearance or a defect so slight that the person's concern is obviously excessive. People who have been of normal weight for years and yet think about their weight endlessly despite the protests of loved ones and doctors are considered to have body dysmorphic disorder.

WHAMMY #1: STRESS

To one extent or another, all anxiety disorders have a basis in the Triple Whammy, but especially in Whammy #1, stress. In "The Chemistry of Stress" (p. 5) we talk in detail about the stress response. It's what happens to all animals, humans included, when we're confronted with anything the brain registers as a threat. A mild stress, like an upcoming exam or deadline, is pretty much confined to an emotional level, with an overall feeling of worry or dread. If the stressor becomes actually threatening, though, like a mugger sticking a gun in your back, the stress response instantly throws your body into overdrive. The hormone primarily responsible for the stress response is adrenalin, triggered by distress signals from the brain. It's this stress response that allows a woman to lift a car off her trapped husband or child. The stress response can be very useful.

People actually thrive on mild forms of the stress response. We all perform a bit better when our stress response has us charged up, say presenting a new idea to the boss. Millions of us jump-start our day at Starbucks, receiving a daily blessing of caffeine, which acts in our bodies like a small dose of adrenalin. But when the stress response is triggered without any real stress, the situation is vastly different.

If you have an anxiety disorder and explore in some depth just why you're feeling anxious, you'll probably uncover an underlying basis for it—there's almost always an identifiable triggering event followed by a stress response that has spun out of control. With a condition like generalized anxiety disorder, it's almost as if your whole system has been reset, and you feel a sense of worry about everything and anything.

In various anxiety disorders, the threat that triggers the stress response can be old stuff, like an unpleasant memory, or a future threat that may never even occur. Neither is as immediately dangerous as the mugger, but your body's response is just the same. As a result, there's some justification in calling the triggering event of any anxiety disorder an empty threat. Consider how impressive the power of your mind is in producing negative changes in your body, in this case triggering stress in response to an empty threat. When it comes to getting well, you can use this same mind-body power in reverse to heal yourself. Even though your mind sent you into an emotional overdrive, you can, through skills such as meditation, self-hypnosis, and guided imagery, turn off your stress response and calm yourself down.

WHAMMY #2: LOW SEROTONIN

Women are most affected by anxiety disorders because you are underserved by stress-buffering serotonin. And like other Triple Whammy conditions, anxiety disorders often run through families, via female family members. Psychiatrists are well aware of the relationship between serotonin and anxiety disorders. The medications that boost serotonin levels in the brain—antidepressants—are at the front line of therapy. Patients with anxiety, panic, OCD, and PTSD are occasionally surprised to receive an antidepressant prescription, but you now understand that it's Whammy #2, low serotonin, that's being shored up. And antidepressants are safer than antianxiety drugs like Xanax (alprazolam) or

Ativan (lorazepam), which for some people can cause serious psychological dependence.

WHAMMY #3: HORMONES

In women susceptible to anxiety disorders, the close relationship between estrogen and serotonin levels often causes anxiety symptoms to worsen in the weeks or days before your period starts. If you're in perimenopause, you're also more vulnerable as your estrogen slowly declines, taking serotonin right along with it. At the other extreme, if you're pregnant, your estrogen levels are at their peak and you may enjoy a respite from your anxiety and panic.

THE TRIPLE WHAMMY APPROACH

– **STRESS** Remember that your anxiety disorder is actually an exaggerated stress response and that your goal is to survive (and thrive!) between visits to your psychotherapist. Now's a good time to turn to page 197 and review the entire "Stress Less" chapter. Especially helpful for anxiety disorders are the *chi* (pronounced "chee") based energy therapies, like yoga, t'ai chi, chi gong, and Reiki. Learn breathing exercises (see p. 217) and hold a positive thought. Most anxiety disorders can be brought under good control in just a few weeks or months.

– **SEROTONIN** You need to apply everything you've learned about raising your serotonin (p. 55). Get out in the sunlight; walk daily; and have high-quality complex carbs with every meal. Some foods for you to especially avoid: caffeine (you need coffee nerves AND panic attacks?); alcohol (which causes changes in your brain that can lead to panic attacks and also lowers your inhibitions generally, making you more defenseless to your underlying anxieties. Alcohol also causes rapid changes in blood sugar levels. A quick drop in blood sugar triggers your body to release a burst of adrenaline, which may start your heart thumping and trigger a panic attack in the process); sugar, sugary foods, and refined foods (these cause swings in blood sugar and bursts of adrenalin when your blood sugar falls too low). And don't forget the serotonin-enhancing vitamin B complex and fish oil.

- **HORMONES** Most of my patients with an anxiety disorder who are still menstruating tell me that their PMS days are the worst. What's happening, of course, is that your serotonin is being dragged down by declining levels of estrogen. If you've wondered about the involvement of your hormones, track your anxiety disorder symptoms on a calendar along with your PMS and period. Review the PMS healing path (p. 153) and follow the recommendations there, cleaning up your diet and taking the hormone-balancing herb chasteberry. If you and your doctor decide that a tranquilizer or antidepressant would be helpful, tell her about the chasteberry. There are no known interaction problems between chasteberry and these drugs.

MEDICATIONS

The number of different medications used for the cornucopia of anxiety disorders is extensive, and every one of them, in one way or another, will work. For severe and incapacitating anxiety symptoms, most doctors employ a "one-two" strategy of calming with a fast-acting tranquilizer from the benzodiazepine group, such as alprazolam (Xanax) or lorazepam (Ativan), while at the same time starting an antidepressant to raise serotonin. It usually takes a month for the serotonin-boosting antidepressants to take full effect, and once you feel better, you can take your tranquilizer only when you need it. The problem with tranquilizers is you can get so tranquil you can crash your car. They can also be habit forming. Our health care system occasionally loses sight of the patient and seems willing to renew both tranquilizer and antidepressant prescriptions without consultation for years. This long-term use isn't necessary and is in fact not good for you. Most people with anxiety disorders are able to taper off SSRI antidepressants after several symptom-free months.

NUTRITIONAL SUPPLEMENTS

You can follow the same general one-two strategy as is used with prescription drugs by choosing nutritional supplements that act as mild anti-anxiety tranquilizers and others that boost your serotonin. Definitely discuss their use with your therapist. My suggestion is that you simultaneously start a natural anti-anxiety supplement (like valerian or GABA) to deal with your immediate symptoms along with supplements to raise your serotonin (St. John's wort, 5HTP); these take three to four weeks to reach their full effect. If you also include such anxiety-busters as meditation, yoga, or massage therapy, you'll probably find yourself taking fewer anti-anxiety supplements each day.

– **VALERIAN** Researchers aren't exactly sure how valerian works, but increasing your level of GABA (see below) is a possibility. No matter what the mechanism, valerian is an effective daytime tranquilizer. Increasing your dose at bedtime makes it an excellent sleep aid. **DOSE:** (as a tranquilizer) 300–400 mg two or three times a day as needed; (as a sleep aid) 800–900 mg at bedtime.

– **GABA** GABA (gamma-aminobutyric acid) is your body's natural tranquilizer. It's an amino acid that functions as a brain chemical by keeping anxiety-related signals at bay. Low levels of GABA in your brain can lead to anxiety and can also cause irritability, insomnia, and even seizures. Taking GABA promotes relaxation and sleep and is probably why many drugs used for anxiety, Valium among them, target GABA receptors in the brain. Unlike prescription tranquilizers, GABA is not habit forming and usually doesn't make you drowsy. But take your first test dose of GABA on your own turf rather than while on the expressway. **DOSE:** 250–500 mg two or three times a day.

– **ST. JOHN'S WORT** Although primarily known for its use in treating mild to moderate depression by raising serotonin, St. John's wort (p. 20) is helpful for any of the anxiety disorders. Like the SSRIs, St. John's wort takes four to six weeks to build up the serotonin in your brain, so you need to be patient with it. If you're going to start taking a prescription antidepressant, tell your doctor you've been on St. John's and then stop taking the herb. Taking both may give your brain too much serotonin and cause symptoms of poor sleep, anxiety, and a sense of feeling "wired." **DOSE:** Start with 450 mg twice a day for three weeks. If you think things are improving but more would be better, increase the dose to three times a day.

– **5HTP** This amino acid is a building block of serotonin and works nicely in combination with St. John's wort to pump up that serotonin. If you start taking an antidepressant, discontinue taking 5HTP. **DOSE:** 5HTP has a slightly sedating quality, so take your dose (100 mg) at bedtime. You can use a smaller dose (50 mg) during the day, for daytime anxiety.

ALTERNATIVE THERAPIES

Practitioners of alternative medicine that uses the subtle energy called *chi* believe that energy imbalances are at the heart of most psychological disorders, including anxiety disorders and depression. They work on your whole body to bring these energies into balance.

– **TRADITIONAL CHINESE MEDICINE (TCM) AND ACUPUNCTURE** Both chronic anxiety and acute panic attacks can respond nicely to acupuncture. For longer-lasting treatment, regular acupuncture sessions combined with Chinese herbal formulations can be very helpful. A regular schedule of psychotherapy along with TCM (p. 285) might even be able to keep you off prescription medication, but if this doesn't work, don't be stubborn. Get appropriate prescription therapy. By the way:

if you're combining conventional and alternative therapies, let each practitioner know about the other in order to prevent any adverse herb-drug interactions. These, as it happens, are extremely rare when using Chinese herbs.

– **ACUPRESSURE** There's a good panic-attack button on your wrist, two thumb widths below the bottom of your palm. If you press this spot firmly with your thumb, close your eyes, and take several slow deep breaths, you'll feel an immediate sense of calm over your entire body. To enhance this effect, keep your thumb in place and, using the middle finger of the hand being pressed, press the spot between your eyebrows at the center of your forehead. See page 207 for more.

– **MASSAGE** Regular massage (p. 236) and other bodywork therapies, like Reiki (p. 239) and reflexology (p. 223), can be extremely effective in reducing stress and improving your overall sense of well-being. Your muscles can store unpleasant memories, so don't be surprised if you suddenly feel tearful, or some unexpected memories appear during a session. Your bodywork therapist is used to this reaction and can offer commonsense counseling and advice.

SELF-CARE

You can use each of these self-care approaches safely with other therapies. The first is essential.

– **NUTRITION** Two cardinal rules apply: first, you need to eat some high-quality carbohydrates—not candy bars—to facilitate serotonin production throughout your day. Second, you don't want your blood sugar levels to swing all over the place, so avoid sugar, processed foods, bakery goods, caffeine, and alcohol (although a glass of red wine with dinner is fine, and will not cause significant blood sugar changes). Don't skip meals and do have a small bedtime snack. See the Triple Whammy Food Plan (p. 245) for more.

– **AROMATHERAPY** The five soothing oils most often recommended for anxiety and stress are geranium, bergamot, melissa, lavender, and ylang-ylang. You can use each alone or mix them together. Put a few drops of each into a warm bath (see p. 211), dim the lights, close your eyes, and try to discern each flower separately. Carry a handkerchief with your favorite oil drizzled lightly and breathe in its calming essence when anxiety starts to surface.

– **FLOWER ESSENCE THERAPY** Mild, safe, and gentle, drops of homeopathic flower preparations placed under the tongue are designed to help with a variety of emotional problems. Aspen is frequently recommended for anxiety accompanied by a sense of dread. Use larch when you feel an inability to cope and red chestnut when you're excessively concerned about the welfare of others. A flower therapist will be familiar with dozens of combinations and her remedies can enhance your counseling sessions. Flower essence therapy is discussed on page 220.

6

CHRONIC FATIGUE SYNDROME

At its most severe, chronic fatigue syndrome (CFS) is the worst of the Triple Whammy disorders. In the thirty years I've practiced medicine, no single illness has been more confusing to the health care system—at the expense of patients—than this one. Physicians first argued over whether the condition was real, and to this day an unfortunately large number of them still question its validity. And the many doctors who do accept its existence continue to disagree on what causes it and how to treat it.

The group of symptoms we use today to define CFS has been around for more than a century. The condition and the symptoms are genuine. CFS patients are not hypochondriacs; they feel terrible and are truly exhausted. They are not "just depressed." There is no evidence that any infection causes CFS. There are no positive lab tests or X-ray results, except occasional evidence of adrenal gland fatigue (p. 10), although adrenal fatigue is present with many other chronic illnesses. The best evidence seems to show that CFS is an extreme form of the fatigue component that accompanies fibromyalgia (p. 88).

A successful understanding of CFS will ultimately be based on the links among mind, body, and the immune system. Currently, CFS researchers would like the condition to be positioned in the diagnostic lexicon as an extreme version of a group of conditions called "affective spectrum disorder," a mind-body diagnostic umbrella that includes fibromyalgia, irritable bowel syndrome, chronic headaches, and PMS, among others. If these sound a lot like some of our Triple Whammy Disorders, you're absolutely right. My only problem with this thinking is that the researchers separate what they call "emotional" disorders, such as depression, anxiety, and panic, into a distinct psychiatric arena, seemingly in denial of the connections between mind and body.

Reducing stress and boosting serotonin by any means helps all the so-called affective spectrum disorder conditions—not only anxiety, depression, and panic, but also irritable bowel, sleep disorders, and migraines. Therefore, a better term, but truly a mouthful, might be "multiple emotional and physical manifestations of low-serotonin disorder which, when occurring in women, are also influenced by cyclic sex hormone shifts."

Yes, a little awkward. The Triple Whammy may be more efficient a description—and a more vivid one.

WHAT CFS FATIGUE FEELS LIKE

Let's talk a little about the fatigue of CFS. We've all been tired. In fact, most of us—especially any woman caring for a family or extended family—have at times in our lives been really wiped out. But unless you have severe CFS yourself, or

WHAMMY #1 AND THE TRIGGERING OF CFS

CFS almost always follows a period of significant stress. This may include an emotional "crash" such as a marriage ending, the death of a loved one, or being incredibly overworked on a job only to be passed over for a promotion. The stress can also be a physical one: a mugging or rape, severe flu, or exposure to chemicals. Interestingly, it almost doesn't matter what kind of chemical—the chemical is the last straw in a series of other stresses or insults to the body and mind. Many, though not all, CFS patients lived relatively unhealthy lifestyles before their illness started, usually a combination of overworking, eating poorly, rarely exercising, and sometimes drinking too much alcohol or overusing other recreational drugs.

All people who go through similar stresses don't get CFS. If they have enough serotonin to buffer the stress, they don't get CFS, but often do have other Triple Whammy symptoms or disorders.

know someone who does, you can't begin to imagine how hopelessly exhausted affected people can feel.

Here's what it's like: it's dawn, and you're lying in bed. You've just awakened from a night during which you didn't sleep well, and it feels as if you could use a few more hours of shut-eye. But you have to pee. Your blankets feel heavy as you try to pull them off your body and you struggle—actually struggle—to free yourself. You know just getting the blankets off your body will start to tax your energy reserves. You have to concentrate to force your legs to swing over the bed onto the floor. Your muscles feel stiff and achy. En route to the bathroom, you use furniture you've arranged to support yourself as you walk. In fact, you may have moved your bed closer to the bathroom simply because the walk was too tiring. You finally reach the toilet, relieve yourself, and stagger back to bed, turning on the TV as you pass it. You'll be watching TV all day because there's really nothing else you can do. You gave up reading because you can't concentrate. Your arms get too tired for an activity like knitting. This has been your life for over a year now.

Fortunately, most patients with CFS don't experience this degree of exhaustion. But some do, and thousands of people with CFS are struggling through their work days, desperately trying to earn a living, care for their families, and maintain relationships as they wonder how long their nightmare is going to last. "It may sound funny, but what I'd really like to do is go bowling," one of my patients with CFS told me. "That's all. You know, after work, meet some friends. Instead, I barely make it home, heat up a TV dinner, and fall into bed." And from another CFS sufferer: "I'd like to start up a flight of stairs without wondering if I'm going to make it to the top."

CFS: A CLASSIC TRIPLE WHAMMY DISORDER

The exact cause of CFS is not known. Like other Triple Whammy disorders, there's probably a genetic predisposition and possibly a family history of other Triple Whammy disorders. Lacking enough serotonin to act as a buffer, neither the sufferer's body nor her mind can handle the unremitting stress. Whammies #1 (stress) and #2 (low serotonin) are at the center of this CFS business.

Through extensive psychological testing, researchers are aware of other aspects of CFS patients. For example, many were hyperactive Type A's before the onset of the illness, usually overworking themselves, never having learned to say "no" to the requests of others. Not infrequently, along with a smorgasbord of external stressors (work, family, finances), internal demons also existed beforehand, such as childhood abuse, unmet life expectations, and low self-esteem. Overwhelmed by stress, with inadequate reserves, seemingly unable to make healthful lifestyle changes, all their systems crash. The last straw may be a bad case of the flu, an injury such as an auto accident, an emotionally traumatic event such as being robbed, or even (paradoxically) a prolonged vacation with the thought of going back to work at a terrible job.

What I suggest to patients is something like this: If you review the year before the start of your chronic fatigue, it's likely your stress level was high and you weren't taking particularly good care of yourself. With a high level of stress, you taxed your stress glands—the two adrenals and your thyroid. The constant stress, which went unchecked because you lack sufficient serotonin to act as a stress buffer, exhausted these glands and compromised your immune system. You became fatigued, and an infection that normally you'd cast off like a mild cold overwhelmed you.

Imagine yourself as an upright line of dominoes. A confluence of events knocks down the first domino, and now the entire row is just . . . lying there. That leaves us with the big question: can someone with chronic fatigue syndrome ever get well? The answer is a firm "it depends."

CFS: THREE WORDS TO GET BETTER BY

Doctors who specialize in treating patients with CFS generally use three words when trying to determine who will improve and who won't: motivation, adaptation, and compliance. (And, actually, these three ideas could apply to anyone with a serious illness.) Because of your complexity as an individual with CFS, some of this probably won't apply to you. But please read it anyway and consider whether you're knowingly or unknowingly sabotaging your healing process. By this I don't mean you're not permitted to have horrible days where you're completely down in the dumps. No way. CFS is a huge challenge, and I ask only that you try to see your efforts at getting better as clearly as possible.

- **MOTIVATION** Those who love and care for a person with CFS (doctors included) want to believe with all their hearts that their patient wants to get well, especially someone suffering the fatigue and pain of CFS. But the human mind is extraordinarily complex, and there may be problems for the patient associated with getting well. What if, for example, the CFS began after a period of intense physical and emotional stress—so intense, in fact, that on a subconscious level, the body understands that getting well means a return to those bad old days? Being sick not only keeps you from confronting the previous stressors, but also provides the added benefits of having fewer demands made on you. In fact, you may want to ask yourself consciously if there are any other benefits you get from being sick—are you able to keep people close to you because of your illness? Does it keep you from having to deal with people you don't want to see? There can be all kinds of reasons. Consciously, of course, the person does want her health restored. But in the labyrinth of the subconscious, getting well may be another matter altogether.

– **COMPLIANCE** Many doctors who work with CFS patients report that a disproportionate number of those patients manage to come up with reasons to say no to proffered therapies. By far the most common sentence I hear is "I can't take that, it gives me side effects." Now, I do cut slack here, because all my Triple Whammy patients have low serotonin and that makes them very sensitive to drugs and chemicals. But when every medicine or supplement—no matter how small the dose—is rejected, your health worker's optimism can fade. When alternative therapies are equally refused ("My insurance won't cover it," "I had a terrible reaction to acupuncture," or "I don't trust chiropractors"), my hope sinks. During the past two years, I've been referring CFS patients into a research study at nearby DePaul University. If a patient paid for it herself, the study would costs thousands of dollars, but this one is totally free. In addition, the success rate is very high for those willing to make a several-month commitment. Yet fully half of those I referred into the study came up with reasons not to participate. This is not a blame-the-patient stance, but shows the sheer complexity and power of mind-body interactions with regard to chronic illness.

– **ADAPTATION** A quality that has been shown to be decisively effective when coping with CFS is the ability to adapt to the challenges brought on by illness. Good research reveals that a form of counseling (p. 232) called cognitive-behavioral therapy, which teaches you the whys and hows of CFS, including lifestyle changes and stress reduction techniques, can be most helpful. By identifying and changing self-destructive behavior patterns, patients start heading to the heart of the matter and press the Forward button to wellness. Not the Fast Forward button by any means, but definitely progress. Great patience is called for, but by adaptation, most people with CFS ultimately get a big chunk of their lives back, and learn a great deal about themselves in the process.

TREATING CFS

In addition to the Three-Week Cure (except for the twenty-minute daily walk), here's what works:

LIFESTYLE CHANGES

The term "lifestyle changes" is used to describe everything from redecorating to getting a puppy. In the context of CFS, making the following changes can take on life-altering meaning.

EXERCISE. Through exercise you can break the cycle of fatigue, muscle-wasting, decreased cardiovascular performance, and diminished interest in movement of any sort and counter the rising desire for more and more rest.

- **START TODAY** by walking outside for three minutes and do this each day for a week.

- **ONE WEEK FROM NOW,** walk for six minutes every day.

- **THE FOLLOWING WEEK,** walk for nine minutes every day.

- **EACH WEEK THEREAFTER,** add three minutes to your daily walk.

Stay carefully within the allotted time frames. It's easy to overestimate what you can do and overexercise, leading to a "crash" the next morning, which will exhaust and ultimately discourage you. Take a watch so you know exactly how far you can go before you need to return—for example, on your three-minute walk, walk for a minute and a half in one direction before turning around and heading back to home base. If you have health insurance, ask your doctor for a referral to a physical therapist for a graded exercise program. Call several physical therapists until you find one who has worked with CFS patients.

WHAMMY #1: STRESS REDUCTION. The trigger for this whole CFS mess was some sort of major stress to your entire self, mind and body. Seriously consider the following.

- **PROFESSIONAL COUNSELING** (p. 232) can help you explore the wrong left turn that got you into this pickle.

- **READ ABOUT STRESS** on page 197 and select one or more activities from the Stress-Relief Menu that appeal to you and that you can do every day, along with your walking. Many of the options I've included there are ideal for CFS patients, including do-at-home guided imagery, meditation, biofeedback, aromatherapy, self-hypnosis, and yoga postures.

DIETARY CHANGES. Many of my CFS patients have inadvertently neglected a good nutrition program. The Triple Whammy Food Plan (p. 245) is a highly nutritious way to get back on course. It's important for you to avoid swings in your blood sugar, so "grazing" throughout the day may be a good choice for you. Avoid foods that will tax your adrenal gland, including those containing sugar or caffeine. CFS patients should avoid adding sugar to anything, and stay far away from caffeine, alcohol, fruit juices, sugary drinks, and even diet drinks. Carbo timing (p. 263) will provide energy and increase serotonin. In addition:

- **ENJOY MEDIUM-SIZED MEALS,** with high-quality protein (poultry, fish), high-quality carbohydrates (legumes, whole grains), fruits, and green veggies.

- **DRINK AT LEAST 64 OUNCES** of water per day.

- **TAKE A HIGH-POTENCY MULTIPLE VITAMIN/MINERAL COMBINATION DAILY.** You can tell a high-potency supplement from a one-a-day variety because the recommended dose will be higher (like two capsules daily) and the RDA numbers will all be greater than 100 percent. Once you're in the high potency group, the different brands are really all alike. And don't worry about doubling up on B vitamins by taking this supplement in addition to the B complex recommended in the Three-Week Cure. Your body will eliminate what you don't need because B vitamins are water soluble, meaning you excrete any extra via your urine. However, this does not apply to fat-soluble vitamins (A, D, E, and K). Any extra you take of these can slowly build up in the fat cells of your body and stay there a good long time—not recommended.

MEDICINES FOR CFS

Since there's no prescription cure for CFS, these medicines address symptoms. Many people with CFS are extraordinarily sensitive to drugs, so start with the smallest feasible dose. Tell your doctor that you're very sensitive and ask if she minds if you start with the lowest dose possible and then work up to a higher dose if needed. Almost no doctor will argue with you about this. Cut your tablets into quarters and, if the medicine comes in capsules, just be sure you've got the lowest dose available.

- **MUSCLE PAIN** Unless your muscle and joint discomfort is severe (not usually the case in those with CFS), milder medications can work for you. Start with acetaminophen (Tylenol) or an anti-inflammatory such as ibuprofen (Motrin), and consider taking it in a longer-acting prescription form, such as diclofenac (Voltaren). A muscle relaxant such as cyclobenzaprine (Flexeril) has the benefit of improving sleep when taken at bedtime. Tramadol (Ultram) or tramadol with acetaminophen (Ultracet) also can help for muscle pain.

- **INCREASING SEROTONIN** Some doctors working with CFS patients recommend older antidepressants such as amitriptyline (Elavil) to boost serotonin because the drugs also improve sleep. Many of my patients find the side effects unacceptable. The SSRI antidepressants (p. 19) Lexapro and Zoloft will increase your serotonin. The newer Cymbalta is unique in that it simultaneously increases both serotonin and norepinephrine. This dual effect may be especially helpful for both fibromyalgia and CFS patients by increasing energy, ehancing mental clarity, and reducing muscle pain.

- **SLEEP** Along with regular exercise, efficient and refreshing sleep can help break your endless fatigue cycle. Although muscle relaxants and antidepressants can double as sleep aids, you may want to ask your doctor to prescribe Ambien or Restoril (see Sleeping Pills, p. 176).

- **STIMULANTS** Two medications for attention deficit disorder (ADD)—methylphenidate (Ritalin) and amphetamine (Adderall)—can improve fatigue. The ADD medications work by increasing brain levels of norepinephrine, and as it rises the brain fog of CFS often improves as well. Start low with Adderall or Ritalin, no more than 2.5 mg or 5 mg once or twice a day, and gradually increase every few days. Each is available in a long-acting form that can be taken once a day. The newer medication Provigil, originally designed for the daytime sleepiness of narcolepsy, can also boost energy levels. Provigil comes in 200 mg tablets that can easily be cut in half. Start with 100 mg each morning. This may be plenty for you and will reduce your prescription cost considerably.

- **ADRENAL SUPPORT** Because adrenal gland fatigue (see p. 10) frequently accompanies and may even precipitate CFS, blood tests for adrenal gland function may be abnormal. This does not mean your adrenals are diseased, but rather "exhausted." Low doses of the prescription adrenal hormones cortisol (5 mg once or twice a day) and fludrocortisone (0.1 mg each morning) may be helpful. Don't be surprised if your doctor is unwilling to prescribe adrenal hormones for CFS, as this is still considered by some physicians to be controversial. In any case do take an adrenal support formula (see adrenal complex supplements, p. 76), whether or not you have been prescribed actual adrenal hormones.

- **FOCUS AND CONCENTRATION** With your pain, sleep, and fatigue issues addressed by lifestyle changes and prescription medication, you'll generally experience an improvement in memory, focus, and concentration. Because you need adequate levels of serotonin and norepinephrine for optimal brain function, raising these neurotransmitters using an SSRI antidepressant and a stimulant like Adderall will generally alleviate your brain fog. If you're reluctant to use prescription medications, several nutritional supplements can help brain fog, including acetyl-L-carnitine (p. 76), phosphatidyl serine (p. 76), ginkgo biloba (p. 116), and pregnenolone (p. 95) taken in a dose of 10 mg per day.

- **HORMONAL CONCERNS** Based on experience with my patients, I believe the effect of fluctuating hormones month-to-month may play less of a role in CFS than in other Triple Whammy disorders. I think this is because women with CFS feel so crummy every day that they don't perceive a PMS component to their CFS. If your symptoms worsen during PMS days, address this by using chasteberry (175 mg to 225 mg daily) or progesterone. Remember, though, that chasteberry affects hormone levels, so don't use it if you're taking hormone replacement therapy or birth control pills (it can lessen their effectiveness), or if you're pregnant or nursing.

- **THYROID FUNCTION** The involvement of the thyroid gland in CFS has been the subject of some controversy. Generally, blood tests for thyroid function are completely normal in people with CFS, which should mean your thyroid gland is working well. But some doctors, myself included, are skeptical. If your basal temperature (armpit temperature, taken when you awaken in the morning; see p. 75) is below 97.6, you might benefit from a small dose of natural thyroid replacement, usually in the range of one half grain to 1 grain daily, available by prescription, to improve your

HOW TO TAKE YOUR BASAL
BODY TEMPERATURE

You might ask, and quite sensibly: what is a basal body temperature? "Basal" means "base," and your basal temperature is your body temperature taken the very first thing in the morning before you've moved out of your sleeping position. Once you get out of bed, the movement of your muscles heats up your body, so it's essential that you follow these instructions closely to get an accurate reading. To take your basal body temperature:

- Use an old-fashioned mercury thermometer.

- Shake down the mercury before going to sleep and place the thermometer on your bedside table with paper and pen.

- When you awaken, place the bulb of the thermometer in your armpit and leave it there for ten minutes. Lie back and relax, keeping your armpit closed over the thermometer.

- After ten minutes, record your temperature.

- Repeat for five days and then take an average. (You remember this from grade school, right? Add the five numbers and then divide by five to get the average.)

If you menstruate, measure your basal body temperature on the second day after your period starts. Ovulation, which occurs later in the month, increases your temperature and thus won't give an accurate reading.

energy. A note: the blood test for thyroid function—TSH (thyroid stimulating hormone)—actually measures levels of a hormone produced by the pituitary, the "master" gland in your body. High TSH levels mean low thyroid function. A TSH of 3.5 (not 5.0, as once believed) should mean the thyroid is functioning normally. However, even if your TSH is normal, if your basal temperature is low a trial period of hormone replacement is definitely worth trying.

ALTERNATIVE THERAPIES AND CFS

Although I'm extremely fond of alternative medicine, if you have a limited budget I think the two steps with the most bang for your buck are counseling—especially cognitive-behavioral therapy—and hiring a personal trainer or physical therapist familiar with the needs of CFS patients. Beyond that, consider the following:

- **IF MUSCLE PAIN IS AN ISSUE,** add a massage therapist (p. 236) or Reiki practitioner (p. 239) to your list of caregivers.

- **TO HELP YOU DISCOVER HOW YOUR CFS GOT STARTED,** traditional Chinese medicine (p. 285) or homeopathy (p. 277) can be helpful as you unravel the complex story-of-your-life issues that started this mess. Read "Looking for Clues in Your Life Story" on page 33 to get an idea of what we're talking about.

- **IF YOU'RE IDEOLOGICALLY AVERSE TO ALL PRESCRIPTION MEDICATIONS** (let me politely disagree with your stance), consider a licensed naturopathic physician (p. 281).

NUTRITIONAL SUPPLEMENTS

The following supplements can help relax muscles and raise serotonin levels.

- **ST. JOHN'S WORT, 5HTP, B COMPLEX, AND FISH OIL** all increase serotonin levels in your brain, ease depression, aid concentration, and improve tolerance to pain. The 5HTP, B complex, and fish oil help your brain manufacture more serotonin by providing raw materials and speeding along the metabolic processes that turn 5HTP into serotonin, while St. John's wort prevents serotonin breakdown. The result is a slow but steady rise in serotonin. If you start taking prescription antidepressants, stop the St. John's wort and 5HTP. **DOSE: ST. JOHN'S WORT** 450 mg twice a day, taken with meals to avoid upset stomach. **5HTP** 100 mg at bedtime; after a week add another 50 mg in the morning (discontinue the morning dose if it makes you sleepy). **B COMPLEX 100** One capsule daily. **FISH OIL** 1,000 mg twice a day.

- **COENZYME Q10 AND NADH** may help your fatigue symptoms. Each of these is involved in maintaining the mitochondria, the energy producing units of your cells. **DOSE:** 50–100 mg of Co Q10 twice a day; NADH 5 mg twice a day, taken on an empty stomach to enhance absorption.

- **PHOSPHATIDYL SERINE AND ACETYL-L-CARNITINE** are involved in healthy brain function. For severe brain fog, they're taken separately and in substantial doses. Several combination products containing these supplements are available. **DOSE:** Phosphatidyl serine 100 mg twice a day; acetyl-L-carnitine 500 mg twice a day; combination product taken according to package directions.

- **ADRENAL COMPLEX SUPPLEMENTS,** typically containing ginseng, licorice, and vitamin B-5, are an excellent addition. A blood test for adrenal exhaustion (p. 11) looks for low levels of DHEA, an adrenal "pre-hormone" that converts to other adrenal hormones. If your DHEA levels are low, DHEA itself is available at most health food stores. **DOSE:** DHEA (women) 10–25 mg per day until levels return to normal; adrenal combination taken according to package instructions.

- **LICORICE AND LOW BLOOD PRESSURE** Related to weak adrenal function, many people with CFS have abnormally low blood pressure that may contribute to their fatigue. In fact, some researchers believe that adrenal exhaustion leading to low blood pressure is the actual trigger for the fatigue itself. The herb licorice has been used for over a century for symptoms of exhaustion and is a part of many adrenal support formulas. If you have very low blood pressure, you can get virtually the same effect as licorice by simply being generous with your table salt and eating salty foods.

SELF-CARE TECHNIQUES

Any or all of these self-care steps can be quite beneficial and safely used with other CFS therapies. Read more about them starting on p. 204.

- **ACUPRESSURE/REFLEXOLOGY** These techniques unblock stagnations and imbalances of your vital energy, called *chi*. You may be pleasantly surprised to feel enhanced energy and clarity of thought when your *chi* is flowing smoothly through your body.

- **AROMATHERAPY** Try the following to help with CFS: tea tree oil (immune stimulation); bergamot, neroli (general uplifting of spirits and vitalizing); thyme, lemon grass (muscle fatigue); valerian, Roman chamomile, lavender (insomnia).

- **FLOWER ESSENCES** The developer of flower essence therapy anticipated the mind-body connection in illness and believed that the first step in treating illness was to begin on the emotional level. See page 220 and consider these extracts: rock rose (sense of never recovering); hornbeam (exhaustion at the thought of performing any task); mustard (depression without known cause); olive (chronically tired).

- **SUPPORT GROUPS** Consider joining a local support group, but please be discerning. You want a group that's positive about healing, not a pity-party affair that preoccupies itself with relating whose symptoms are the worst and endlessly telling anecdotes about uncaring physicians and insurance companies. While a brief sharing of these experiences can be helpful, the continual review of the negative is extremely counterproductive to healing and often serves to entrench the illness further. Join a support group only if it's being led by a health professional familiar with CFS.

- **T'AI CHI AND YOGA** The gentle movements of these health-enhancing, stress-reducing, and strength-developing exercises are ideal for anyone who has CFS. The people who lead these classes are extremely sensitive to individual ability, so if you have to rest between movements or positions, they will be understanding and support you.

7.

DEPRESSION

Grief and sadness are among those emotions that define us as human beings. When you respond to an upsetting event in your life, or to a painful memory, by feeling blue, having the blahs, shedding a few tears—this is you as a person feeling more. As the poet wrote, "Better to have loved and lost than never to have loved at all." When we drizzle tears at the end of a movie, we know this is a good emotion to have experienced. In fact, we may feel a little uncomfortable around someone who claims not to have felt a thing.

But just as sadness is part of good emotional health, so is acknowledging and understanding it, and seeing beyond it. When grief or sadness last and last and are accompanied by a persistently empty feeling, then we're entering the dark land of depression. In this dismal place, we encounter extreme feelings of dejection, melancholy, hopelessness, helplessness, and despair. Unlike grieving or sadness, in which we're feeling *more*, with depression we're actually feeling *less*. Activities we once enjoyed, such as socializing, eating, and sex, do nothing for us. During depression, you go through the motions of life without really feeling anything along the way. To me, one of the real tragedies about depression is that to this day, some people still believe it's a sign of personal weakness—a flaw in their characters—and that if only they tried harder or were more worthy they could snap out of it. This could not be further from the truth.

WHAMMIES 2+1 AND DEPRESSION

Your susceptibility to depression is very much related to Whammy #2, feel-good serotonin, and the other neurotransmitters in your brain. In general, women have periods of major depression far more frequently than men because - they're born with less available serotonin. But just like other serotonin disorders, depression runs in families, so a daughter of two parents with depression is especially vulnerable. But even though a genetic predisposition makes you vulnerable, it usually takes one or more stressful life events to trigger depression. For women prone to it, depression often surfaces at different points in their lives and, like other Triple Whammy disorders, usually is triggered by Whammy #1, stress. The stressful event varies widely by individual but can include experiences as diverse as divorce, surgery, job loss, retirement, or a child leaving home.

Factors other than stress can set off depression. For example, sunlight is needed for the brain to make serotonin. So for some people—again mainly women—the autumnal shift to shorter, dimmer days and longer dark nights may set off the depression of seasonal affective disorder (SAD, p. 164). Postpartum depression (p. 146), initiated by dramatic hormonal shifts and an attendant drop in serotonin, affects some women. Susceptible women also seem vulnerable to the symptoms of depression during PMS days. Some prescription medications, such as birth control pills or high blood pressure medicines, can trigger depression.

Nutritionally oriented physicians (and I am one of them) believe that lifestyle choices—including excessive caffeine or sugar, alcohol, tobacco, or a generally unhealthful diet—can also leave susceptible women vulnerable. Since a steady intake of good-quality carbohydrates (see Carbohydrate Timing, p. 263) is essential for maintaining adequate serotonin levels, a low-carb eating program can be troublesome, especially for women with genetically low serotonin levels. Prolonged carb restriction can set off a pervasive snarkiness if you're deprived too long.

THE HEALTH CARE SYSTEM, COUNSELING, AND ANTIDEPRESSANTS

I'm convinced that the U.S. health care system does not treat depression in ways that meet the best interests of the depressed patient. There are three reasons:

- Antidepressants are overused by overworked physicians who have no business prescribing them. Counseling and lifestyle changes can often work more effectively.

- Antidepressants are underused by non-physician psychotherapists who aren't
  trained in their use, are forbidden by law to prescribe them, and may keep their
  clients engaged in ineffective talk therapy for years for depressive symptoms that
  could disappear after a month of medication.

- Very few mental health practitioners, doctors and non-doctors alike, tell their patients about alternatives, such as the herbs and nutritional supplements of the
  Three-Week Cure, Chinese medicine, relaxation, and bodywork therapies.

The result is that people who believe they are depressed need to be extremely
proactive—even feisty and demanding—in order to get the best care they can afford. And they have to do this, of course, when depression itself is making them
feel less than able to do so.

Like many physicians, I have mixed emotions about antidepressants. On the
one hand, after a few weeks of antidepressant therapy, many patients report that
the black veil of their depression lifted and life is good again. And side effects can
be substantially reduced or avoided when medication is given correctly in the
lowest effective dose. Antidepressants are quite safe. They are not uppers, not
habit forming, and when given to a person without a serotonin disorder, nothing
really seems to happen. But too many physicians and patients are taking a complex condition like depression and trying to simplify it with a pill. Antidepressants address the biochemistry of depression—your low serotonin—but nothing
else. People are complex beings, and how they respond to a crisis varies considerably. So before taking a medicine that changes your brain chemistry, I'd like
you first to explore some vital issues and learn some strategies to handle stressors
as life hands them out. As a patient, you won't get much counseling in a ten-
minute office visit with your overworked HMO primary doc. But unless you in-
sist on more than a prescription, what you receive will be, pardon the expression,
pretty half-assed mental health care.

My second issue with antidepressants is that the tens of thousands of
psychologists, therapists, and clinical social workers who actually counsel depressed patients for a living are taught next to nothing about medications and,
because they're not MDs, can't prescribe. As a result, they're often not aware of
when medication intervention can bring to a successful halt months of less-than-
effective talk therapy. Each year here in the Chicago area, about five hundred
people trained to treat mental illness graduate from training programs. Of these,

ANTIDEPRESSANTS

When correctly and appropriately prescribed, antidepressant medicines are extremely helpful. If you're suffering significant depression or unremitting anxiety, antidepressants can put your life back on track. Before antidepressants existed, hundreds of thousands of people lived in relentless despair. Suicides were common. State mental hospitals were filled with people diagnosed with "chronic melancholia." Our knowledge of brain chemistry, and the creation of an extraordinarily safe family of medications, changed that. The number of people actually hospitalized with severe depression drops every year. So if you think, "Whatever happens, I won't go on antidepressants," I ask that you keep an open mind. When antidepressants work, you'll get your life back.

Although one drug may be different from another because of which neurotransmitter it affects, in actual fact each one will work to some degree. No antidepressant is better than another, but all take as long as a month to kick in because it takes time to increase neurotransmitter levels in the gaps (synapses) between your brain cells. Please keep in mind that your first prescription may not be the best. You have a 65 percent chance that the first antidepressant selected for you will actually lift your depression. You might have to switch drugs a couple of times, or even combine two, before you find the right treatment. And since low-serotonin Triple Whammy disorders run in families, if you happen to know which antidepressant helped your mom or your sister, let your doctor know. It's a good place for you to start.

only about fifty (the psychiatrists) can write prescriptions for antidepressants. As a result, there's an extremely ineffective shuttling of patients back and forth between their therapists for talk and their primary care physicians for medication. After a few months, when a person's mental health insurance benefits run out, she stops seeing her therapist. At the same time, her primary care doctor is encouraged by the health insurance company to write automatic renewals for her antidepressants a year at a time. By doing so, the physician loses track of the patient. So it's not uncommon for someone to be on antidepressants for years without any medical or psychological support whatsoever.

The bottom line? When it comes to using antidepressants, proceed with some sensible caution.

SO NOW LET'S TALK ABOUT HOW TO APPROACH DEPRESSION

Let's say you've been feeling especially glum and it's lasting a lot longer than you know is good for you. You aren't suicidal (if you are, you need to see your doctor *pronto*), but, still, life seems to have lost its joy and you're functioning on automatic pilot. If you've been depressed in the past and know you need to be on medication, obviously call your doctor. If depression is new to you, arrange for counseling first and see if you can work through these dark times using talk therapy and the Triple Whammy tactics described below without taking any medication at all.

COUNSELING (see also p. 232). If you've got health insurance, take a quick glance at your mental health benefits and see if it includes a list of therapists approved by your plan. "Approved" doesn't mean they're any better than other therapists; but selecting from among them won't cost you an arm and a leg. If you don't have health insurance, check your bank balance and spend a little money on yourself. If you ask, many therapists will charge you the same rate they receive from health plans, which means a substantial discount on their published fees. Negotiate. If you don't have a bank balance, consider a neighborhood mental health clinic.

TRIPLE WHAMMY TACTICS. Like other Triple Whammy disorders, depression is the three whammies gone into overdrive. In your genes, you're predisposed to problems with neurotransmitters such as serotonin. And if you have PMS or are menopausal, there's likely a hormonal component to your depression, given what we know about the parallel ups and downs of estrogen and serotonin. Finally, stress kicks the whole depression into gear—or up a notch. Let's quickly review the steps from the Three-Week Cure (p. 45) that will address the depression challenge: increasing serotonin levels to ease depression, getting hormones balanced, and taking an honest look at the stresses in your life. If you're depressed, I recognize these steps may be challenging for you, but please make your best effort to start doing each of these now and continue with them:

- **WALK BRISKLY OUTDOORS** During the daytime, walk for twenty minutes a day. The exercise will raise your serotonin and so will the daylight.

- **GO INTO THE LIGHT** Your brain needs sunlight to make more serotonin, and your daily walk is a good start. In addition, pull back curtains and rearrange furniture so you're always bathing yourself in sunlight. See Chapter 15 for more ideas.

- **TAKE FISH OIL AND B COMPLEX** Fish oil helps your brain manufacture more serotonin by providing raw materials; some of the B vitamins, especially B_6 (pyridoxine), are necessary for enhanced production of serotonin.

- **EAT WELL AND TIME YOUR CARBS** You need good nutrition and you need carbs to make serotonin. Timing your carb intake will keep your serotonin levels up throughout the day. Learn more on page 263.

- **BALANCE YOUR HORMONES** Follow the steps in the Three-Week Cure. If PMS or menopause applies to you, read their healing paths.

- **STRESS REDUCTION** You need to release as much stress as possible. Learn about this starting on page 197.

NUTRITIONAL SUPPLEMENTS

European doctors wonder why American physicians feel so compelled to prescribe antidepressants when nutritional supplements like St. John's wort, 5HTP, and SAMe have been proven to work by many clinical studies. Maybe we write so many antidepressant prescriptions as a response to the endless barrage of advertisements. In one week, I'll be visited by at least five antidepressant salespeople ("pharmaceutical representatives") who leave me piles of free samples, at least a dozen really nice ballpoint pens, paperweights, wall clocks, and note pads. I'll be invited to dinners at some of the city's best restaurants for a canned "educational seminar." When I open any medical journal, frowning out at me will be the glum face of a depressed woman, and on the next page, her beaming happy face, the obvious effect of medication. (We assume she didn't get so joyful because she changed her life, got rid of her jerky boyfriend, or won the lottery.)

My suggestion: if you feel you may have mild depression, start the following supplements at the same time you're undertaking the Triple Whammy tactics. The supplements, plus counseling, plus working on your whammies, may reverse your depression faster than the month it takes for most antidepressants to take effect.

- **ST. JOHN'S WORT** This herb is extremely popular among European physicians for mild-to-moderate depression. It's very gentle and acts like most antidepressants in that it slowly raises your serotonin. If someone (like your doctor) tells you St. John's wort (p. 20) doesn't work for depression, she's likely remembering that the herb was indeed shown not effective for *severe* depression. JAMA, the Journal of the American Medical Association, published an article about St. John's wort that largely dismissed the twenty positive St. John's wort studies as inadequate and instead focused on a study funded by an antidepressant manufacturer. (The manufacturer was considering beginning to sell St. John's wort and said it wanted to test it before doing so.) The subjects of the study had extremely severe depression and to most critics of the study, doses were totally inadequate for this severely depressed population. Based on the JAMA article, "Failure of St. John's wort" has been etched into the brains of America's physicians, who have largely ignored dozens of studies attesting to its benefit. If your depression is severe, don't use the herb in place of a prescription antidepressant. If your depression isn't severe, try it. This is especially important considering a 2005 study in the British Medical Journal (see p. 20) that unequivocally showed that St. John's wort was equally good if not better than the widely used antidepressant Paxil—and had fewer side effects. **DOSE:** To use St. John's wort correctly, you want to take enough of it. Start with 450 mg twice a day and give it at least three weeks. If you think you're a tad better, but not yet over your depression, increase to three times a day. However, if after these first three weeks of St. John's wort you're not at all better—or you're worse— ask your doctor about antidepressant medicines. Discontinue the St. John's wort if you start taking antidepressants because they act similarly on brain chemistry.

- **5HTP (5-HYDROXYTRYPTOPHAN)** This amino acid is a building block of serotonin. It has a slightly sedating quality, so take your dose before bed. 5HTP (p. 20) works nicely with St. John's wort to pump up your serotonin. If you start taking an anti-depressant, discontinue 5HTP to avoid making too much serotonin. **DOSE:** 100 mg at bedtime. You can use a smaller dose (50 mg) during the day, for daytime anxiety.

- **B COMPLEX AND FISH OIL** Both are needed to help your brain make serotonin. **DOSE:** Follow the Three-Week Cure dosages for these supplements (p. 50).

- **SAMe (S-ADENOSYL METHIONINE)** This amino acid derivative was shown in clinical studies to be as effective as many prescription antidepressants. Oddly, SAMe is also helpful for arthritis. **DOSE:** SAMe comes in 200 mg and 400 mg tablets. Most of the European studies using SAMe for depression were in the range of 800–1,200 mg per day. Start with 400 mg tablets, taken twice a day. In order to maximize absorption, take SAMe on an empty stomach. To do so, take your first immediately on rising and the second about one hour before lunch. Make sure you take the full, recommended dose.

ALTERNATIVE THERAPIES

I am impressed by how well alternative therapies that involve manipulating our energy can be used to treat depression. Do I know exactly how these work? No, but I suspect that somehow balancing the flow of these energies opens the mind to new insights and balances brain chemicals. It will take more than this lifetime for me to really understand what healing is all about. After treating one of our patients, the Reiki therapist I work with told me, "We were able to release the blockages around her heart. It was quite a breakthrough. We both cried. I think she's going to do just fine." Women have amazing powers to heal. Be willing to try an energy treatment that works even if you don't fully understand it. Eastern medicine has been healing people for centuries longer than Western.

- **TRADITIONAL CHINESE MEDICINE (TCM)** Acupuncture and Chinese herbal formulations can be extremely helpful in relieving depression and bringing about a sense of calm and better sleep. If you're taking an antidepressant, let your practitioner

MANIC DEPRESSION/BIPOLAR DISORDER: NOT A TRIPLE WHAMMY DISORDER

If you think you may have bipolar disorder, you need to put the Triple Whammy self-care suggestions on hold until you get a thorough professional evaluation and perhaps start on appropriate medication. On page 295 I've included a questionnaire designed by a team of psychiatrists to help you determine if your symptoms indicate bipolar disorder, also known as manic-depressive disorder or simply manic depression. The questionnaire is not meant to diagnose the condition, but if after completing it you believe you may have bipolar disorder, please schedule an appointment with your physician or, better yet, a psychiatrist for a complete evaluation.

Bipolar disorder is defined by unexpected and dramatic shifts in mood. You may have symptoms that sound like depression, such as lasting sadness and lack of energy, and then shift gears a few days later into the land of mania, where you're a bundle of energy, with racing thoughts, grandiose ideas, impulsive actions, and not much insight into how your mood changed so quickly. It's estimated that up to one-third of people diagnosed with depression and anxiety actually have bipolar disorder. As far as diagnosing any illness—from appendicitis to warts—making an incorrect diagnosis on every third patient is a pretty high failure rate. Surveys among people with bipolar disorder reveal it can take up to ten years of seeing doctors, usually for symptoms of depression, before one of them finally stumbles on the correct diagnosis.

One of the key ways to diagnose bipolar is to see what happens if you take antidepressants. Whether the therapy is natural, like St. John's wort, or a prescription antidepressant, the medication may set off a period of manic behavior, with racing thoughts and boundless energy. Rule out bipolar disorder with your physician before you start any kind of therapy for depression.

know so she can make sure no adverse herb-drug interactions will occur. (TCM is discussed on page 285.)

- **MASSAGE** Regular massage (p. 236) and other bodywork therapies, like Reiki (p. 239) and reflexology (p. 223), can be extremely effective in reducing stress and improving your sense of well-being. Because your muscles can act as storehouses for unpleasant memories, you may suddenly feel tearful or be reminded of past events during a session. Bodywork therapists are used to this, and can be a great support with counseling and advice.

SELF-CARE

These two self-care items are fully within your control and essential in managing depression.

- **NUTRITION** Two rules apply here. One: you need a small amount of high-quality carbohydrates (p. 266) throughout your day to facilitate serotonin production. Two: you don't want your blood sugar levels to swing all over the place; this taxes your adrenal glands, the stress glands of your body. When your adrenals are exhausted, you will be too. Therefore, avoid sugar, refined carbs such as bakery goods and other white-flour products, processed foods, and excess caffeine and alcohol, all of which can cause havoc with your blood sugar. Don't skip meals. Have a small bedtime snack. Read the Triple Whammy Food Plan starting on page 245 for details on carbo timing and healthful eating.

- **EXERCISE** If you aren't moving, you're not generating free serotonin, which is produced when you exercise. Start with the twenty-minute brisk walk outside every day and gradually add to it. If you can't do more, be religious about getting your twenty daily minutes.

STRESS REDUCTION

Work with the suggestions in Chapter 20, "Stress Less," but here are a few selections that can be especially helpful for depression.

- **AROMATHERAPY** (p. 210) The floral scents are most often recommended for depression. Jasmine is quite nice, as are neroli, rose, melissa, and ylang-ylang. Add a few drops to your bath and take a luxurious soak. Put a couple of drops in a handkerchief and take a deep whiff before a stressful event. Ask your massage therapist to make a massage oil with one of these.

- **FLOWER ESSENCE THERAPY** (p. 220) Mild, safe, and gentle, these homeopathic flower preparations are designed for calming emotional turmoil. Wild rose is frequently recommended for depression when everything seems a total blah. Mustard has been the flower essence of choice for depression for over sixty years.

- **GUIDED IMAGERY** (p. 214) My patients speak highly of the guided imagery recording for depression produced by psychologist Belleruth Naparstek. Listen to it just before going to sleep at night and incorporate its wisdom into your dreams.

- **T'AI CHI OR YOGA** The gentle movements of these disciplines can be powerful allies as you work to overcome depression, relieving stress and opening up your body's vital energy, or *chi*. Find a class that's convenient, enroll, and attend regularly. Read more about t'ai chi on page 228 and yoga on page 230.

Q & A: ANTIDEPRESSANTS FOR LIFE?

Q. I had several Triple Whammy symptoms (depression, PMS, fatigue) that all disappeared when my doctor placed me on a small dose of antidepressants. The only problem is that whenever I try to go off the antidepressants, my symptoms return. Does this mean I have to stay on medicine for the rest of my life? Or, worse yet, does this mean I've gotten addicted to them?

A. A pair of great questions, and I'll answer the second one first. Needing maintenance antidepressants definitely does not mean you're addicted to them, any more than a diabetic is addicted to the insulin needed to control her blood sugar. What it does mean is that basically you were born a quart short of serotonin (sorry about the car comparison) and that you need medication to bring your level up to what's normal for your needs. Keeping in mind that serotonin is your stress buffer, and that your depression, PMS, and fatigue well may be your emotional and physical responses to stress, you may find your need for medication to support your serotonin lessens as you control the stressors in your life. More important, as you follow the lifestyle changes in Triple Whammy Cure (supplements, diet, exercise, sunlight, carb timing), you may ultimately create enough serotonin on your own so that going off medications becomes a real possibility. Obviously, you'll work with your doctor on this. In the end, though, some people, despite their best efforts, do need to stay on antidepressants, and after decades of use, they remain extremely safe. Just be glad they're available!

8

FIBROMYALGIA

The most important piece of information you can hear if you have fibromyalgia is that real relief is possible. Your pain level can drop from a 10 to a 1 or 2, your fatigue can melt away, and you can actually sleep through the night and awaken refreshed.

Fibro is a classic Triple Whammy disorder and to get well you must take total charge of each whammy: stress, serotonin, and your hormones. But first, you need to get your symptoms under control because the untreated, unremitting pain of fibromyalgia is probably your single greatest source of stress.

When it comes to understanding the range of medical conditions caused by the Triple Whammy, I always start with fibromyalgia because once you understand it, you'll really grasp how the Triple Whammy works. I'm going to devote more space to fibro than any of the other Triple Whammy disorders because it's one of the most complex, misunderstood health challenges, affecting more than fifteen million people, primarily women. To treat fibro successfully, you must pull out all the stops, trying conventional medicine, alternative medicine, vitamins, minerals, herbs, changes in your diet, and self-care therapies for relaxation and reducing stress.

The word *fibromyalgia* means simply "muscle pain" in Greek, but fibromyalgia defies what doctors were taught in medical school about disease. When you visit your doctor with a symptom such as pain, she'll examine you and order a diagnostic workup, like blood tests and X-rays, that looks for evidence that something's wrong in your body. The big problem with fibro (just like other Triple Whammy disorders) is that the results of all tests and X-rays are negative and there's no evidence of disease. And because all your test results are negative, your doctor's "I can't find anything wrong" sort of lets her off the hook. In fact, for many years, fibro patients faced a lingering prejudice that the condition didn't exist at all.

TENDER POINTS AND OTHER SYMPTOMS

The main symptoms of fibromyalgia are singularly unpleasant: widespread muscle pain, profound fatigue, inefficient sleep that fails to provide any refreshment, and "brain fog," a peculiar lack of focus, poor concentration, and even memory impairment. Ironically, because people who have fibro often look quite healthy, they are frequently told, "Well, there's really nothing *wrong* with you" or "There's nothing that can be done." With support like this, you can well understand why depression often accompanies the other symptoms.

When fibromyalgia is high on a doctor's suspect list of conditions to look for, the diagnosis is straightforward. Added to the triad of unrefreshing sleep, fatigue, and widespread muscle pain (lasting at least three months) are so-called tender points. There are eighteen of these points, located in a symmetrical pattern on the body, mainly in areas where fibrous tissues attach muscles to bones. Tender points are located at the base of the skull and on the neck, shoulders, upper chest (just below the collarbone), inner elbows, inner knees, outer thighs, lower back, and buttocks. When firm fingertip pressure is applied to a tender point, the person with fibromyalgia experiences pain (not discomfort, but PAIN) that persists for some minutes after the pressure is removed. If you have a severe case of fibro, the fingertip pressure can bring you to tears or make you feel dizzy and lightheaded.

In addition to muscle pain and fatigue, people with fibro frequently have other Triple Whammy disorders, such as irritable bowel syndrome (p. 103), temporomandibular joint dysfunction (TMJ, p. 181), migraine headaches (p. 136), chronic anxiety (p. 59), and depression (p. 78). And just like fibromyalgia, the physical symptoms of these conditions are very real and often quite incapacitating, yet again, diagnostic tests are usually normal.

WHAMMY #1: STRESS, THE FIBRO TRIGGER

Fibromyalgia affects women more often than men, especially women between twenty and fifty. Most often, the trigger is severe, prolonged emotional stress ("It began after the worst year of my life"). Less often, fibro is triggered by physical trauma, such as a whiplash injury or an extremely severe case of the flu. But whatever the stress trigger, it's a situation that your body can't handle. The state of having fibromyalgia seems to be a consequence of changes the body undergoes when physical and emotional components of the stress response (also called the fight-or-flight response) continue unchecked for an extended time.

If you consider how unconsciously we all tense up our muscles when we're under emotional pressure, it's easier to understand how chronic stress can bring about fibro muscle pain. Just imagine keeping your muscles constantly tense, day in and day out, and you're setting the stage for fibromyalgia. Add to this the additional stresses of fatigue, poor sleep, and visiting doctor after doctor with an undiagnosed or unsatisfactorily treated medical condition. Sadly, after just a few months, the misery of fibromyalgia settles in to become a way of life.

One of most cheerless studies I ever read showed that a disproportionate number of women with fibromyalgia had been physically or sexually abused as children. A little girl would tense her muscles, folding in on herself, trying to protect herself. Later, as an adult, whenever confronted with stress, she'll unconsciously protect herself by assuming a less obvious version of that same childhood posture.

WHAMMY #2: LOW SEROTONIN, THE CAUSE OF FIBRO?

Although the exact cause of fibromyalgia is not known, many scientists relate the disorder to low levels of serotonin. A feature of all Triple Whammy disorders, serotonin abnormalities seem to run in families (p. 38) and can manifest themselves in different forms (which you'll note by looking at all the Triple Whammy disorders in this section) among the women of the same or multiple generations. It's possible that women's lack of serotonin is responsible not only for fibro muscle pain but also for symptoms such as "brain fog," extreme sensitivity to odors (like perfumes or chemicals), and extreme sensitivity to the side effects of medications. It speaks poorly of the medical profession that patients complaining of chemical sensitivities and "side effects to everything" are generally categorized as neurotic.

SUBSTANCE P AND THE HPA AXIS

More recently, some attention has been paid to a second brain chemical, called Substance P, which plays a role in the transmission of pain messages from the body to the brain. Very high levels of Substance P may lead to the abnormal sensitivity to pain that people with fibromyalgia experience. Whether high levels of Substance P occur because of the constant muscle contraction or are the cause of the pain itself is not known. One of the newer treatments for pain relief, applying small amounts of capsaicin (cayenne pepper) cream to each tender point several times a day, is thought to work by depleting the accumulated Substance P surrounding the tender point. A second factor in fibromyalgia research involves a body system called the hypothalamic-pituitary-adrenal (HPA) axis. The hypothalamus acts as a connecting link between our emotions and our endocrine glands. The hypothalamus sends messages to the pituitary, the master gland that controls the thyroid gland, adrenal glands, and sex glands (ovaries and testicles). It's within this HPA axis that Whammy #3, your hormones, comes into play.

WHAMMY #3: THE HORMONE CONNECTION

Remember that, as a woman, your levels of serotonin are very much related to your levels of estrogen. As I described on page 17, these hormones are like a two-car roller coaster, with estrogen as the lead car, dragging serotonin behind. During the few days to a week before your period, estrogen slowly drops and continues to drop until your first day of flow, when the next cycle begins and estrogen starts rising again (usually toward the end of your period). As estrogen drops, so follows serotonin, and you enter PMS Land, where you are irritable, moody, and cry at Hallmark commercials.

If you have PMS plus fibromyalgia, all your symptoms may get dramatically worse before your period. In fact, some women with fibro say that the week after their period ends, when estrogen and thus serotonin are on the rise (at the top of the roller coaster), is the only time of the month their fibro actually seems to improve.

But let's get back to your pituitary, part of the HPA axis. Your pituitary not only controls your sex hormones, it's also in charge of hormones coming from your adrenal glands, dubbed the "stress glands" because when we're stressed the emotional signal is relayed from the brain (hypothalamus) through the pituitary to the adrenal glands. This is the HPA axis.

Adrenal hormones, including adrenalin and cortisol, trigger our physical responses to stress (the flight-or-fight response) and command our muscles to run or fight. This response is meant for emergencies only. The system is built to turn on quickly and then turn off quickly. But if the stress (Whammy #1) is nonstop, the constant contraction of muscles becomes painful. And in time, the adrenal glands, left in the "on" position, become exhausted. With chronic stress, the adrenals shift their output from adrenalin, which is generally reserved for immediate dangers, to cortisol, and your reserves of cortisol are limited. Understand that in fibro, your adrenal glands are not diseased in any way, but "exhausted" (see p. 10). Their depletion may be partially responsible for the fatigue of fibromyalgia.

But remember that your pituitary as the master gland affects your thyroid as well. The thyroid is best described as your gas pedal, controlling the rate of chemical and metabolic processes everywhere (and I mean everywhere!) in your body. If it's stimulated constantly by your pituitary, your thyroid starts getting fatigued too, and you may start experiencing some symptoms of underactive thyroid. Your blood test (TSH) might be normal, but your basal temperature readings (an older way of testing for underactive thyroid; see p. 75) may be a clue. Again, remember your thyroid isn't diseased, but exhausted.

TREATING FIBROMYALGIA

To be able to walk away from the pain, fatigue, and general misery of fibro, you have to first deal with your symptoms and get them under reasonable control, and then deal with each of the whammies. The connection between low serotonin and fibromyalgia is so well known that many conventional physicians routinely prescribe serotonin-boosting antidepressants right at the start. I'll review here the medications generally used for fibro. But please understand that many (though certainly not all) women see good results after a few weeks of using nutritional and herbal supplements (p. 98). Whether you choose conventional medicine, alternative medicine, or a blend of the two, your goals are fourfold: relieving pain, promoting efficient and restful sleep, easing severe fatigue, and ending brain fog.

RELIEVING PAIN

Because fibromyalgia is a chronic pain syndrome, it needs aggressive treatment. You've got to break the cycle of pain/impaired sleep/fatigue/increased stress/increased pain. As much as I like using alternative therapies whenever possible, alternative medicine has little to offer that has a lasting effect on pain. The results obtained from chiropractic, acupuncture, and massage, although excellent sources for temporary relief, can get expensive. Nutritional or herbal remedies are just not strong enough to stop the fibro pain cycle.

Prescription muscle relaxants and pain medications are your best bet to break the pain cycle. If you're reluctant to use prescription drugs, be aware that because of your low serotonin levels you are likely extremely sensitive to medicines of any kind. This means that much of your pain can be diminished dramatically with very low doses. Two groups of medicines almost always work without fail: muscle relaxants and painkillers (analgesics).

- **MUSCLE RELAXANTS** If taken during the day, muscle relaxants such as Flexeril (cyclobenzaprine) and Zanaflex cause most users to walk around in a drowsy fog. This side effect can be used to your advantage, however, when you take them at bedtime because they promote deep, efficient sleep. In fact, many of my patients starting muscle relaxants report their first good night's sleep in years. For daytime use, ask your doctor about prescribing a very tiny dose of Flexeril (like one-half or even one-quarter of a 5 mg tablet). At bedtime, start with a 5 mg tablet. If you feel groggy the next morning, take the Flexeril earlier than you did the night before.

- **PAINKILLERS** Using painkillers for the chronic pain of fibromyalgia has been mired in an unnecessary controversy over drugs that may be habit forming or potentially addicting. I agree that medicines such as tramadol (Ultram, Ultracet) and the opioids (codeine, oxycodone, and others) require close monitoring by you and your physician. But in fact, among patients with severe and chronic pain, actual addiction is extraordinarily rare. People prefer a pain-free life over one stuck in constant pain, and all my pain patients quite sensibly ask, "Can I ever go off my pain medication?" The answer is most commonly yes, because, taken for a period of time, usually for six to twelve months, the medicine does manage finally to break the pain/stress/more pain cycle.

The newly released antidepressant Cymbalta (duloxetine) may allow many fibromyalgia patients to avoid painkillers altogether. Cymbalta acts by increasing brain levels of serotonin along with a second neurotransmitter, norepinephrine. Clinical studies have shown this dual effect reduces chronic muscle pain and, although the FDA has not yet approved Cymbalta specifically for fibromyalgia, it seems to be one of the most promising medications on the horizon.

The pain of fibromyalgia can virtually melt away with very small doses, like half-tablets of Ultram (tramadol) or Vicodin (hydrocodone), taken two or three times a day. However, each of these is short-acting and will wear off in about three hours. To avoid swings in and out of pain, I prescribe low doses of pain medications that are released slowly but steadily into the bloodstream, like

OxyContin (oxycodone) or the Duragesic (fentanyl) skin patch. OxyContin tablet sizes range from 10 mg to 160 mg. The 10 mg size can provide dramatic relief for the vast majority of fibromyalgia patients.

Physicians involved in pain management have loudly protested any government banning of these medicines, fearing they'll lose some of the best means they have of helping their pain patients live comfortably. I frequently hear from my patients that good pain control allowed them to live their lives again. Although side effects at these low doses are uncommon, fibro patients are so medication-sensitive that they can occur. The two most common are drowsiness and mild nausea, both of which disappear as your body acclimates itself to the medication. Take your pain med at bedtime for a few days and then take your first daytime dose on a weekend morning. Doing this will considerably reduce your chances of an uncomfortable side effect.

Most women who are skittish about prescription meds have had some bad experience with side effects. I believe this occurs because they were prescribed doses far too high, and that includes the standard starting dose recommended by the pharmaceutical company. Unless you're dealing with a medical emergency, like a life-threatening pneumonia, fibro patients should ask their doctors if they can start them out on pediatric-sized doses.

PROMOTING SLEEP

People with fibromyalgia make dramatic improvements when they sleep well. Some researchers even believe the basis of fibro is a chronic sleep disorder. Many patients respond well to natural sleep therapies, such as melatonin (1 to 3 mg) or valerian (400 to 900 mg), or a combination of the two along with guided imagery audio tapes (p. 214), self- hypnosis (p. 226), and even gentle aromatherapy (p. 210).

Others require something stronger, like the prescription medications Ambien (5 to 10 mg) or Restoril (7.5 to 15 mg; see Sleeping Pills, p. 176). The correlation between poor sleep and the severity of fibro pain is so strong that your doctor may recommend you treat mild fibromyalgia using just one medicine, an older antidepressant called amitriptyline (10 to 25 mg). By taking advantage of amitryptiline's side effect of intense drowsiness, when you take this medication at bedtime you sleep deeply and feel better in the morning. A few weeks later, as with other antidepressants, the steady rise in serotonin will relieve the depression that frequently travels with fibro.

EASING FATIGUE

Usually the combination of pain control, efficient sleep, and restoring adrenal function (see Adrenal Support, p. 98) brings a dramatic improvement in fatigue. However, some people who have fibro are "fatigue-dominant" and require additional therapy. Although nutritional supplements such as ginseng and nicotinamide adenine dinucleotide (NADH) can be effective, medications are sometimes necessary. I've found that Ritalin and Adderall—and especially the newer Provigil—effectively relieve a constant, debilitating sense of exhaustion. (Provigil was originally designed for narcolepsy.) Ritalin and Adderall are used primarily for youngsters with attention deficit disorder.

ENDING BRAIN FOG

As you take steps to ease your pain, sleep problems, and fatigue, you'll experience considerable improvement in memory, focus, and concentration. Interestingly, serotonin is well-known as a necessary substance for brain cells to grow and mature, so as your serotonin increases, you'll also feel smarter. Some fascinating research has shown that nutritional supplements can also improve brain fog. These include acetyl-L-carnitine, phosphatidyl serine, ginkgo biloba, and pregnenolone. Acetyl-L-carnitine appears to work by increasing levels of the neurotransmitter acetylcholine, needed for focus and memory. Phosphatidyl serine is needed for the smooth transmission of nerve impulses in the brain. Ginkgo increases blood flow to the brain, while pregnenolone seems to improve the efficiency of serotonin as a neurotransmitter.

Prescription drugs for debilitating brain fog include piracetam and selegiline. Piracetam improves communication between the left and right sides of the brain. Selegiline (deprenyl), a medicine used for Parkinson's disease, in low doses raises levels of another neurotransmitter, dopamine.

ANTIDEPRESSANTS

With justification, many of my patients comment that they wouldn't be depressed if they weren't in so much pain. Antidepressants increase low serotonin levels. In "Whammy #2: Serotonin, Powerful Stress Buffer" (p. 12), I discussed the close connection between serotonin and pain and serotonin's role as a pain buffer. I often think people might feel better about taking antidepressants if they were renamed "neurotransmitter enhancers."

At my office, we first try natural alternatives to raise serotonin, like the fish oil and B complex that are a part of the Triple Whammy Cure. Other serotonin boosters include St. John's wort (900 to 1,350 mg per day) and 5HTP (100 to 150 mg per day), turning to prescription medications only if these fail.

Prescription antidepressants and their usual starting doses for fibro include Elavil (10 mg), Cymbalta (20 mg), Prozac (10 mg), Lexapro (5 mg), and Zoloft (12.5 mg). Many doctors would argue that these doses are too low to be effective, but because Triple Whammy patients are more drug sensitive than others, a little dose goes a long way. After a few days, you'll know if you can tolerate the medication and, with your doctor's supervision, you can start inching upward by, for example, increasing the amount of Lexapro you take by 2.5 mg each week. Cymbalta acts by increasing brain levels of serotonin and with another neurotransmitter, norepinephrine. The drug is the first antidepressant to be promoted for its pain control effect, and an increasing number of patients have been reporting good results.

ALTERNATIVE THERAPIES AND FIBROMYALGIA

After years of treating many hundreds of fibro patients, I can report that there is no universal formula for matching the best alternative treatments to the patient. Every person is unique, and a big part of what will work for you depends on what you're open to and how the condition affects you day to day. To determine which is the best for you and devise an individualized treatment plan, consider the following:

IF STRESS IS A SIGNIFICANT FACTOR, and you can track a strong link between events in your life (p. 33) and symptoms, consider psychotherapy (see Counseling, p. 232) along with some of the self-care relaxation techniques listed under Self-Care Remedies on page 100.

IF MUSCLE PAIN AND STIFFNESS PREDOMINATE, especially along your neck and spine, work with a good chiropractor (p. 275).

IF YOU ACHE ALL OVER, schedule regular time with a massage therapist (p. 236).

IF YOU HAVE A COMBINATION OF PAIN, FATIGUE, AND EMOTIONAL ISSUES that dates back years, consider adding traditional Chinese medicine (p. 285) or homeopathy (p. 277) to your treatment.

IF YOU ARE PHILOSOPHICALLY OPPOSED TO USING MEDICATION of any kind, connect with a naturopathic physician (p. 281) who is knowledgeable about fibro and can offer a variety of non-drug treatments including herbs, acupuncture, manipulative therapies, and counseling.

For everyone with fibro, the following alternative approaches can make a real difference:

- **CHIROPRACTIC** Chiropractic (p. 275) research has shown that some fibromyalgia comes about as a consequence of misalignment of the spine, especially in the neck. A condition called "posttraumatic fibromyalgia," in which fibro symptoms can be dated to a physical injury such as a whiplash auto accident, often responds especially well to chiropractic manipulation plus serotonin-enhancing supplements and medications.

- **TRADITIONAL CHINESE MEDICINE** (TCM, p. 285) In virtually all fields of alternative medicine, disease occurs due to imbalance in a person's "vital force," or *chi*. Acupuncture and Chinese herbal combinations selected by an experienced practitioner are aimed at balancing your energy and can provide significant relief.

- **MASSAGE** Deep tissue massage (p. 236), performed regularly, can have a dramatic effect on symptom control. Adding some aromatherapy (p. 210) can be very helpful as well.

- **HOMEOPATHY** Your homeopath (p. 277) will take an extremely detailed history of your life and your symptoms before choosing a natural remedy. Her ultimate goal will be to unravel the multiple contributions that brought on your ill health and make you completely well again.

- **HEALTH SPAS** Many people with fibro make a real breakthrough when they discover the connections between their symptoms and long-standing stressors in their lives. Many of my fibro patients have discovered that their symptoms dramatically decrease during an extended vacation or after a job change. When a patient's schedule and income allow it, I frequently prescribe a week or two at a health spa. After the fifth day of healthful eating, yoga, massage, and walking, many realize they feel well for the first time in months or years. They're finally "getting it"—the message that's in their fibro, which is they've got too much stress. If, after they come home and get back into their routine, their symptoms start to return . . . well, it may be time to consider making some significant life changes to reduce stress levels (learning to say "no" is a good place to start), and a little professional counseling (p. 232).

  If money or time commitments make this spa idea impossible, plan a spa weekend at home. Ask family or friends to take the kids for a few days. Turn off the home phone and tell people the cell phone is only for emergencies (use it yourself to call your kids). Do no chores. Make one shopping trip to stock up on fresh fruits and veggies. Open this book to the Three-Week Cure, read through the steps and begin by listening to a stress-reducing audio tape. Then write in your journal; visit a massage therapist or Reiki practitioner; listen to an entire Beethoven symphony without interruption; keep the TV off; and have an aromatherapy bath (p. 211). Are you beginning to get my drift?

NUTRITIONAL AND HERBAL SUPPLEMENTS that relax muscles and raise serotonin levels, combined with regular aerobic exercise, massage, and relaxation techniques, can help control your symptoms.

– **MAGNESIUM,** a mineral and natural muscle relaxant, is often deficient in people with fibro. Several products combine magnesium with malic acid to enhance absorption. In one preliminary study, fibromyalgia sufferers reported less pain and reduced muscle tenderness after two months on a treatment regimen that included high doses of magnesium and malic acid. **DOSE:** Magnesium 400–800 mg per day with 1,200–2,400 mg malic acid (sold in numerous combination products).

– **ST. JOHN'S WORT, 5HTP, AND FISH OIL** all increase serotonin levels in your brain, which helps ease depression and improve tolerance to pain. The 5HTP and fish oil make more serotonin, while St. John's wort prevents its breakdown. The result is a slow but steady rise in serotonin levels. If you start prescription antidepressants, stop both the St. John's and 5HTP because of the nervous side effect of making too much serotonin. Taking B complex supplements, timing your carbohydrate intake, getting more sunlight, and exercising are simple serotonin enhancers (see the Three-Week Cure, p. 45, for details). **DOSE:** St. John's wort 900–1,350 mg per day divided into two doses and taken with meals; 5HTP 100–150 mg per day, taken at bedtime for its mildly sedative effect.

– **COENZYME Q10** and **NADH** may help fatigue symptoms. Each is involved in maintaining the mitochondria, the energy-producing unit of your body's cells. A study from the University of Texas found NADH very helpful in reducing the fatigue of fibromyalgia. **DOSE:** Take 50–100 mg of coenzyme Q10 twice a day; take 5 mg of NADH twice a day on an empty stomach (about one hour before or two hours after eating).

– **PHOSPHATIDYL SERINE AND ACETYL-L-CARNITINE** are involved in healthy mental functioning. For brain fog, these are taken separately and in substantial doses. Several products containing combinations are available. **DOSE:** Phosphatidyl serine 100 mg twice a day; acetyl-L-carnitine 500 mg twice a day. For combination product follow package directions.

– **MELATONIN OR THE HERB VALERIAN** can help you get to sleep more easily. It's virtually a rule of thumb that a poor night's sleep yields pain the following day. Deep sleep means a much lower level of discomfort. **DOSE:** Melatonin 1–3 mg about a half hour before bedtime; valerian 800–1,000 mg about one hour before bedtime.

– **ADRENAL SUPPORT COMBINATION PRODUCTS** are helpful when fatigue is a dominant symptom. A readily available blood test for adrenal exhaustion looks for low levels of DHEA, an adrenal "pre-hormone" that converts to other adrenal hormones. If your DHEA levels are low, DHEA is available at most health food stores.

CANDIDA, FOOD SENSITIVITIES, AND FIBROMYALGIA

Two controversial diagnoses associated with fibromyalgia are food sensitivities and candida overgrowth syndrome (p. 290). Sometimes food sensitivities or an intestinal overgrowth of candida (yeast) can aggravate a Triple Whammy disorder. Although various theories have been proposed for this, in my opinion each of these situations—candida or food sensitivities—becomes yet another stressor against a body already in overdrive. If, for example, every time you eat a seemingly harmless food like a bagel, your body reacts as if it's been attacked by a harmful substance like a virus, this can cause discomfort and pain. Your immune system will churn out antibodies literally against the bagel and then, when the antibodies latch onto the wheat molecules, the combination can land in a vulnerable area, like your joints. Here are two clues to determine if you should explore either of these issues:

TRY THE FOOD SENSITIVITY ELIMINATION DIET on page 109 for two weeks. If your symptoms are exactly the same, you probably aren't sensitive to the foods that commonly cause allergic reactions. If, however, you feel significantly better after eliminating the suspect foods for two weeks, follow the reintroduction instructions to help pinpoint the guilty party.

IF YOU'D TAKEN ANTIBIOTICS REGULARLY in the years before your fibro started *and* you seem to get one vaginal yeast infection after another, candida overgrowth syndrome may be a problem.

Eliminating certain foods or clearing yourself of candida is not going to solve everything about your fibro. Sometimes these are aggravating factors, but they seldom turn out to be responsible for everything. But addressing these possible problems *will* help you feel better—and you need every little bit of help you can get.

Understand, though, that a little DHEA goes a long way, so limit your use to two months or less, unless you're working with a practitioner who is familiar with DHEA and can retest your levels periodically. Some DHEA may convert to the male hormone testosterone, and if you experience a flare-up of acne or even some facial hair growth, you've obviously taken enough DHEA and should stop taking it. Read more about adrenal fatigue and exhaustion on page 10. **DOSE:** Adrenal support products are formulated with slight differences. Follow the package instructions.

– **CAPSAICIN CREAM** This cream, made from capsaicin—the "hot" in hot peppers—is sold over the counter. It was originally developed to relieve the pain of shingles, but a study demonstrated its unequivocal effectiveness in relieving fibromyalgia pain. To use the cream, locate your most painful tender points with fingertip pressure. Mark each with an X and then, several times a day, rub a pea-sized amount of the cream into each X. After several days, this will reduce the pain-causing Substance P (p. 91) located around each tender point. This treatment can be continued indefinitely, and you'll likely discover that once or twice a day is sufficient for maintenance. Be sure to read the precautions on the package and do not touch your eyes, nose, or other mucous membranes (including your genitals) before thoroughly washing the cream off your hands.

– **CHASTEBERRY** If you discovered a PMS component to your fibro, taking chasteberry or a PMS herbal combination can help. A series of articles in the conventional medical literature has confirmed what herbalists have known for years: that chasteberry balances hormones and reduces physical symptoms of PMS. **DOSE:** Chasteberry 175–225 mg each morning *or* one of the PMS herbal combinations. Select one that contains some chasteberry and follow the package instructions. Chasteberry affects hormone levels, so don't use it if you're taking hormone replacement therapy or birth control pills (it can lessen their effectiveness), or if you're pregnant or nursing.

SELF-CARE REMEDIES

– **EAT SMALLER, MORE FREQUENT MEALS AND TIME YOUR CARBS** Carbohydrates are important because they'll increase your shaky levels of serotonin. To maintain a steady supply, eat five smaller meals during the day instead of three large ones (or eat three meals and a couple of the carb-containing snacks). Foods made of sugar and refined flours are perceived as stress by your body because they raise, then lower, your blood sugar levels. You don't need more stress. Read the Triple Whammy Food plan (p. 245) for details on carbo timing and start eating the Triple Whammy way.

– **APPLY HEAT** To relieve pain and stiffness, reduce inflammation, and increase circulation, soak in a very hot bath to which you've added up to one or two cups of Epsom salts (magnesium sulfate) just before bed. Test the temperature of the water with your foot, not your hand, to make sure it's hot enough. Keep adding more hot water from the tap while you're soaking. While still warm from the bath, go immediately to bed. Having the bed prewarmed with an electric blanket or hot water bottle may allow a restful sleep and result in less pain when you rise. On days you awaken with a lot of discomfort, go immediately to a hot bath, take a hot shower, or apply a heating pad. See the recipe for a relaxing bath on page 211.

- **EXERCISE REGULARLY** Begin a gradual program of aerobic exercise. Instead of taxing already sore muscles, aerobic exercise seems to help ease the symptoms of fibro. If you haven't been exercising, consult your doctor and then start with low-impact activities such as walking, swimming, or bicycling. Be very careful not to overtax yourself or you'll experience a worsening of symptoms the following day. Start with fifteen minutes a day and build steadily, increasing your daily workout by fifteen-minute increments each week. If you have health insurance, ask your doctor to write a physical therapy prescription for: (1) myofascial release, a form of massage therapy especially good for fibro patients; and (2) graded exercise. You'll be able to start a slow but steady exercise program under the supervision of a physical therapist who will likely be more knowledgeable about fibro than a personal trainer.

- **GET PLENTY OF SLEEP** Studies have shown that the severity of fibro pain during the day is directly proportional to the lack and/or quality of sleep the previous night. Try to get at least eight hours of sleep every night. Stick to a regular sleep schedule, even on weekends. Many of my patients report dramatic relief from those pressure-relieving foam-type mattresses that conform to your body's shape.

- **DO SELF-MASSAGE** Applying pressure to tender points can relieve pain and soreness. An S-shaped massage tool sold at health-food stores is useful for pressing the difficult-to-reach tender points of your neck, shoulders, and upper back, points that hold the greatest tension in many people. Read the section on acupressure (p. 207) for more information.

- **TRY MEDITATION, SELF-HYPNOSIS, OR YOGA** Practiced consistently, these techniques can help relieve muscle tension and improve sleep. Yoga (p. 230) will also help you become stronger, so you won't tire as easily. Once you've learned meditation (p. 215) or yoga from an instructor, practice at home, morning and evening, for at least fifteen minutes. Self-hypnosis is discussed on page 226.

- **AROMATHERAPY (P. 210) AND FLOWER ESSENCES (P. 220)** Add some lavender oil to your hot bath or put a few drops of ylang-ylang into a handkerchief. If you're "stuck" on certain issues in your life, a flower essence practitioner can prepare a flower formula that's suitable for your emotional needs. You can also read up on these essences and learn to prepare your own formula.

FIBROMYALGIA AND CHRONIC FATIGUE SYNDROME

The relationship between fibromyalgia and chronic fatigue syndrome (CFS, p. 67) has been debated for years. Currently, most researchers agree that the two conditions are different manifestations of the same disorder. In fact, researchers now include irritable bowel syndrome, migraines, and other stress-related conditions under an umbrella diagnosis of "affective spectrum disorder," which is medical jargon for acknowledging that the state of your emotions can trigger a variety of significant, quite real symptoms. On the plus side, by naming what's going on, conventional doctors are more willing to treat people with fibro and CFS respectfully, rather than labeling them neurotic as they used to. On the minus side, the word "affective" (which means "emotional") continues to categorize both conditions as basically psychiatric, when they have enormous physical symptoms. Yet your insurance coverage and disability benefits almost always place restrictions on treatments for psychiatric diagnoses. Far more descriptive but unwieldy would be "multiple manifestations of low serotonin disorders aggravated by stress and hormonal shifts." This would remove the burden of a psychiatric diagnosis and point toward a more acceptable (and "insurable") metabolic disorder, like diabetes or high cholesterol. Of course, we can save a lot of extra words by calling them Triple Whammy Disorders.

9.

IRRITABLE BOWEL SYNDROME (IBS)

Irritable bowel syndrome (IBS) is very high on the list of truly annoying and exasperating Triple Whammy conditions. A syndrome is a collection of symptoms but not truly a disease, which is an accurate way to describe IBS. All that discomfort you feel—the bloating, cramps, diarrhea, pain, constipation—occurs within perfectly normal intestines. That's why your blood tests, X-rays, stool analyses, colonoscopies, biopsies, and abdominal scans are almost always normal.

Typical of most Triple Whammy disorders, IBS afflicts more women than men. Most flare-ups can be related to stressful periods in the sufferer's life, and also seem to have a hormonal component—IBS often worsens during PMS days. IBS, in fact, is among the leading symptoms of PMS.

The relationship of IBS to stress and serotonin is interesting. Keep in mind that during the sudden fight-or-flight stress response, in addition to speeding up your heart rate and tightening your muscles, the stress hormones pouring out of your adrenal glands change the way blood flows through your intestines. This in turn can cause symptoms ranging from gas and bloating to constipation and diarrhea. Maybe you've experienced a sudden urge to move your bowels right before a big job interview. With enough serotonin in your brain, acting as a buffer against stress, you can reduce the odds of one of these get-to-the-bathroom-or-else events.

The nerves inside your intestines also contain a large amount of serotonin—

so much, in fact, that some physiologists regard the intestines as sort of a primitive brain. Gut feelings can often give you quicker information than your rational mind. Serotonin signals the intestines either to contract or not contract, depending on the receptor site it lands on. Chronic stress probably leads to mixed messages being sent, and the large intestine gets irritated from too many or too few contractions, causing IBS symptoms of either painful cramps and diarrhea or sluggish constipation.

Serotonin is very important when we discuss a little later the new medication Zelnorm (tegaserod) for constipation-dominant IBS. Tegaserod actually blocks the "do not contract" intestinal receptor sites, leaves the "contract" sites open, and starts sluggish intestines moving. The fact that Zelnorm is one of the only medications that works primarily for women suggests low levels of serotonin throughout the body are needed for best results.

Taking control of your IBS definitely requires a lot of initiative on your part. Identifying and resolving the role of serotonin, stress, and hormones in your IBS is a big part of this healing path. Also, think about whether your IBS is constipation-dominant, diarrhea-dominant, or split evenly between the two. Some aspects of your treatment will depend on which is your dominant type.

FIRST STEPS: JOURNALING AND PERIOD-TRACKING

As a preliminary, you'll need to begin a month of fairly extensive journaling:

- **KEEP A FOOD JOURNAL** Although there's some disagreement among physicians about the role food sensitivities play in IBS, in my experience there's enough of a correlation between many gastrointestinal disorders and irritating foods that investigating them is definitely worth your time. Not all IBS is triggered by the low-serotonin/stress combination. Record what you eat over the next month to determine if there's any correlation between food and your IBS symptoms. Be aware that there may be a twenty-four-hour lag time between a culprit food and symptoms. By keeping your journal in conjunction with following the three-week Food Sensitivity Elimination Diet (see p. 109), you may see patterns emerge more quickly.

- **TRACK YOUR MENSTRUAL CYCLE FOR A MONTH** If you're like many women with IBS, your symptoms go into high gear during the week before your period starts. Using a wall calendar, highlight the days of your period and record your daily symptoms throughout the month. Since more than one hundred separate symptoms have been linked to PMS (p. 153)—including, of course, IBS—you may find yourself correlating not only a flare-up of IBS to the days before your period, but also other problems you hadn't paid much attention to, like an acne outbreak or low back pain. Even if you're in perimenopause or menopause, there may still be some slight cyclic component to your symptoms, so try this calendar tracking for a couple of months.

TEST FOR OTHER CAUSES

Ask your doctor to check you for the possibilities listed below. If she's never heard of these tests, you can get them through most holistic and nutritionally oriented physicians (p. 295) as well as many chiropractors (p. 275). Diagnostic tests for these conditions are often covered by health insurance:

– **COMPREHENSIVE STOOL DIGESTIVE ANALYSIS WITH OVA AND PARASITES** You send three stool specimens via overnight mail to a lab, which determines if you're deficient in any digestive enzymes, have an imbalance of intestinal bacteria, or have a parasite infection. The parasite *Blastocystis hominis* is very common and produces symptoms indistinguishable from IBS.

– **FOOD SENSITIVITY PANEL** The doctor mails a small sample of your blood to a lab, which tests it to see if your immune system is creating antibodies against any of ninety-six commonly eaten foods. A high level of antibodies against a food is very suggestive of a sensitivity to that food, which you can then eliminate from your diet.

  Sometimes, and for unclear reasons, there may be an inconsistency between your test results and what you noticed during the food sensitivity elimination diet (see p. 109). For example, your blood test will be positive for a food that doesn't give you any problems or vice versa—you're really bothered by a food that shows up negative on the blood test. Don't stew about this. Just eliminate any food that gives you symptoms when you eat it.

Your doctor will be familiar with these two tests:

– **GLUTEN SENSITIVITY (CELIAC DISEASE)** This intestinal condition is a peculiar reaction to gluten, a protein found in certain grains, like wheat, rye, and barley. If your IBS is diarrhea-dominant, two blood tests with utterly unpronounceable names will rule out this condition: anti-gliadin antibodies and anti-endomysial antibodies. Jot them down and hand the paper to your doctor.

– **LACTOSE INTOLERANCE** Lactose intolerance is an inability to digest lactose, the sugar found in dairy products, and it occurs in many people of both sexes as they get older and also with greater frequency in certain ethnic groups, including African Americans and Latinos. It's not the same as a food allergy to milk or sensitivity to milk. Following the food sensitivity elimination diet (p. 109) can give you a hint that your IBS may actually be lactose intolerance. If, after reintroducing dairy products, you feel really bloated and gassy, with abdominal cramping, your problem may be lactose intolerance rather than IBS. Your doctor can also order blood and breath analysis tests to confirm this diagnosis.

  The immediate way to stop your symptoms if you are lactose intolerant is to stop eating all dairy products. Some people can still tolerate yogurt even though they have problems with other forms of dairy. Alternatively, you can buy Lactaid, a concentrate of the enzyme lactase that you're lacking, and add a couple of drops to milk so the lactose is predigested for you. Lactaid Ultra is a chewable tablet of lactase you take before eating a dairy-containing dish. Lactaid brand milk is also available.

TRIPLE WHAMMY APPROACH TO IBS

WHAMMY #1: STRESS Because IBS is a Triple Whammy disorder, triggered when you "internalize" your stress, it's well worth comparing your IBS symptoms against your Stress Journal (p. 198) to find your stress triggers. If your IBS is triggered by stress, take some positive steps, such as practicing another stress reliever from the Stress-Relief Menu (see p. 204). More dramatic stress-relievers might include getting rid of the roommate from hell or leaving your much-hated job.

WHAMMY #2: LOW SEROTONIN Your stress buffer, serotonin, is integrally involved in IBS. Use the natural ways from the Three-Week Cure (p. 45) to boost serotonin: exercise, sunlight exposure, the supplements fish oil and B complex, and carbohydrate timing. But make sure you're not sensitive to any of the grains in these carbs.

WHAMMY #3: HORMONES If your IBS flares during the week before your period, heed this PMS warning and start taking chasteberry (p. 52) or any good PMS herbal combination when you're not menstruating. If you have a smorgasbord of other PMS symptoms, remember that PMS itself is a Triple Whammy disorder; read and follow the PMS healing path on page 153.

LIFESTYLE CHANGES

– **EAT SMALLER AND MORE FREQUENT MEALS** Larger meals can trigger intestinal contractions. Review the Triple Whammy Food Plan on page 245 and start eating the Triple Whammy way.

– **DRINK PEPPERMINT TEA ONCE OR TWICE A DAY** Consider replacing some of your coffee with it. Peppermint relaxes the muscles of your digestive tract, relieving cramping and gas, and stimulates the flow of digestive juices.

– **CHANGE YOUR EATING HABITS** Increase the fiber in your diet (whole grains, fresh fruits and vegetables) and reduce low-fiber fare like meat, poultry, and foods made primarily with refined white flour. If you're sensitive to gas-forming (but beneficial) foods like beans, lentils, peas, and broccoli, eat smaller amounts. One study showed that people with IBS who increased their fish intake reduced their symptoms, apparently because omega-3 fish oil is a natural anti-inflammatory. This underscores the importance of taking the fish oil supplements recommended in the

Three-Week Cure. Some people with IBS are very sensitive to coffee, alcohol, spices, and foods with hydrogenated oils. Check to see if you're among them.

- **GET MORE EXERCISE** Not only is exercise a wonderful way to raise your serotonin and keep you fit, but studies have shown that IBS patients who exercise regularly report a real decline in symptoms. Exercise stimulates digestion and thwarts stress.

- **EAT YOGURT** Yogurt contains probiotics, helpful bacteria like acidophilus and bifidobacter that help restore a balance of good guy bacteria in your intestines. Eat a cup daily, making sure the label indicates that it contains "live active cultures." Most of the pudding and fluffy-style yogurts don't have active cultures, and they're also loaded with sugar. Buy plain low-fat yogurt and add whole fruit or a spoonful of fruit preserves or honey to it. If you're sensitive to dairy, read about lactose intolerance (p. 105) and follow the steps there.

- **GET A CONCENTRATED SOLUBLE FIBER PRODUCT** Psyllium (Metamucil) and any of the fiber formulas available in drugstores and health food stores all act pretty much the same way, absorbing excess water and increasing the bulk of your intestinal contents (there's a euphemism for you). Whether you have constipation or diarrhea-dominant IBS, these products will help by normalizing your bowel movement. (Eating the Triple Whammy way will make this step unnecessary.)

NUTRITIONAL SUPPLEMENTS FOR IBS

- **PEPPERMINT OIL** Peppermint relaxes intestines and aids digestion. Peppermint oil capsules, available in health food stores, may be effective in reducing your bloating, gas, and abdominal cramping. Take them regularly for at least a month to see if they work for you. **DOSE:** Take one or two capsules (make sure they're coated, also called enteric capsules) two or three times a day before eating. Don't use if you're pregnant as peppermint relaxes the uterus.

- **FISH OIL** Not only are the omega-3 essential fatty acids in fish oil needed to bolster levels of your stress-buffering serotonin, they also act as natural anti-inflammatories throughout the body, including your irritable large intestine. **DOSE:** Take 1,000 mg twice a day, adding a third midday capsule if you think it might help.

- **PROBIOTICS** If you're sensitive to dairy or simply aren't thrilled with a daily cup of live-culture yogurt, your health food store has a vast selection of probiotic products. I suggest a combination of lactobacillus acidophilus and bifidobacter, in an enteric (coated) capsule so that the bacteria won't be killed off by your stomach acid. Try to find one that doesn't need refrigeration (otherwise you'll put them in your refrigerator, forget they're there, and find them years later when you clean). **DOSE:** Follow package instructions.

ALTERNATIVE MEDICINE

- **TRADITIONAL CHINESE MEDICINE** (TCM, p. 285) Both acupuncture and Chinese herbals have been clinically proven to control IBS.

- **HOMEOPATHIC MEDICINE** A classically trained homeopath (p. 277) would interview you at considerable length before developing a specific remedy to address your IBS symptoms and also the aspects of your personality that bring on symptoms.

SELF-CARE

- **RELAXATION AND MEDITATION** Virtually any of the techniques described in the Stress-Relief Menu will help your IBS. High on the list of those with proven benefit are yoga (p. 230), t'ai chi (p. 228), biofeedback, meditation, and guided imagery (p. 214).

- **FLOWER THERAPY** (p. 220) Most IBS sufferers internalize anger and frustration, so vervain might be a nice remedy to start. Others include cerato for relief of self-doubt, crab apple to help rid the mind of negative thoughts, aspen for panic and anxiety, and impatiens, perfect for those whose intestines churn when caught in traffic.

- **AROMATHERAPY** (p. 210) The relaxing oils, like lavender and melissa, can be helpful. An aromatherapist might also suggest bergamot to encourage good digestion, and a few drops of grapefruit oil mixed into a carrier oil and gently massaged into your abdomen to calm painful intestinal cramps.

CONVENTIONAL APPROACH TO IBS

Both conventional and nutritionally oriented holistic physicians begin any treatment of IBS by increasing fiber in the diet. No one argues with the benefit of psyllium and other fiber concentrates (Metamucil and many other brands) taken on a daily basis. But following the Triple Whammy Food Plan (p. 245), with its emphasis on fruits, vegetables, and whole grains, is a better way. Doctors frequently prescribe antispasmodic drugs like Bentyl (dicyclomine), Donnatal (belladonna/phenobarbital), or Levsin (hyoscyamine), all of which work by blocking nerve impulses from your brain to your intestines. I try to avoid prescribing these medications, even though they are occasionally (but not spectacularly) effective, because the side effects are so unpleasant: dry mouth, blurred vision, low libido, and difficulty passing urine.

- **IF DIARRHEA IS YOUR MAIN PROBLEM,** ask your doctor about low doses of Lomotil (diphenoxylate/atropine), a prescription medicine that slows intestinal movement.

Although the usual prescribed dose is six to eight tablets per day, my Triple Whammy patients are usually very sensitive to Lomotil, and as small a dose as one or two tablets a day can stop intestinal churning and bring diarrhea to a screeching halt.

– **IF YOUR IBS IS CONSTIPATION-DOMINANT,** ask about Zelnorm (tegaserod), a prescription drug that initiates intestinal contractions and gets sluggish, constipated bowels moving again. A similar drug, Lotronex (alosetron), is generally reserved for the most severe cases because of potentially dangerous side effects.

Lastly, don't be surprised if your doctor recommends an antidepressant, even if you aren't feeling particularly depressed. The older tricyclic antidepressants, like Elavil (amitriptyline) or Tofranil (imipramine), act on your brain to block the nerve impulse that causes intestinal spasms. They also block pain receptors in your intestines from relaying pain messages to your brain. You can get by with very small doses of either of these, and by doing so you will generally avoid the side effects of dry mouth and sleepiness.

FOOD SENSITIVITY ELIMINATION DIET

This self-test will help you discover whether or not certain foods are responsible for your symptoms. Sensitivities to foods have been linked to problems such as IBS, inflammatory bowel diseases like ulcerative colitis and Crohn's disease, migraine, chronic fatigue, skin rashes, joint pain, chronic sinusitis, and even a general sense of chronic ill health.

The most common food irritants are dairy, eggs, corn, wheat, and citrus. If dairy is setting you off, you may have lactose intolerance (see p. 105).

Although blood tests for food sensitivities are available, this test is one of the most useful tools because you do it yourself, and you're also in charge of interpreting your body's response. This diet is also sometimes called "elimination and challenge," because first you eliminate foods and then you reintroduce them, in a sense challenging your body to respond. Let's get started.

FOR SEVEN DAYS (DAYS 1–7) eliminate all foods that contain dairy, wheat, corn, eggs, and citrus. If you're still eating prepared foods (see the Triple Whammy Food Plan on page 245 for reasons not to), you'll have to read labels to check for these ingredients:

– **DAIRY PRODUCTS,** including milk, cream, yogurt (you can use dairy-free probiotics, available at health food stores), ice cream, sour cream, cheese. If it comes from a cow, eliminate it.

- **EGGS,** including foods containing eggs.

- **CORN** and corn products (you'll really have to be vigilant about checking labels for corn syrup).

- **WHEAT** (definitely the most difficult to eliminate).

- **CITRUS.**

Now before you imploringly ask, "But what am I going to eat?" believe me, no one has ever starved to death with full access to all grains except wheat. Remember rice? Barley? Buckwheat? Oats? This is a fine opportunity to try some new whole grains. Also, you can have any vegetables, including potatoes, and all meat, poultry, fish, and fruit (*except* citrus).

You may be a little surprised to discover how much you eat from one particular group. For example, many people eat products containing wheat (waffles, pancakes, doughnuts, scones, sandwiches, pasta) several times a day for years and years.

After you've eliminated these potential culprits for a full week, do a sort of body scan. Do you sense an improvement in any of your long-standing symptoms, or even a general sense of feeling better? If you feel exactly the same after a week of food elimination as you did before, you probably don't have an issue with food sensitivities and you can resume your normal eating habits.

If, however, one or more of your symptoms has improved, or you just generally feel better, then you may be onto something important. "Better" is, of course, vague, but it's your body and you're the one most intimately acquainted with how you feel. For you, "better" may mean less gas and bloating, less muscle aching and fatigue, clearer sinuses, anything. If you fall in this category, start to reintroduce each food group as follows:

DAYS 8–10: Reintroduce dairy in any quantity you're comfortable with. Monitor yourself for a return of any symptoms. If none appears, dairy is not a problem and you can return to having dairy and reintroduce the next food group. If, however, some symptoms return, stop having dairy altogether.

DAYS 11–13: Reintroduce eggs, watching carefully for symptoms. If you have any, stop eating eggs altogether. If no symptoms, you can now continue to eat eggs and at the same time move on to the next group.

DAYS 14–16: Reintroduce corn.

DAYS 17–19: Reintroduce wheat.

DAYS 20–21: Reintroduce citrus.

After three weeks, you may have learned something about how your body responds to the foods you eat. Food sensitivities are annoying but not a serious risk, unlike food allergies, which can cause your body to go into a major, sometimes life-threatening shock after eating an offending food, such as shellfish. If you "cheat" and indulge in one of the foods you're sensitive to, expect a return of your symptoms, but nothing dangerous to your health.

10.

MEMORY LOSS AND BRAIN FOG

Problems with clear and productive thought—and by this I mean focus, concentration, and memory—occur often with Triple Whammy disorders and also on their own. Each of the whammies, taken individually, is intimately involved with how efficiently your brain functions.

A change in your cognitive skills may become more noticeable to you during your mid-forties, and could be a result of declining levels of estrogen and neurotransmitters like serotonin. Of course, the brains of men age, too (as you may have noticed). But probably because of women's lower levels of serotonin and the need for estrogen for good brain function, women seem to experience this problem at an earlier age than men. Research has shown that some, but certainly not all, women experience a change in memory and focus with menopause, and that some of these women, but again, not all, find they improve with hormone replacement therapy (HRT).

And, of course, the "A" word looms large when you've had too many senior moments. "Could it be early Alzheimer's?" you wonder anxiously. Let's look at the facts. Although people with significant age-related memory problems are at greater risk for developing Alzheimer's disease, the key word here is "significant."

I suspect that doctors rarely inquire about mental functioning because they incorrectly believe that not a whole lot can be done for mild memory loss or other cognitive impairments. Conventional doctors are pretty clueless about the documented value of nutritional medications like ginkgo and acetyl-L-carnitine. Because numerous medications are awaiting FDA approval, many physicians are unaware or unwilling to prescribe the memory-enhancing medications marketed in Europe but also available in the United States. And in the wake of the Women's Health Initiative (WHI) study, many doctors have completely abandoned HRT, or prescribe it only for severe menopause-related symptoms, allowing a woman stumbling through the mental fogginess of peri-menopause to pretty much fend for herself.

The Triple Whammy approach to memory loss and other thinking impairments will help women in any age bracket. Some aspects of it, like bioidentical hormone replacement therapy, are obviously geared for a women going through the menopause transition. And although the other aspects are obviously not a cure for Alzheimer's disease, they may help people of both sexes suffering from this condition.

WHAT CAUSES MEMORY LOSS AND OTHER THINKING IMPAIRMENT?

You might be surprised at how long the list of causes is. On the plus side, many of these factors are under your control. You can actually do quite a bit to improve your brain's performance, both now and in the years to come. To begin with, no matter what you've heard, your brain cells aren't dying off, they're just shrinking, which may not affect brain function at all. Indeed some areas of your brain continue to generate new cells even as you age, so although aging itself is inevitable, declining brain function is not. There are some very (very!) smart ninety-year-olds out there, a lot of them brighter, more creative, and funnier than you or I will ever be.

Let's review some of the factors that can affect mental function:

- **CIRCULATION TO YOUR BRAIN** can diminish with age, and if your brain receives less blood, this adversely affects your mental functioning. Remember, too, that saturated fats clog your arteries. To maintain healthy circulation to your brain, reduce the amount of saturated fat you eat (the Triple Whammy Food Plan, p. 245, can help). Even more important is to keep your blood moving: exercise regularly—and at least occasionally, vigorously. Your twenty-minute walk outside each day is an excellent start. Keep it brisk to keep the blood pumping to your brain.

- **HIGH CHOLESTEROL, HIGH BLOOD PRESSURE, AND DIABETES** all damage arteries, including those in your brain. If you have any of these, work with your doctor to bring them under control.

- **ALTERED OXYGEN MOLECULES CALLED FREE RADICALS** have been implicated in chronic brain disorders such as Parkinson's disease and Alzheimer's disease. Cigarette smoking is a major source of free radicals, and damages your arteries, too, so if you value your brain, give it up (p. 177). Start taking a high-potency multivitamin blend and also antioxidant nutritional supplements to mop up free radicals. The Triple Whammy Food Plan is loaded with antioxidant foods. Antioxidants are so effective that conventional neurologists now include high doses of the antioxidant vitamin E as part of their treatment plan for Alzheimer's. In one research study, rats fed a diet rich in blueberries (which are high in antioxidants) performed better in remembering a complex maze than those who were not.

- **EXCESSIVE SUGAR (INCLUDING TOO MUCH ALCOHOL)** is not brain food. When you eat any food rich in sugar, including refined foods, the glucose (sugar) level in your blood rises and quickly comes crashing down. Low blood sugar, called hypoglycemia, can damage healthy brain cells. Likewise, alcohol beyond moderate consumption is toxic to the brain, though all studies on longevity show that a single glass of red wine daily has nothing but positive health benefits.

- **NUTRITIONALS NEEDED FOR HEALTHY BRAIN CELL STRUCTURE** include B vitamins to help your brain manufacture neurotransmitters, including serotonin. Helpful fats, the omega-3s found in fish oil and the omega-6s in flaxseed (among others), are necessary for good brain cell structure. If you're following the Three-Week Cure, you've already started on B complex 100 and fish oil and you're working with the Triple Whammy Food Plan.

- **CHRONIC NEGATIVE STRESS,** our Whammy #1, works mightily against clear mental function. Studies have shown that the adrenal gland hormone cortisol, which is generally released only under chronic stress, actually interferes directly with the brain's ability to remember details and think analytically. On the other hand, positive stress, like cramming for an exam or facing a new but interesting challenge, such as a difficult crossword puzzle, is a virtual aerobics class for your brain.

- **DECLINING LEVELS OF NEUROTRANSMITTERS,** including Whammy #2 serotonin, but also dopamine and acetylcholine, definitely affect the efficiency of your brain. My patients with Triple Whammy disorders like depression and chronic anxiety often report terrible memory and focus problems. These dramatically improve when serotonin levels rise, whether through the natural methods outlined in the Three-Week Cure, by taking the herbs St. John's wort or 5HTP, or in response to antidepressant medications. So it isn't surprising that the new medicines for treating Alzheimer's disease do so by raising neurotransmitter levels.

- **WHEN YOUR SEX HORMONES SHIFT,** either during premenstrual days or in perimenopause, you may experience mild to moderate impairment of thinking. Remember that when estrogen rises, so does feel-good serotonin, which you also need for clear thinking. With PMS, brain fade can occur when your falling estrogen drags down serotonin. During perimenopause, your brain faces a steady fall in estrogen and serotonin.

Let's finish this considerable list with three frequently overlooked sources of memory loss:

- **HYPOTHYROIDISM** Thyroid hormone is vital for efficient brain function, and even a mildly underactive thyroid can impair cognitive skills. Taking thyroid replacement hormone can dramatically improve your focus, concentration, and memory.

- **PRESCRIPTION DRUGS** Many drugs cause side effects like drowsiness and fuzzy thinking. Read your package inserts.

- **UNTREATED CHRONIC CONDITIONS** Liver, kidney, or lung disease all affect brain function in different ways and can cause problems with clear thinking. Heart and lung disease can deprive your brain of adequate oxygen. The liver and kidneys are needed to remove potentially toxic wastes from your body, so when they're not working your brain is poisoned by the normally excreted end products of your metabolism.

TREATING MEMORY LOSS AND OTHER COGNITIVE IMPAIRMENTS

In this section, I'll be introducing you to an array of supplements and prescription medications, but we'll first tackle your Whammies. I generally recommend prescription medication only if working on the Whammies and using these supplements isn't as effective as you'd like.

WHAMMY #1: STRESS I can't overemphasize the negative effect of chronic stress on brain function. Let's say you're in a terrible job, with a supervisor from hell, and every night you go home horribly dispirited. Thinking about this job dominates your mind, interferes with your sleep, and sucks the joy from life. You find you can't concentrate enough to balance the checkbook, you forget your parents' anniversary, or you can't follow the plot of the mystery you're reading. This can all happen because of other stressors, too. If you have chronic stress in your life, read chapter 20 on limiting stress (p. 197) and get to work.

WHAMMY #2: LOW SEROTONIN Your naturally lower level of serotonin isn't necessarily a problem unless you're faced with stress. Stress and low serotonin make you susceptible to all Triple Whammy disorders including cognitive impairment. Everything you learned in the Three-Week Cure (p. 45) about boosting serotonin applies. If you haven't begun the serotonin-boosting steps, please start today and stick with them.

WHAMMY #3: HORMONES Pay attention to your body to see if there's a hormonal component to your memory and focus issues. If you're menstruating, your symptoms will most likely occur during the week or two before your period. If you have fuzzy thinking before your period, get those hormones balanced with the advice in the PMS healing path (p. 153). If a change in your overall sharpness started in perimenopause or menopause, review the Menopause Transition healing path on page 120. Your brain function may benefit from small doses of bioidentical hormones. Most women need hormones only briefly.

NUTRITIONAL SUPPLEMENTS FOR MEMORY ENHANCEMENT

Once you're in full swing against the three whammies, you should very definitely begin with a nutritional supplement program for memory enhancement before resorting to medications. Supplements are safe and surprisingly effective. If you're interested in knowing more, you can spend a little time on the Internet and unearth articles about the supplements that have appeared in conventional medical journals, written by good clinical researchers.

- **START WITH A HIGH-POTENCY DAILY MULTIPLE VITAMIN.** Start taking a high-potency multivitamin blend, something beyond the "minimum-wage," one-a-day product you bought on sale at the dollar store. You can recognize the high-potency blend by dose (you take two tablets a day), and because the percentage of minimum daily requirements (MDR) or recommended daily allowance (RDA) is well beyond the basic 100 percent that simply staves off a vitamin deficiency disease but has little value in preventing chronic disease. Don't worry about doubling up on B vitamins by taking a multiple vitamin in addition to the B complex recommended in the Three-Week Cure. Your body will eliminate what you don't need because B vitamins are water soluble, meaning you excrete any extra via your urine. This, however, does not apply to fat-soluble vitamins (A, D, E, and K). Any extra you take of these can slowly build up in the fat cells of your body and stay there a good long time—not recommended.

- **REMEMBER THE TWO IMPORTANT ESSENTIAL FATTY ACIDS.** You get omega-3 in your 2 grams of fish oil per day as part of the Three-Week Cure. Add also omega-6, another EFA, in the form of capsules containing borage oil or flaxseed oil. Flaxseed oil is also available as a liquid; take one tablespoon daily or mix it into your food or juice. It's also featured in some bread spreads.

- **FOLLOW THE TRIPLE WHAMMY FOOD PLAN** (p. 245). It includes foods that will dramatically increase your intake of all nutrients, antioxidants, and phytochemicals. Eating the Triple Whammy way provides you with a nutritionally sound foundation for better memory. Timing your intake of complex carbohydrates (p. 263) also helps memory because your brain needs a periodic infusion of carbs to create serotonin, which improves focus and concentration.

NEXT, THE SUPPLEMENTS

The main challenge with the following list of nutritional supplements is that you end up taking a lot of pills every day. However, several nutritional manufacturers combine most of the following supplements into a single product. To keep yourself sane, I suggest using a combination product such as Brain Sustain, Cognitex, or Neurotone, among others.

If you do a little label reading, you'll notice that some combination products contain B vitamins that replicate the B complex 100 you're taking for the Three-Week Cure. If you find yourself taking a lot of B complex, such as in a high-potency multiple vitamin and also a brain mix combination, don't worry. Your body will eliminate via your urine what it doesn't use, though you may choose to stop taking your B complex 100 capsule.

Most of the combination products are a blend of three or more of the brain-enhancing supplements listed below. Whether you want to use individual supplements or a preformulated blend is up to you. The blend will be more economical, but you can achieve higher doses using individual supplements. However, you certainly don't need both individual supplements *and* a well-formulated blend.

- **GINKGO BILOBA** Ginkgo has been shown in dozens of studies to enhance memory by improving circulation to the brain. **DOSE:** 60–80 mg two or three times a day with food to avoid stomach irritation.

- **ACETYL-L-CARNITINE** Involved in brain function by carrying fuel into the mitochondria, the energy centers of brain cells (and all cells), and removing the waste products of brain cell metabolism. **DOSE:** 500 mg two or three times a day on an empty stomach to enhance absorption.

- **CO-ENZYME Q-10** Co Q10 acts on mitochondria in the brain (and throughout the body) and is fundamental for optimal brain cell energy. **DOSE:** 50–100 mg twice a day with food to enhance absorption.

- **DMAE (DIMETHYL AMINO ETHANOL)** Available for more than thirty years, DMAE was originally developed for attention deficit disorder and is widely used for improved focus and concentration. Some studies showed that DMAE stabilizes the delicate membranes surrounding brain cells and increases levels of the neurotransmitter acetylcholine, a brain chemical involved in focus, concentration, and memory. It's sold as Deanol in Europe. **DOSE:** 150 mg twice a day on an empty stomach to enhance absorption.

- **PHOSPHATIDYL SERINE** Like DMAE, phosphatidyl serine is involved in maintaining healthy brain cell membranes so that brain cells can effectively communicate with each other. **DOSE:** 100 mg two or three times a day on an empty stomach to enhance absorption.

- **LIPOIC ACID** Also called alpha-lipoic acid, this is a newer, very potent antioxidant that protects the brain from free radical damage. **DOSE:** 100–120 mg twice a day, with or without food.

PRESCRIPTION MEDICATIONS FOR MEMORY ENHANCEMENT

Some conventional doctors shy away from what is called off-label prescribing, which is when a doctor writes you a prescription for a medication whose intended use is different from its FDA-approved use. For example, doctors were prescribing the blood pressure medication propanolol to prevent migraines several years before the FDA finally approved its use for this condition. The recommendations I've listed below are all off-label. Basically, you'll have to ask your doctor for a prescription for these medications and keep your fingers crossed. Some doctors have no problem prescribing off-label; others will adamantly refuse to do so. With a little hunting on the Internet, you can probably find a doctor in your area who is a member of one of the alternative medical associations, like the American Holistic Medical Association, the American College for the Advancement of Medicine, or the American Academy of Anti-Aging Medicine. Physician members in these organizations keep up on the latest advances in nutritional medicine, and often use the products themselves.

- **GALANTAMINE (RAZADYNE),** derived from daffodil bulbs, is now FDA-approved for treating Alzheimer's disease. It's been available over the counter for years as a memory enhancer and is sold at health food stores or online. Of course, if you can get a prescription from your doctor, your health insurance may pay for it. **DOSE:** Reminyl 4–8 mg or Galantamind (sold over the counter) 8 mg once or twice a day.

- **SELEGILINE (ELDEPRYL)** is used primarily to treat people with Parkinson's disease but has been shown to enhance memory and focus. It works by increasing levels of the neurotransmitter dopamine, which helps the body move smoothly and enhances focus and memory. **DOSE:** 2.5 mg daily or every other day.

- **ERGOLOID MESYLATES (HYDERGINE)** was initially developed for Alzheimer's disease because of its ability to improve blood flow to the brain. It's now used worldwide as a memory enhancer by mimicking a substance in the brain called nerve growth factor. The drug increases the number of connections (called dendrites) your brain cells make with other brain cells. **DOSE:** 1 mg two or three times a day.

- **HORMONE REPLACEMENT THERAPY (HRT)** Read about the Women's Health Initiative (WHI) study on page 122. I believe using HRT (ideally with bioidentical hormones) for three years or less is safe. Estrogen itself has several very positive effects on the brain: it increases neurotransmitters like serotonin and acetylcholine. Estrogen also increases receptor sites to which neurotransmitters attach; it maintains the health of brain connections called dendrites; and it works with several nerve growth factors (molecules that protect the brain from free radical damage) to maintain the structure of brain cells.

  Current thinking by conventional doctors limits HRT use to the relief of symptoms such as hot flashes, night sweats, and interrupted sleep during the perimenopausal years only. I agree with this, but would add memory and concentration problems to the list of symptoms meriting an HRT prescription. **DOSE:** The dose for memory and concentration problems is variable. Read more about bioidentical hormones on page 129 and talk to your doctor.

- **THYROID HORMONE THERAPY** An underactive thyroid interferes with brain function, but you should take thyroid replacement only if you've been diagnosed with this condition. Be aware that the "normal" value of thyroid tests has changed and if you were borderline low-thyroid in the past, you should be retested. Doctors are not in agreement about the existence of a condition called subclinical hypothyroidism, in which blood tests are normal but the person seems to have low thyroid function, including lack of energy, dry skin and hair, feeling cold all the time, fuzzy thinking, mild constipation, and a low (97.6 or lower) basal temperature (p. 75). If you're borderline low-thyroid, ask your doctor for a prescription for a trial period of thyroid hormone to see if your symptoms improve. **DOSE:** Start with a low dose 1/2 gram (30 mg) of natural thyroid. Natural thyroid is extracted from livestock (cattle, pigs) and many physicians believe this form more closely resembles human thyroid than the synthetic version. Your doctor may opt to increase your dose to 1 gram (60 mg) as needed.

SELF-CARE TREATMENTS FOR ENHANCING BRAIN FUNCTION

An often-heard comparison of your brain to your muscles is reasonable: use it or lose it. Keep your brain challenged and keep it free from stress. Keep it busy and it will continue to perform well.

- **LEARN TO MEDITATE** People who meditate regularly report improved focus and concentration as well as enhanced creativity (not to mention reduced stress). Learn more about meditation on page 215.

- **STIMULATE YOUR BRAIN TO FORM NEW CONNECTIONS** Break away from routine. Walk backwards for an increasing distance each day or brush your teeth using your other (nondominant) hand. Learn a new card or board game. Do the *New*

York Times crossword puzzle a couple of times a week. Balance your checkbook without using a calculator. Play Scrabble.

– **CHALLENGE YOURSELF** Learn a new language, a musical instrument, a new computer program, or something you always considered difficult, like algebra or astronomy. Undertake a research project, such as learning everything about an artist and then viewing her work at a gallery or museum. Keep a difficult jigsaw puzzle on your dining room table and work at it a little each day.

– **GET YOUR LIFE BETTER ORGANIZED** You won't keep losing your keys if you install a key rack and when you walk in the door say aloud, "I am now going to hang my keys on my new key rack." Keep an appointment book, have a calendar on which you can jot down birthdays and anniversaries, and maintain a daily things-to-do checklist.

– **REVIEW YOUR PRESCRIPTION DRUGS** If you're taking any prescription medicines, make a complete list of them and then work with your doctor to see if any can be lowered or even discontinued. Medicines for pain, depression, anxiety, high blood pressure, and allergies can all cause brain fog. You'd think that taking an antidepressant would help brain function because it boosts serotonin, and it does in most people, but some people react adversely and develop fuzzy thinking.

ALTERNATIVE THERAPIES

– **TRADITIONAL CHINESE MEDICINE (TCM)** Acupuncture and Chinese herbs may be of benefit in the hands of an experienced practitioner. A Chinese herb called huperzine A, derived from a species of moss, has been shown to enhance brain function by raising levels of acetylcholine. TCM is discussed in greater detail on page 285.

11.

MENOPAUSE TRANSITION

Menopause is not a disorder, Triple Whammy or otherwise. It's a passage in every woman's life and I use the word transition to underscore the fact that perimenopause and menopause take place over a period of time. For some lucky women, perimenopause and menopause are a walk in the park. One month you don't get a period and you're pretty certain you're not pregnant. Then a couple of period-free months go by, and that's it. Most women, however, don't get off so lightly.

Like other Triple Whammy–related conditions, you're unique when it comes to what you'll experience during the menopause transition. Think of it as a process. Your ovaries started producing estrogen and progesterone when you were about ten years old, changing the shape of your body, making you aware that boys had some yet undiscovered potential beyond annoyance. A couple of years later, when these hormones reached a certain level, they triggered your menstrual cycles. In your late thirties, your sex hormones began a slow decline until finally, by your late forties or early fifties, they reached a point where they could no longer trigger your periods.

Beforehand, you may have noticed that your periods had shortened or become irregular. And because levels of estrogen are intimately linked with Whammy #2, the feel-good neurotransmitter serotonin (estrogen up = happy, estrogen dropping = not so happy), if you had PMS during your regular periods, you may have noticed it getting a little worse. Premenopause/perimenopause refers to the months or years when you're still having some periods but also experiencing indications that your hormone levels are dropping, like a change in the timing or amount of menstrual flow or occasional hot flashes. You've arrived in menopause, on the other hand, when a year has gone by without a period, regardless of symptoms.

Women with severe premenopause symptoms feel a rightful sense of injustice. "I mean," as one of my patients told me, "If I've got to be peeling off my clothes during hot flashes or waking up drenched with night sweats, give me a break and let's stop it with these periods already." Not knowing myself what any of this feels like, I can only sympathetically nod and tell you most men I know couldn't handle it. On the plus side, menopause symptoms relent on their own after a few years. This is only guardedly comforting; a few years of night sweats and hot flashes is still a very long time.

YOUR MIND, ON MENOPAUSE

The menopause transition can bring other symptoms too, and those that affect my patients' minds are often the most distressing. Women who suddenly start experiencing unpredictable emotional swings, poor concentration, fuzzy thinking, and lapses in short-term memory (see Memory Loss and Brain Fog, p. 111) feel powerless against these unexpected and totally disconcerting symptoms, not to mention anxious about what will happen to their minds in the future. The reason these symptoms occur is best illustrated by the many positive ways that estrogen—now dropping—acts on the brain. Estrogen increases your brain's level of all neurotransmitters, including serotonin, and it improves the overall efficiency of each brain cell by increasing the number of neurotransmitter receptor sites. Estrogen also maintains and encourages the growth of part of the brain cell called the dendrite, which permits multiple connections with other brain cells.

The premenopausal downward shift in estrogen (and with it serotonin) can make a smart, emotionally stable woman feel as if her brain is turning to mush. You might find yourself forgetting names and appointments or be horrified to discover that balancing your checkbook has become an exercise in higher mathematics. You might scream an obscenity at a cabdriver who's picked up another fare or feel like tossing your partner into the Cuisinart for forgetting to pick up bread on her way home from work. One of my patients, whose father had died of Alzheimer's, dropped off her husband for a short appointment in downtown Chicago with the understanding that she'd circle and return in ten minutes. She discovered to her horror that she'd forgotten the location of the drop-off/pick-up. She knew something was very much wrong with her mind, and wondered if she was destined for a steady decline into dementia at age fifty-three. (Hormone replacement restored her memory; more on that next.)

SEX DRIVE

A declining interest in sex occurs for many, though certainly not all, women during the menopause transition. Vaginal lubricants may make the mechanics of intercourse less uncomfortable, but to give yourself enough oomph to participate in sex with enthusiasm, I recommend adding some testosterone to your bioidentical hormone replacement (p. 129). Most of my patients who have done this report very (very!) positive results. My surefire formula for an enhanced postmenopausal sex life is Viagra for him and testosterone for you both.

HORMONE REPLACEMENT AND THE WOMEN'S HEALTH INITIATIVE STUDY

Until recently, the solution to this mess was apparently easy. The ever-helpful pharmaceutical industry stood poised to give women what they "needed": hormones. In the first years of hormone replacement therapy doctors were encouraged to prescribe estrogen alone. Several years and quite a few deaths later, it became apparent that women receiving "unopposed" estrogen (i.e., without progesterone) were susceptible to developing uterine cancer, also called endometrial cancer. This particular risk disappeared when women received a second prescription for progesterone, later combined with estrogen in Prempro.

Before the Women's Health Initiative (WHI) study was published in 2002, approximately fifteen million women were using HRT. Six months afterward, that number was reduced by half, with most of this group not telling their physicians that they'd stopped taking hormones. Fearing for the well-being of their patients, and concerned about an anticipated barrage of malpractice suits, many doctors simply stopped prescribing hormones. This left whole communities of women adrift in the symptom-infested waters of menopause.

Briefly, what the WHI study actually said was this:

- HRT does relieve symptoms of menopause (hot flashes, night sweats, vaginal dryness, mood and memory disturbances).

- The downside of taking HRT is an increased risk for developing breast cancer.

- Long-term use of HRT, originally thought to protect against heart disease and stroke, actually slightly increased the risk for developing these conditions, mainly in women who already had risk factors for heart disease (high cholesterol, high blood pressure, diabetes) rather than low-risk women.

- And finally: if you take HRT for symptom relief, use the lowest possible dose for the shortest time period.

It's equally important to get the other side of the picture, however. Many researchers didn't agree with the conclusions of the WHI study. Contrarians felt the warnings about HRT were prematurely released (the five-year study being far too short) and resulted in unnecessarily frightening and misinforming women and their doctors. After all, they said, should we ignore the previous evidence that HRT combinations other than Prempro actually did protect women from developing depression, memory problems, and heart disease? This group thought that the study simply didn't provide enough evidence to compel eight million women to stop their hormones.

Take, for example, the issue of the increased breast cancer risk with hormones. The contrarian researchers say that if a woman is diagnosed with breast cancer, those cancer cells will have been in her breast several years before the lump is felt or seen on a mammogram. Thus, if the average woman in the WHI study developed breast cancer after she had been on HRT for three years, this means she may have entered the study with an undiscovered breast cancer well before she started taking hormones. And, in fact, if you look at other studies using milder estrogen, there is some evidence that correctly administered HRT might actually protect a woman from developing breast cancer, or improve the outlook of a woman who develops breast cancer while on hormones.

Comparable data showed that estrogen does help the brain, heart, and blood vessels and that the villain in this whole affair may have been the synthetic progesterone (medroxyprogesterone) used in the HRT that was administered. Bioidentical progesterone has not been studied because it cannot be patented by a pharmaceutical company, which would receive no financial gain in underwriting the cost of tests. And lastly, no one disputes the evidence that HRT protects a woman's bones from developing osteoporosis without her having to resort to prescription drugs like Fosamax.

My point is that the WHI conclusions are anything but the final word on the subject of HRT.

Many of the eight million women who stopped their hormones had such a severe resurgence of symptoms that they simply returned to their HRT prescriptions, shrugging off the WHI conclusions and telling themselves, "Life's too short to suffer like this." Other women who stopped taking hormones were pleasantly surprised to find their symptoms had become milder over the years or had abated altogether. Apparently, they'd weathered the worst of menopause and now it was over.

I suspect a majority of the eight million women who quit their HRT are still wondering what's best for them. In addition, each week thousands of women now entering perimenopause and menopause are experiencing their first major hot flash or are awakened by their first night sweat. About forty million U.S. women will go through the menopause transition over the next twenty years, and they are wondering what path to take.

Now that you've read these conflicting views, you might be thinking, "What does all this mean for me? What exactly should I do?"

THE ABC TRIPLE WHAMMY APPROACH TO MENOPAUSE

Nowhere in medicine does the phrase "one size fits all" apply less than in addressing the symptoms of perimenopause and menopause. Our Triple Whammy approach looks at three groups with different menopausal symptoms. See if you can locate yourself:

- **GROUP A,** with virtually no symptoms at all, can get away with doing nothing in particular. If you fit here, you're a winner in the menopause transition lotto. Of course, just because you've lucked out, you don't have permission to ignore your health. Continue the obvious: follow the basic Three-Week Cure steps and add some calcium for bone health (see Eight Ways to Prevent Osteoporosis, p. 133). Please also follow Step One: Lifestyle Changes on page 125.

- **GROUP B** Women in this group have mild to moderate symptoms that include occasional hot flashes and night sweats, with one or two nights a week of disturbed sleep. You may have some mild vaginal dryness or occasional mood/memory problems, but generally you're functioning and feeling well. If you see yourself here, follow the steps in the Three-Week Cure, in the Eight Ways to Prevent Osteoporosis, and also the suggestions in Step One: Lifestyle Changes. In addition, review Step Two: Nutritional Supplements (p. 126), and, based on your symptoms, begin taking one or more of the suggested supplements to address them. Although you may cruise through menopause using this combination of lifestyle changes and nutritional supplements, if your symptoms become more disruptive, be open to bioidentical HRT (p. 129).

- **GROUP C** has industrial-strength menopause from hell and requires something more. If you're in this group, your symptoms are everything just described with the volume turned up: you can't count the number of hot flashes during the day and you have nightly drenching sweats. You can't remember the last time you slept solidly and woke up refreshed. The word exhausted was invented for you. Depressed? Libido? Don't ask. Clear thinking? You draw blanks on the names of dear friends and your computer is covered with sticky tags.

   For you, an extra-strength Triple Whammy Cure Plus is in order. Using a combination of lifestyle changes, bioidentical hormones, and, only rarely, some additional prescription medication, you should be feeling dramatically better in two to three weeks.

   Here's the action plan for Group C:

   1. Continue following recommendations in the Three-Week Cure (p. 45) and Eight Ways to Prevent Osteoporosis on page 133.
   2. Read and begin Step One: Lifestyle Changes, below.
   3. SKIP Step Two: Nutritional Supplements.
   4. GO DIRECTLY to Step Three: HRT, the Facts, and My Advice (p. 127), and also read step four.

   Remember, neither HRT nor any recommended medication is permanent. I advise my patients on this plan to reduce their doses periodically just to see if the hormonal landscape has changed. Some day, believe me, the tumultuous ride of menopause will be over and you'll be very much alive. Your exhaustion due to poor sleep should dramatically improve once you calm your night sweats, but please also review the Sleep Problems healing path that begins on page 170.

STEP ONE: LIFESTYLE CHANGES

- **CHANGE YOUR DIET** to keep hot flashes at bay. Increase your intake of phytoestrogens (see Adding Soy, Phytoestrogens, p. 263), which are found in soy and have estrogen-like effects. You might get enough estrogen effect from phytoestrogens to eliminate your hot flashes. My wife avoids hot flashes with a daily large soy latte from one of the major coffee chains, but you can also make these easily yourself with coffee and soy milk. Phytoestrogens can also protect you from estrogen-stimulated cancers. If you've had breast cancer in the past and were warned about the dangers of pharmaceutical estrogen, you might receive some protective benefit from phytoestrogens. And while you're paying attention to your eating habits, get rid of the junk food and eat more dark greens for their calcium and numerous other benefits. Read the Triple Whammy Food Plan (p. 245) and start following the basics of healthful eating.

- **EXERCISE REGULARLY** for all the expected advantages. Start with your twenty-minute daily brisk walk, which not only raises your serotonin but gets your metabolism cooking at a higher rate for the day. Weight-bearing aerobic exercise (jumping rope, alternating walking and running, dancing!) strengthens your bones and improves cardiovascular fitness. Unless you're 100 pounds or more overweight, I recommend exercise instead of dieting (see Weight Loss Agonies, p. 188). During the menopause transition, a little extra weight will keep your bones healthier (see Eight Ways to Prevent Osteoporosis, p. 133) and your estrogen levels higher than those of thin women. Muscle weighs more than fat, so start with your daily walk and then expand your exercise program.

- **PRACTICE STRESS REDUCTION** every day to reduce the number and severity of hot flashes. Keep in mind that your serotonin is low because your estrogen is declining. Stress, our Whammy #1, can be quite destructive without your serotonin buffer. To prevent hot flashes, perform the Breathing Out Stress exercise (p. 217) for ten minutes twice a day. If you're in an acceptable location during your hot flash, taking a few slow deep breaths will shorten its duration. Read Chapter 20 on stress (p. 197) and sample some of its suggestions for managing stress. It will make a real difference in your symptoms.

STEP TWO: NUTRITIONAL SUPPLEMENTS

With the WHI studies scaring the bejeesus out of many women, conventional medicine is finally taking a serious look at herbal remedies.

- **BLACK COHOSH** has been in continuous use for hundreds of years. The first choice among European physicians for menopause, it has not impressed many American doctors, who tend to rely on pharmaceuticals. Solid clinical research studies have shown that this herb, which acts by increasing the efficiency of your remaining estrogen, relieves hot flashes better than a placebo. Remember that even though you're in menopause and having symptoms, this doesn't mean that you have zero estrogen; you just don't have enough. Black cohosh enhances estrogen just enough to get rid of hot flashes for many women. **DOSE:** 20 mg to 40 mg capsules (available as Remifemin), one or two capsules once or twice a day, either alone or in combination with chasteberry. Alternatively, take whole root freeze-dried black cohosh in 550 mg capsules, once or twice daily.

- **CHASTEBERRY** (p. 51), also called vitex, is used primarily to keep premenstrual symptoms in check, but European doctors add chasteberry to black cohosh as part of their herbal approach to hot flashes. Chasteberry acts on the pituitary gland, the "master gland," balancing your remaining levels of estrogen and progesterone. Because chasteberry affects hormone levels, you shouldn't use it if you're taking hormone replacement therapy or birth control pills (it can lessen their effectiveness), or if you're pregnant or nursing. **DOSE:** 175–225 mg once a day, alone or in combination with black cohosh.

- **DONG QUAI AND HERBAL MENOPAUSE COMBINATIONS** protect your body against stress. Dong quai, also known as female ginseng, by itself doesn't seem to be particularly effective against hot flashes. However, most herbal combinations for menopause are a blend of black cohosh, chasteberry, and dong quai with occasional additional "female" herbs included based mainly on their historical use or the clinical experience of the herbalist. From the reports of the many women in my practice, most of the menopause blends are similar and act equally well, so don't worry about how many milligrams of each herb are present in the product you select. Or, you can follow the keep-it-simple principle and stick with black cohosh. **DOSE:** Use dong quai in a menopause combination that also contains black cohosh and chasteberry

- **ST. JOHN'S WORT** (p. 20) will help ease the emotional turmoil that can accompany menopause by raising levels of Whammy #2: serotonin. In fact, the largest-selling herb in Europe (and available in the United States), called Remifemin, is a combination of black cohosh and St. John's wort. **DOSE:** 450 mg twice a day, taken with food to avoid upset stomach.

STEP THREE: HRT, THE FACTS, AND MY ADVICE

When you give serious thought to hormone replacement therapy, free from the panic of the headlines, it seems a sensible solution to menopausal symptoms. After all, we don't bat an eye about taking thyroid replacement hormone, and some diabetic people have used the hormone insulin since childhood, so what's the problem with taking sex hormones?

A small but vocal group of physicians believes the problem with HRT has a great deal to do with the source of the hormones themselves. Premarin, the most commonly prescribed estrogen, comes from the ovaries of a horse. It's not the same molecule as your human estrogen. If you're going to restore your levels of sex hormones, you need to use hormones that are identical to your own—hence the term bioidentical hormones. These are also called "natural" hormones, since they are derived from plants such as soybean and wild yam, but bioidentical is really a more exact description.

How, you may ask, are yam/soybean hormones any more identical to mine than horse hormones? The utterly inedible wild yam contains the molecule diosgenin and the soybean contains beta sitosterol. Both can be can be converted in a laboratory to molecules identical to human estrogen and progesterone. (Even though soybeans have some mild estrogenic properties of their own, the actual conversion of yam or soybean to bioidentical hormone must be done in a lab.)

Let's return to the type of hormones used in the WHI study. For the study, researchers used Prempro, a combination of Premarin (conjugated equine estrogens) and medroxyprogesterone (a synthetic progesterone). Note that Premarin contains conjugated *equine* estrogens. For a pharmaceutical company to use the word "equine" instead of "horse" reminded me of how circus owner P. T. Barnum got everyone out of his circus tent with the alluring sign "This Way to the Egress," which sounded like some exotic animal. The unsuspecting who didn't know that egress is another word for exit were unceremoniously ushered out of the show. So, if you didn't know "equine" meant "horse," don't feel bad. It was planned deliberately by the pharmaceutical industry to keep you in the dark about where your Premarin was coming from.

PREMARIN AND THE TORTURE OF HORSES

To the surprise of many women, Premarin stands for PREgnant MARe urINe, and there's probably no product manufactured on Earth involving greater cruelty to animals. Animal rights activists have been petitioning its manufacturer to come up with something more humane for years. But why should they bother to curtail the cruelty? Until sales plummeted in the wake of the WHI study, profits from Premarin were in the billions. Here's how they make Premarin. If you have a weak stomach, definitely skip the two paragraphs that follow:

At the very peak of Premarin use, approximately 100,000 mares were confined to narrow stalls for their adult lives. (With declining sales, this number has dropped.) The mares are artificially impregnated and a tube is inserted into their bladders to collect their urine. The estrogen levels of all mammals increase during pregnancy. In order to get the greatest concentration of urinary estrogen, the mare is perpetually deprived of adequate water and kept in a constant state of dehydration.

The company itself would not reveal what happened to the colts but the animal rights activists investigated this and discovered that the colts were slaughtered and the meat shipped to Europe and Japan, where it's considered a delicacy. The fillies were saved for future Premarin production and the aged mares were slaughtered for dog food. Most of the Premarin farms are up in Canada. A mare is re-impregnated until she simply dies from exhaustion. In the fifty-eight years of Premarin manufacture, approximately one million horses have been slaughtered. Recently, when Premarin sales plummeted, tens of thousands of mares were slaughtered as well. (Interestingly, Reiki practitioners and others who work with energy say they can sense negative energy in each tablet of Premarin.)

WHY HORSE ESTROGEN IS WRONG

Here's why horse estrogen isn't right for you. Human female estrogen consists of three separate molecules: estrone (10–20 percent), estradiol (10–20 percent), and estriol (60–80 percent). Premarin, on the other hand, is mainly estrone (75 percent) and equilin (25 percent), the latter found only in horses. Although Premarin may act like a replacement for human estrogen, just the fact that the estrone content is three times that found in women means the match is far from perfect. And of course equilin is a totally foreign molecule altogether.

BIOIDENTICAL HORMONES

Because human molecules cannot be patented, there's little incentive on the part of the pharmaceutical industry to spend funds on research. And in the absence of clinical studies, using bioidentical hormones is based more on common sense and faith rather than hard evidence. For this reason, without the blessing of the Food and Drug Administration, and being pathologically skittish of potential malpractice suits, a majority of conventional physicians remain reluctant to prescribe them.

We know for certain that bioidentical hormones effectively relieve menopause symptoms. What we don't know for certain is how effective they are when it comes to preventing osteoporosis. Logically, they should work just as efficiently as Premarin and other replacement hormones, but they haven't been tested for this.

Doctors who prescribe bioidentical hormones can be located through the compounding pharmacies that fill the prescriptions. Both College Pharmacy (www.collegepharmacy.com) and Women's International Pharmacy (www.womensinternational.com) offer a free "Find a Physician" service online. The physician you choose may recommend "Tri-Est" (consisting of all three estrogens) or "Bi-Est" (which doesn't include the weakest one, estrone) in addition to progesterone. Some will suggest you cycle the hormones, taking them three weeks out of every month. Others will suggest you take them daily.

An even more exact cycling would be Bi-Est during the first two weeks of a month, Bi-Est plus progesterone during the third week, and nothing during the fourth week, although I think this makes something simple into something unnecessarily complicated. The amount of hormone per capsule can be adjusted based on your symptoms. Doctors sometimes also add a small amount of the male hormone testosterone to each capsule. This can enhance the effect of the estrogen (without needing to increase the amount of estrogen) and can bolster a faltering libido if this is among your symptoms.

A typical prescription reads: "Estriol 1 mg/Estradiol 0.125mg/Micronized oral progesterone 40 mg/Testosterone 1.25 mg." Another way to write this is: "Bi. Est 1.125/MOP 40 mg/Test. 1.25 mg." Now, since all this is placed into a single capsule, you can see why they're called compounding pharmacies. Your local chain store pharmacy simply doesn't want to bother with the work it requires. (Believe me, I've asked.)

Bioidentical hormones are available from compounding pharmacies throughout the United States, and are mailed to you after they receive the telephone order or written prescription from your doctor. Because bioidentical hormones are sold by prescription, they're eligible for insurance reimbursement from your health plan. You mail them a paid receipt, though you might have to rattle their cages a bit in order to receive your payment.

The "official" risks of bioidentical hormones are the same as drugs like Premarin—that is, gallstones, increased susceptibility to blood clots, and stimulation of existing estrogen-sensitive breast cancers. But we who work with bioidentical hormones virtually never see these problems, probably because the hormone exposure is lower and the product is matching exactly what you already have in your body.

Since I am not wildly impressed by the WHI conclusions, I don't recommend that you stop using HRT if your symptoms are being controlled, but rather that you talk to your doctor about switching to a bioidentical hormone formulation. On the other hand, if you've been using HRT of any kind for a year or two, it's worth stopping the hormones for a month or so to see if your menopause symptoms are still present. You can always get a prescription for bioidenticals and get your symptoms back under control. Ultimately, the choice of taking any HRT is yours. Most women don't need HRT after five years, but some plan to take bioidentical hormones for life.

IF YOU'VE HAD A HYSTERECTOMY

Women who have had a total hysterectomy (both uterus and ovaries removed) need immediate replacement of their hormones. Otherwise, most will feel pretty crummy from being plummeted into instant menopause. My suggestion is to replace exactly what has been surgically removed—both estrogen and progesterone. Understand that most physicians will say that you really don't *need* progesterone along with the estrogen because you don't have to worry about cancer of the uterus. But really, these hormones have widespread effects in the body, and you should restore what's been eliminated. I suggest bioidentical estrogen and progesterone, perhaps with a dollop of testosterone if you're concerned about sex drive.

MEASURING HORMONE LEVELS

Women frequently ask me if they should have their hormone levels measured before starting therapy. I've never found this particularly helpful because hormone levels are constantly changing. As a side note, the tests are very expensive and often not covered by health insurance. I would base your initial prescription mainly on the intensity of your symptoms, starting with the lowest dose I believe would be effective (the one suggested just above). Later, your dose can be adjusted upward according to your needs.

STEP FOUR: MEDICATION

Remember that whenever estrogen falls, as it does during perimenopause and menopause, it takes feel-good serotonin along with it to give you a Double Whammy. Until recently, researchers believed the rises and falls of estrogen correlated directly with serotonin, but now there is some evidence that the reverse is true as well—that increasing your levels of serotonin may enhance the effect (but not the actual blood levels) of your remaining estrogen. This may be helpful if you can't take estrogen (if you've had estrogen-sensitive breast cancer, for example), you choose not to take it, or you don't want to push your current estrogen dose any higher. A 2003 clinical study confirmed what doctors suspected for some time: that antidepressants, by raising serotonin, could dramatically reduce a woman's hot flashes. Although the study used Effexor-XR, other antidepressants work as well. Without having to take HRT, 60 percent of women with hot flashes got considerable relief.

ALTERNATIVE MEDICINE FOR MENOPAUSE

If you want nothing at all to do with HRT, follow the Three-Week Cure, the lifestyle changes in Step One, the nutritional supplements of Step Two, and the self-care remedies below. Many women feel considerably better by making these simple changes. The following alternative medical systems can also be helpful.

- **TRADITIONAL CHINESE MEDICINE** If you're still suffering hot flashes and night sweats, seek out a practitioner certified in TCM (p. 285). The combination of acupuncture and Chinese herbal formulations is extremely effective—and totally hormone free.

- **HOMEOPATHY** Although harder to find than practitioners of TCM, classically trained homeopaths (p. 277) can also provide good relief for menopausal symptoms.

SELF-CARE APPROACHES

I recommend you use one or more of these three self-care techniques with any of the remedies described earlier:

- **AROMATHERAPY** The most popular essential oil for hot flashes is clary sage. Use an aromatherapy (p. 210) diffuser in your home or just place a few drops in a handkerchief and inhale whenever you feel a hot flash coming on.

- **REFLEXOLOGY** Look at a reflexology (p. 223) foot chart and find the reproductive, pituitary, and adrenal gland points. At the onset of a hot flash, go for these points using the thumb-walk technique described on page 225. Do reflexology in the morning to prevent flashes during the day or at bedtime to prevent night sweats.

- **FLOWER ESSENCE THERAPY** (p. 220) Some women experience emotional upheavals during perimenopause and menopause. Consider walnut (life changes), scleranthus (mood swings), mustard (depression), and mimulus (fear of growing old).

EIGHT WAYS TO PREVENT OSTEOPOROSIS

You're already taking several of these steps by following the Three-Week Cure. The first six are for all women; add the last two if you're fifty or over.

1. TAKE A GOOD CALCIUM/MAGNESIUM/VITAMIN D SUPPLEMENT. Look for one that provides you with at least 1,500 mg of calcium, 750 mg of magnesium, and 400 I.U. of Vitamin D (which helps you absorb and retain calcium). I recommend OsteoPrime Forte (made by PhytoPharmica), two capsules twice a day if your diet contains other sources of calcium (dairy) and magnesium (green veggies). If your diet doesn't, or you're dealing with early osteoporosis, add Cal Apatite with Magnesium (Ethical Nutrients), one tablet twice a day. These are available online and at most health food stores.

2. DO REGULAR WEIGHT-BEARING EXERCISES like walking, dancing, lifting weights, or aerobics.

3. WALK IN THE SUNLIGHT to increase your Vitamin D.

4. STOP SMOKING—as if you need another reason.

5. LIMIT YOUR ALCOHOL to two drinks per day.

6. EAT CALCIUM-RICH FOODS like low-fat dairy foods (skim milk, low-fat yogurt), broccoli, almonds, dark leafy greens, and canned salmon and sardines.

7. GET THIS QUICK AND PAINLESS TEST. Ask your doctor to write you a prescription for a bone density test after you reach age fifty. Repeat the test every three to five years depending on your doctor's recommendation.

8. IF OSTEOPOROSIS RUNS IN YOUR FAMILY, talk to your doctor about the results of your bone density test and ask her about bone-building medications like Fosamax or Evista.

MENOPAUSE TRANSITION

*When it comes to menopause, many women know
a whole lot more than their doctors.*

Leslie was a new patient who had driven down to my Chicago office from the suburbs. She began by telling me that several years earlier she'd been looking forward to menopause, her periods having long since worn out their welcome. In her teens and early twenties, her period was accompanied by severe exhaustion and breathtakingly painful menstrual cramps. When she read in college about menstrual huts, where women congregate during their periods, she wanted one of her own, preferably in Tahiti.

After four children, her cramps had eased up, but her PMS, which had begun as a mild single-day event, increased over the years into a two-week epic. Now, turning fifty, Leslie knew the end of all this was on the horizon. Her periods had become irregular, she'd read several books about what to expect, and she was ready to spend several cramp-less, PMS-less decades as one of the wise women in her suburban development.

But within a month of her birthday, things changed. Her first hot flash had arrived innocently enough ("Honey, you're turning red"), but she was puzzled. After all, she was still having some periods, so this couldn't be the start of menopause. But, sure enough, these were hot flashes and, looking in the mirror, she saw beads of sweat across her brightly flushed Irish skin. Then she started waking up at night drenched in sweat, blankets askew, sleep shot to hell. Her husband complained it was like sleeping with a space heater and was not happy with the bedroom window open wide in the middle of a Chicago December. She also started feeling tired during the day, definitely grumpy, and, to her utter horror, increasingly forgetful and absent-minded. "I was getting so scatterbrained," she said. "Maybe the PMS wasn't so bad after all."

At least her periods were down to an irregular trickle. Her gynecologist agreed that she was in perimenopause and tore off a preprinted prescription for the hormone replacement Prempro. (This was a year before the Women's Health Initiative Study was released, terrifying many women into believing that hormone replacement was a prescription for breast cancer.) Within a month of starting the hormones, Leslie felt almost normal. No hot flashes or night sweats, better sleep, mood and energy good. She even could remember the names of all her grandchildren—"no small feat for an Irish Catholic," she told me.

But when she read about the hormone study, Leslie checked and rechecked her breasts for lumps and, joining millions of women, tossed her hormones into the john and braced herself. She was back to square one in three weeks.

At that point, she decided she was going to try some of that natural stuff she'd read about. She started her day with soy milk on her cereal and grimly set about learning to cook with tofu. She bought a family-sized bottle of black cohosh at the warehouse club, some "menopause vitamins," a jar of progesterone cream, and crossed her fingers. Within a month, she felt a tad better. Her hot flashes had dropped from twenty a day to only a dozen, and she was even sleeping some nights. Her brain still felt like oatmeal and she said she had the sex drive of a cold potato.

When Leslie was done with her story, I told her I thought she'd been doing an admirable job on her own, despite the fact that she still felt pretty awful. I then took a deep breath and started my explanation of bioidentical hormones. This proved unnecessary. She'd already read a book about them and was way ahead of me. Her own gynecologist didn't prescribe them, and that was precisely the reason for her visit.

"Are you going to measure my hormone levels?" she asked. I told her I thought we could safely assume they'd be low, given her symptoms.

"Good. I didn't want to wait anyway. Now does your compounding pharmacy use FedEx? I want these overnight."

Well, that was a short visit, I thought to myself.

Off the herbs, and on the bioidenticals, Leslie's symptoms improved substantially, but after two months, she still wasn't out of the woods. She was convinced now that she had the worst menopause in North America. None of her friends was anywhere near as miserable. She felt depressed, irritable, and just plain dumb at times. And she was still having enough night sweats to disturb her sleep twice a week, and some hot flashes every day. Back in my office, she was angry with the menopause gods and asked me if I had any other ideas.

It was my cue to suggest a small dose of a prescription antidepressant to raise her serotonin levels. Normally I'd recommend St. John's wort and 5HTP first, but Leslie needed help fast. I was about to launch into my serotonin-estrogen lecture (estrogen low at menopause = low serotonin) when she stopped me with a wave of her hand. "Oh, I read about depression in menopause already."

I'll tell you, when it comes to menopause, many women know a whole lot more than their doctors.

She added, "Let's start with a small dose. I've actually been feeling very depressed with all this."

Finally—finally!—Leslie had landed on the right combination. Her bioidentical hormones reduced the hot flashes and restored some of her sex drive. The antidepressant erased the last of the flashes, eliminated the night sweats altogether, improved her mood, and returned her brain to full function. She had had one definitely rocky menopause transition.

A lot of women have some really rough going during perimenopause and menopause, but eventually just about everyone gets the right combination of therapies and things settle down. Over the next few years, we'd be monitoring Leslie's symptoms, checking her breasts regularly, and slowly reducing the doses of everything she was taking. After all, you're not in the menopause transition forever.

As Leslie left the office, I heard my assistant laughing as Leslie relayed what her husband had said the night before: "Now that you're feeling better, can we ease up on the tofu?"

12.

MIGRAINE HEADACHES

The exact cause of migraine headaches isn't known, but when you start listing who gets them, and under what circumstances, you can begin to appreciate how migraines are a typical Triple Whammy disorder. The source of migraine pain seems to be chemicals of inflammation released in the brain when something triggers a tiny brain artery to go into a spasm. Migraines run in families, especially among the women, and most women who have migraines report a high frequency of other Triple Whammy disorders among their female relatives.

Like all Triple Whammy disorders, migraine is related to low levels of serotonin, our Whammy #2. Part of conventional medicine's treatment involves manipulating serotonin levels. And since low levels of serotonin increase your susceptibility to stress, it follows that stress—Whammy #1—tops the list of migraine triggers. If you list the most common migraine triggers—insufficient sleep, exposure to bright lights, certain odors, caffeine withdrawal, some foods, changes in blood sugar levels, and sudden changes in barometric pressure—you can see they're circumstances your body regards as stressors.

If you have premenstrual migraines or migraines triggered by birth control pills you know that Whammy #3, your hormones, is a pretty potent trigger. Birth control pills contain a combination of estrogen with a synthetic progesterone. Although you might think the estrogen in the pills would keep up serotonin

FIRST, LET'S BE SURE IT'S MIGRAINE

People endlessly confuse the different kinds of headaches, mistakenly calling their sinus headaches "migraines" or their tension headaches "sinus headaches."

TENSION HEADACHES, also called muscle contraction headaches, are by far the most common cause of head pain. These are extracranial, meaning that all the mischief is taking place outside of the skull (extra = outside, cranial = skull), rather than in your brain or sinus cavities. The muscles covering your skull start in the back of your neck, spread like a cap over the top of your head, and attach to your skull in a band above your eyebrows. If your neck muscles start tightening up—a common response to stress—you'll feel discomfort ranging from tightness in the back of your neck and shoulders to a dull ache and constant pain in your temples or in a band-like distribution across your forehead. Because women's low serotonin levels render them more physically susceptible to stress in general, you get far more tension headaches than men. Tension headaches can be triggered by the same things that bring on migraine: stress, hunger, visual strain, or fatigue. Unlike a migraine, a tension headache can be helped by massaging the back of your neck or shoulders, which loosens up the contracted muscles, and taking some aspirin or Tylenol.

SINUS HEADACHES affect men and women in equal numbers. Acute sinus infection almost always follows a bad cold, and the main symptoms are pain over your cheekbones and behind your eyebrows. Plus, you produce enough mucus to share with everyone. You're blowing your nose a lot, feeling all sorts of unpleasant drainage in the back of your throat, and coughing when you lie down. You generally need to see your doctor for some antibiotics if you want to clear this up. Remember, if there's no mucus, back-of-the-throat drainage, or nose blowing, the likelihood of your headache involving your sinuses is small. The irony is that some people take so-called sinus headache remedies, which are mainly aspirin-based or Tylenol-based. The aspirin relieves a tension headache, but the user then feels her diagnosis of sinus headache has been confirmed.

levels, in reality the progestin wins out over estrogen and some women taking birth control pills get depression as well as migraines. Many of my patients have migraines during their PMS days, when levels of estrogen start to decline, and during perimenopause for the same reason.

MIGRAINE SYMPTOMS

Migraine pain is typically described as "throbbing" and on "one side of the head," although admittedly neither of these is an absolute written in stone. Interestingly, the word migraine itself comes from the Greek *hemicrania,* meaning "one side of the skull." Migraines usually start as a one-sided throbbing pain but can spread over your entire head. Unlike tension headaches, they're sometimes accompanied by nausea, vomiting, and extreme sensitivity to light and noise.

Migraines may be preceded by visual symptoms called auras that can appear as flashing lights, wavy lines, blind spots, and even numbness or tingling on one side of your body. A few fortunate people, like me, have auras but no migraines; I get a few minutes of an internal light show that clears up on its own.

PATH TO A MIGRAINE

If you think about how the following order of events leads to migraine pain, you'll be able to follow how and why all the forms of migraine therapy operate:

A Stressor leads to . . .

B The stress response (also called the fight-or-flight response), which causes the release of stress hormones including adrenaline, commanding blood vessels throughout the body to dilate (open) or contract (close).

C Because of low levels of serotonin in the brain, one susceptible blood vessel in the brain starts to open and close, triggering migraine (and migraine aura) by . . .

D Releasing painful chemicals of inflammation and pain.

THE CONVENTIONAL APPROACH TO TREATMENT

Using the path to a migraine as a general guide, let's look at what conventional doctors recommend to stop it along the way:

A Reduce stress; avoid trigger foods (see p. 143) and situations.

B Use medications that actually block the effect of the adrenalin released during the stress response at the site of the blood vessel itself. These include beta-blockers, such as propanolol and atenolol, and calcium channel blockers such as verapamil.

C Use medications (antidepressants) or nutritional supplements to raise serotonin.

D Use medications that calm brain wave activity (antiseizure drugs such as Topamax, Neurontin, Gabitril). Although the exact mechanism of action is unknown, this whole family of antiseizure medications seems to change the ways several neurotransmitters, including serotonin, act inside the brain.

STOPPING A MIGRAINE ONCE IT'S STARTED

If you aren't able to halt the migraine on its path to fruition, you're stuck with the headache. The tools conventional medicine uses to quell migraine pain include the following:

- For mild migraines, over-the-counter medicines such as aspirin, Aleve, or Tylenol can act in the area where the inflammatory chemicals are released and relieve pain.

- For more severe migraines, the family of drugs called triptans (including Imitrex, Amerge, Maxalt, Zomig, Frova, and Relpax) increase the effect of serotonin around the dilated blood vessel and allow it to contract, stopping the migraine.

- For extreme pain, stronger pain medications such as codeine and Demerol are given, usually in emergency rooms and acute care walk-in clinics.

Having a migraine can be very expensive. Although medications can be quite effective, they are also astonishingly pricey (Imitrex is $15 a pill; the migraine preventer Topamax is $12 a day) and burdened with side effects. If you're among the 45 million uninsured Americans and you have migraines, you should start following the Triple Whammy treatment below. And even if you can afford migraine drugs, wouldn't you rather place a few roadblocks on the migraine's path and prevent the headache altogether rather than treat the headache itself?

PREVENTING MIGRAINE USING THE TRIPLE WHAMMY APPROACH

You have a reasonably good chance of eliminating, or at least reducing, the number of migraines you get by making a full frontal assault on them, including reducing stress, changing your diet, using specific nutritional supplements, and adding herbs for PMS if you believe there is a hormonal component to your symptoms. Alternative medicine is helpful too. Start by spending some time on the following preventive maneuvers. Since stress triggers most migraines, let's start first with some ways to reduce it.

STRESS REDUCTION

- **EXAMINE YOUR LIFE CAREFULLY AND IDENTIFY YOUR SPECIFIC STRESS TRIGGERS.** Chapter 20, "Stress Less" (p. 197), contains lots of ideas to help you with this.

- **GET PLENTY OF SLEEP**—about the same amount every night. Don't build up a "sleep deficit" by burning the midnight oil and getting up early during the week and then sleeping very late on weekends.

- **BUILD SEROTONIN TO PROTECT YOU AGAINST STRESS** Start with the twenty-minute daily walk outdoors in the light and continue with all the other serotonin-boosting steps described in the Three-Week Cure (p. 45).

- **LISTEN TO GUIDED IMAGERY TAPES.** Belleruth Naparstek has an audio tape specifically for headache sufferers, and I recommend it highly.

- **PICK A PRACTICE FROM THE STRESS-RELIEF MENU** (p. 204). Learn meditation, self-hypnosis, or biofeedback; take classes in yoga or t'ai chi; try reflexology. Have a flower essence therapist make a remedy to match the difficult parts of your personality. (Oh, you don't have any? Sorry!)

DIETARY SUGGESTIONS

- **DON'T SKIP MEALS,** as this can cause swings in your blood sugar. The Triple Whammy Food Plan will help you think about food in a new way, with its focus on whole foods and high-quality carbohydrates that you eat throughout the day.

- **AVOID OBVIOUS FOOD TRIGGERS.** These are outlined on page 143.

- **TEST YOURSELF FOR HIDDEN FOOD SENSITIVITIES** using the Food Sensitivity Elimination Diet on page 109.

- **INCREASE YOUR SEROTONIN** This bears repeating. In addition to the fish oil you're taking as part of the Three-Week Cure, eat more oily fish (salmon, tuna, mackerel) to get more of the omega-3 oils that increase serotonin production. See page 254 for some precautions. The B complex included in the Three-Week Cure is also essential for your brain to produce more serotonin. Use carbo timing to help your body produce serotonin throughout the day (p. 263).

NUTRITIONAL SUPPLEMENTS

Because it's always easier to take pills than it is to make significant lifestyle changes, it's human nature to try the pills first, hoping you really don't have to bother with the hard parts. But Triple Whammy disorders, and most especially migraine, require that you do everything—stress reduction, diet changes, and taking supplements—in order to heal your headaches. So if you skipped those other parts, please review them now. For this essential step, schedule a trip to the health food store. Try the following sequence of migraine prevention programs (the dosages are given on pages 141–42), each for at least six weeks. If one program seems to give you partial relief, add a supplement from another. These supplements can all be safely combined without any adverse interactions. You're free to be creative here, and may end up doing a lot better than your doctor. Remember that these supplements are for prevention—not for treating a migraine-in-progress:

1. St. John's wort + 5HTP + Feverfew
2. Butterbur + Riboflavin
3. Co Q10

- **FEVERFEW** Good clinical studies have shown that feverfew, when taken regularly, can act as a reliable migraine preventive. Doctors think it works by permitting Whammy #2, the neurotransmitter serotonin, to operate more efficiently. **DOSE:** Take two 125 mg capsules (for a total of 250 mg) each morning with food to avoid stomach irritation. I can be very specific about what to buy. When several feverfew products were analyzed, most did not contain adequate amounts of the active parthenolide ingredient. Neurologists agreed that the freeze-dried form produced by Eclectic Institute was the best product.

- **BUTTERBUR (PETADOLEX)** is an herbal product that is showing some good clinical results in preventing migraines. Clinical studies conducted in Germany showed that when Petadolex was taken twice a day for four to six months, users experienced a substantial reduction in the number of migraines per month. After four to six months, you can stop taking it for a while because the effect seems to last for a few months afterward. **DOSE:** Take one capsule twice a day with food for migraine prevention.

- **RIBOFLAVIN** Some reports indicate that high doses (400 mg) of this B vitamin can reduce the number of migraines you have. Riboflavin will color your urine an eye-popping yellow, so don't be alarmed if you are dazzled by your toilet water. **DOSE:** Even though you're getting 100 mg of riboflavin in your Three-Week Cure B complex 100 regimen (p. 50), any excess is harmless. Take the extra 400 mg once a day with or without food.

- **5HTP** (5-hydroxytryptophan) This amino acid can increase levels of serotonin in your brain. You can find good research articles on the Internet from Europe and Australia about using 5HTP as a migraine preventive. Don't take 5HTP if you're taking an antidepressant (unless you're under the care of a physician familar with this supplement) because you'll actually end up making too much serotonin, which can produce side effects like nervousness and sleep disturbances. 5HTP and St. John's wort are an excellent combination for migraine prevention. **DOSE:** 100–150 mg at bedtime on an empty stomach to enhance absorption.

- **ST. JOHN'S WORT** This herb will help raise serotonin levels, but don't take it if you're already taking an antidepressant because it will cause your body to make too much serotonin, which can produce side effects like nervousness and sleep disturbances. St. John's wort and 5HTP are an excellent combination for migraine prevention. **DOSE:** 450 mg twice a day with food to prevent stomach irritation.

- **MAGNESIUM** People who have migraines seem to have lower levels of the mineral magnesium than the rest of the population. Naturopaths and nutritionally oriented physicians add magnesium to their migraine prevention regimen, though good control studies for magnesium are lacking. **DOSE:** 800 mg per day.

- **COENZYME Q10** Published studies show that high doses of this cellular energizer are effective in migraine prevention. The exact mechanism is unknown, but Co Q10 is very safe and side effects are minimal. **DOSE:** 100 mg three times a day.

HORMONE BALANCING

Most commonly, it's PMS that triggers a migraine, but the estrogen drop during perimenopause can, too. Migraines are also a side effect of birth control pills and some women can readily date their migraines to the month they went on the pill.

- **THE PMS CONNECTION** To find out if your migraines are occurring regularly before your period, track both your period and your migraines for a couple of months on a calendar. If you see a pattern of migraine symptoms in the days before your period, start taking the herb chasteberry either alone or in a PMS herbal combination. Because chasteberry affects hormone levels, you shouldn't use it if you're taking birth control pills (it can lessen their effectiveness) or if you're pregnant or nursing. If chasteberry fails to give you relief, try progesterone cream instead, as described in the PMS healing path on page 158. It's available at any health food store. You want a brand that contains real progesterone (like Progest-900) and not just wild yam. **DOSE FOR CHASTEBERRY:** 175–225 mg daily with food. **DOSE FOR PROGESTERONE CREAM:** one-quarter teaspoon twice a day (or one-half teaspoon daily), rubbed onto an area where your skin is naturally thinner (such as your inner arm or thigh) during the seven to ten days before your expected flow.

- **IN PERIMENOPAUSE** You want to use an herb that will support your declining hormone levels. Your best bet is black cohosh (p. 51). Some women enhance the effect of black cohosh by adding progesterone cream during the second half of each month. **DOSE FOR BLACK COHOSH:** 20–40 mg daily. **DOSE FOR PROGESTERONE CREAM:** one-half teaspoon daily during the last two weeks of every month, rubbed onto an area where your skin is naturally thinner (such as your inner arm or thigh).

- **EAT THE TRIPLE WHAMMY WAY** To even out the action of your hormones, read the Triple Whammy Food Plan (p. 245) and start adding more healthful choices to your diet.

ALTERNATIVE MEDICINE

As an alternative to conventional medicine's mostly pharmaceutical solution for migraine, explore one or more of these:

– **ACUPUNCTURE AND TRADITIONAL CHINESE MEDICINE (TCM)** I have witnessed acupuncture break an acute migraine headache in less than five minutes, and most well-trained licensed acupuncturists are quite good at this. A comprehensive TCM evaluation and treatment with Chinese herbs can help with migraine prevention. You can read more about both TCM and acupuncture on page 285.

– **HOMEOPATHY** A homeopath can provide excellent remedies for a migraine-in-progress, but generally these remedies work for migraines of the milder sort. Three common remedies sold in most health food stores are *Bryonia alba, Sanguinaria canadensis,* and Glononium. For migraine prevention, consider a more detailed classical evaluation by an experienced homeopathic physician (p. 277).

– **NATUROPATHY** In states that license naturopathic medicine (p. 281), these are the experts at using nutritional and herbal remedies for migraine treatment and prevention.

MIGRAINE FOOD TRIGGERS

If you have migraines, you've probably seen lists of food triggers. Common sense prevails here: if you eat something that regularly triggers a migraine, don't eat it anymore. Foods that can cause migraine include those containing chemicals that have a direct effect on blood vessels or neurotransmitter levels. Culprits include tyramine-containing foods (chocolate, aged cheese, red wine), nitrate-containing foods (bacon, hot dogs, cured meats), and certain food additives (aspartame, food dyes). Although sugar itself isn't known to cause migraines, some people are highly sensitive to changes in their blood sugar levels, and in these people hypoglycemia (low blood sugar) can trigger a migraine. You can avoid hypoglycemia by eating the Triple Whammy way. Some people are simply sensitive to certain food groups that really don't contain obvious migraine triggers. If you sense that food plays a role in your migraines, test yourself for hidden food sensitivities using the plan on page 109.

SELF-CARE REMEDIES TO CALM
A MIGRAINE-IN-PROGRESS

When you know a migraine is imminent . . .

- **DRINK A STRONG CUP OF COFFEE** This can be especially effective if you're not a regular coffee drinker.

- **LIE DOWN AND APPLY ICE** Keep a gel pack called Migraine Ice handy or use an ice bag, preferably in a dark room. Bright light aggravates pain, and darkness can be soothing.

- **TRY ACUPRESSURE** Apply pressure using the tips of your thumbs or other fingers to a pair of points elegantly named Gates of Consciousness (or GB 20 in Chinese medicine). They are located about two inches beneath the base of your skull on either side of an imaginary line down the back of your neck. Since you'll be pressing firmly for two-minute sessions, you'll probably be more comfortable sitting at a table with your elbows propped up. You can read more about acupressure on page 207.

- **USE ROSEMARY OIL** This massage oil, which is regularly mentioned in aromatherapy (p. 210) texts, can help calm a migraine. Prepare the oil by adding a few drops of rosemary to an ounce of a neutral carrier oil, like canola. Massage your neck and shoulders regularly with it. You can also incorporate rosemary oil into a hot bath stress-reliever: use a few drops of the oil in a hot bath and follow the instructions for a relaxing bath on page 211.

TRIPLE WHAMMY CASE STUDY

MIGRAINE

"Six migraines every month, each lasting two days."

Alex was telling me about her migraine headaches. I asked what she thought set them off. "Everything! Nothing! Stress always, foods, perfumes, PMS, changes in the weather, and then sometimes nothing at all."

Alex had tried numerous treatments. At one time or another she had downed virtually every prescription migraine medicine and had taken far too many painkillers for either of our liking.

Six migraines every month, each lasting two days, meant that almost half her month was shot. Alex was willing to try anything to stop her headaches. I explained to her that we had to try to see her headache problem in a more holistic way. When conventional doctors are confronted with a migraine patient, they consider new and different medications, in seemingly endless combinations. Although a pharmaceutical approach can help, if you fail to deal with the migraine triggers, you're missing the point. If you have a headache from banging your head against a wall, you can increase your aspirin dose, put a foam pad on the wall so it hurts a little less, or stop banging your head against the wall. I figured we'd try the last.

We began by reviewing a diet that not only eliminates the standard migraine triggers (including chocolate, red wine, and aged cheese), but also looks for hidden food sensitivities, such as dairy, corn, and wheat. The program totally eliminates foods containing certain chemicals, including sulfites and food dyes. It's described in detail in Dr. David Buchholz's excellent *Heal Your Headache: The 1-2-3 Program.* Dr. Buchholz and I agree that being on painkillers itself can be a migraine trigger.

From there, Alex used a calendar and notebook to track her headaches in relation to her periods and discovered the PMS component to be much stronger than she had thought. Her new migraine-prevention eating program (she followed the Triple Whammy Food Plan) pretty much eliminated junk food, and to that we added the supplements from the Three-Week Cure—chasteberry, B complex, and fish oil.

We then added four migraine-specific supplements: magnesium, the herb feverfew, the B vitamin riboflavin (more than was already in her B complex capsule), and the serotonin-booster 5HTP to improve her stress-buffering system against migraine triggers.

Alex was religious in following other steps from the Triple Whammy program: twenty minutes walking every day in the sun would increase her serotonin without the need for a prescription antidepressant. We also outlined a program of regular exercise. For stress reduction, she chose a guided imagery audio tape and agreed to work with an acupuncturist.

When I saw Alex again, things clearly had improved. "Not gone," she said, "but way better." Her two migraines (down from six) since I'd seen her had been milder, controllable with an ice-filled headache band. Alex showed me a diary of her symptoms. "Look . . . this one was a PMS migraine. Do you think that progesterone cream we talked about can help? And this headache in August? Just an hour after I accidentally put an artificial sweetener in my herbal tea."

She paused. "I think I'm beginning to understand this now. In the past, I left it up to the doctors to take care of everything. But like it or not, they're my headaches, and really it's up to me solve the puzzle."

13.

POSTPARTUM DEPRESSION

Postpartum depression is a Triple Whammy disorder that catches most women by surprise. You've finished nine months of feeling pretty great emotionally, even though during that last month you could safely say the novelty of pregnancy had worn out its welcome. You remember thinking, "I'm definitely ready to have this baby." You wrapped up your childbirth classes, prepared the nursery, and packed your bag. Finally, after some memorable hours in labor, you're presented with the most beautiful baby you've ever seen. Then, thanks to the economic priorities of your health insurance company, you're discharged from the hospital a little too soon. Weak and tired, but definitely happy, you and your partner head home.

BABY BLUES

Despite the joy of one of life's grandest experiences, a majority of women are vulnerable to a condition called the baby blues during their first three days at home with their infant. Based on surveys, between 50 and 80 percent of women feel very tearful, depressed, and edgy for between three days and a couple of weeks. Many have trouble sleeping even though they know they're exhausted. The baby blues are an emotional shift that is so common that now they're considered a normal physiological response after childbirth. My take is that the baby blues are usually a mild, temporary form of depression that usually resolves by itself without treatment. Later on we'll explore what triggers these common blues.

WHEN BABY BLUES GET WORSE

For an estimated 10 percent of women, however, the blues get worse. For some, what began as mild depression now shifts into something deeper. For others, the mild baby blues disappear for a couple of months, then return with a roar. Each of these is a form of postpartum depression, and each is characterized by the sense that you're sinking into an abyss of persistently joyless, negative thoughts, feeling utterly overwhelmed and inadequate, and obsessing that something is wrong with your baby (which maybe you caused) or that you actually might harm your baby.

Experts now consider postpartum depression the most common complication of childbirth, and they've lengthened its name to postpartum mood disorders, which include depression, anxiety, panic, and obsessive-compulsive disorder.

Before doctors had a better understanding of brain chemistry, the general attitude about depression developing after delivery perversely blamed the woman for her problems. In medical school, I actually remember being told that some narcissistic women so enjoyed being in the spotlight when they were pregnant that they became depressed once they delivered because they were no longer the center of attention and simply couldn't deal with the "boring" reality of having a

TRIPLE WHAMMY RECAP: POSTPARTUM DEPRESSION AND BABY BLUES

During the vulnerable weeks and months following delivery the stress, Whammy #1, can be intense. Exhausted by your delivery or C-section, anxious about breastfeeding, and sore from an episiotomy (or really sore from a C-section), you're trying to recuperate while knowing you're responsible for a new life. You're sleep-deprived, perhaps eating erratically, and often don't have a decent support system. Then, just when you need it most, your factory-installed buffer against stress, serotonin—Whammy #2—is pulled out from under you because estrogen is in post delivery free fall—hormonal Whammy #3. This Postpartum Depression healing path will show you how to get the whammies back in sync.

new baby at home. Can you imagine the pain of women who endured that male-dominated health care?

Doctors would later learn that postpartum emotional disorders were of course not a mother's fault, but instead were totally beyond her control, involving massive shifts in the feel-good neurotransmitter serotonin and also her hormones, Whammies #2 and #3. Stress, Whammy #1, need not be described further to any new mom.

WHAT WE KNOW NOW ABOUT POSTPARTUM MOOD DISORDERS

Virtually all women who get postpartum mood disorders have a previous history of some variation of one of the Triple Whammy disorders, including depression, anxiety, or PMS, some diagnosed, some not. Most have female family members with these as well. The intense relationship between serotonin and estrogen triggers most postpartum mood disorders. During pregnancy, your estrogen rises to the highest levels you'll ever experience in your life, and your serotonin rises right along with the estrogen, like the second car of a two-car roller coaster at the top of the tallest hill. In fact, most of my patients with Triple Whammy disorders who have been pregnant remark that they felt relief from them during pregnancy: their moods were more positive, downright cheerful and optimistic. Some report that fibromyalgia pain virtually melted away and migraine sufferers report a nine-month reprieve.

Then, within hours of delivery, levels of both estrogen and serotonin plummet. If you're breastfeeding, your estrogen will remain low, suppressed by other hormones needed for milk production. Only after breastfeeding ends and your periods return do your estrogen levels (and, of course, serotonin) begin to climb again.

The symptoms of postpartum mood disorders are understandably terrifying because they seem so inappropriate to the happy surroundings. New moms with postpartum depression endlessly ask themselves questions like "Why am I so sad? Why can't I stop crying? Why can't I sleep? Why am I so panicky when someone else is holding my baby? Why can't I get the thought out of my head that my baby will be kidnapped, or that I might hurt my baby? This is not like me. WHAT IS WRONG WITH ME?" Many affected women are afraid to tell anyone—even their physicians—about these thoughts, fearing that the so-called authorities will take the baby from them.

PREPARING FOR A GOOD OUTCOME

Depression after childbirth is the disorder most women have read about, but anxiety, panic, obsessive-compulsive disorder, and social anxiety disorder can also occur. If you had a problem with any of the Triple Whammy disorders before you became pregnant, you'll have a period of increased vulnerability when you get home from the hospital. Before you deliver, let your doctor and midwife know about your history. Although the odds are in your favor that everything will be fine, if you do get depressed, everyone will be poised to support you. Here are some steps you can take to prepare for a good outcome. Discuss them with your ob-gyn, too:

– **WHILE YOU'RE PREGNANT,** take especially good care of yourself. Follow the Three-Week Cure (p. 45) with two exceptions—*don't take any herbs during pregnancy* (including chasteberry and St. John's wort) and *don't use progesterone cream.* Otherwise, all the steps will be helpful, including the natural ways suggested to keep your serotonin levels as high as pregnancy can send them.

– **CREATE A SUPPORT SYSTEM,** the best you can arrange. If your family can help, terrific. Remember, even though your mother may not be familiar with the latest pregnancy book, she actually has more experience in all this than you do. I also advocate enlisting the aid of a doula, a woman who has professional training in caring for women and babies both before and after delivery. Doulas are human instruction manuals on how to operate your new baby, and they're not difficult to locate. Start by asking your obstetrician or midwife, or visit the DONA (Doulas of North America) website at www.dona.org.

– **AFTER YOU'RE HOME** with your baby, I can't overemphasize the importance of caring for yourself during the early, vulnerable weeks. Get outside in the daylight with your baby in a stroller (even in winter, I strongly recommend getting out, baby and you bundled up warmly). Since many health clubs now have infant and childcare facilities, take your little one along to your workouts. You'll meet other new moms, exchange information, and get some needed exercise. Happily, your baby will be there in the care center, probably blissfully asleep, after you've finished your class.

– **IF THE SPECTER OF DEPRESSION OR ANXIETY APPEARS,** or if your brain gets locked into unwelcome and obsessive thoughts, don't think twice about getting professional help—*remember, it's your hormones and your serotonin in a grand free fall.* It's not in your head, it's in your whole body. Your obstetrician is well-trained in diagnosing postpartum mood disorders; call her first. She may want to refer you to a psychiatrist for medication, and that's a fine idea. Don't worry if you have a postpartum mood disorder—ask for help.

"MEDICATIONS? BUT I'M NURSING . . ."

Most women with significant postpartum depression or other postpartum mood disorders need medication. The serotonin levels in your brain desperately need to be restored to get you out of this mess. And let's face it, you really want to stop crying and start enjoying your infant. If you need reassurance about antidepressants, I can unequivocally tell you:

– Antidepressants are not "uppers." They simply improve the feel-good neurotransmitter levels in your brain.

– Antidepressants are neither addicting nor habit forming. Many women who take them for postpartum depression discontinue them after a few months by tapering off use. Some women need the boost in neurotransmitters and stay on them. Read more about selective serotonin reuptake inhibitor (SSRI) antidepressants on page 19.

– Studies have shown that although some antidepressants, like Zoloft, do appear in breast milk, levels of the drug in nursing infants are barely detectable and quite harmless. There is no evidence of effect on any infant by a nursing mother using antidepressants, even though more women are being treated with them now than at any time in the past. If you need antidepressants, take them. You will not hurt your nursing baby. If despite these reassurances you don't want to take a drug while nursing but know you need help, you have to bottle feed your baby and take care of yourself by taking a drug you need.

ALTERNATIVE THERAPIES

For postpartum depression and other postpartum mood disorders, conventional medicine is your mainstay. Use the following alternative therapies only in conjunction with—never instead of—conventional medicine. If you have the baby blues, the less serious condition discussed earlier, all of these will be good for you.

– **AROMATHERAPY** For any kind of depression, the floral scents are beneficial. These include jasmine, rose, neroli, ylang-ylang, and melissa. While someone else cares for the baby, care for yourself by taking a luxurious bath (p. 211) with a few drops of oil. Or keep a handkerchief to which you've added several drops of scent; take a deep breath from it periodically throughout the day, and perhaps before breastfeeding, to relax. Your massage therapist can also make a massage oil with one of your preferred scents.

– **MASSAGE** (p. 236) kneads out stress and boosts your sense of well-being. Other types of bodywork therapy such as Reiki (p. 239) or reflexology (p. 223) also help. Your muscles can store memories, and as your therapist works to dislodge tension

BIPOLAR DISORDER AND POSTPARTUM DEPRESSION

Even though bipolar disorder (p. 85) is *not* a Triple Whammy disorder, during the weeks after giving birth, the brain of a woman with bipolar disorder is highly susceptible to shifting hormones and neurotransmitters, including serotonin. For some women, these shifts trigger such intense emotional swings that previously undiagnosed bipolar disorder may finally be correctly diagnosed and treated.

If you are a woman with bipolar disorder, the course of events following delivery is surprisingly predictable. Within a few days, you might enter what doctors call a hypomanic phase, feeling a tremendous surge of energy, eager to talk (and talk!) about the ease of delivery and your utter absence of fatigue ("I can't understand why some women feel tired!"). Then everything changes, and you start slipping into the darkness of depression.

A good psychiatrist will be able to help you see that you've probably been experiencing this pattern for years. You may have had episodes of sadness or even depression that never responded to antidepressants—because antidepressants don't work for bipolar disorder—followed by a sudden lifting of your mood and a sense of great energy and creativity. If you've just delivered your baby and this pattern sounds familiar, see your doctor right now and ask her for a referral to a psychiatrist.

you may feel tearful. It's all part of the release process; bodywork therapists are accustomed to it and can be most supportive.

- **FLOWER ESSENCE THERAPY** (p. 220) Homeopathic flower preparations are a safe, gentle choice for reducing emotional turmoil. For more than sixty years, mustard has been the flower essence used for depression. Wild rose can also be helpful.

- **GUIDED IMAGERY** My patients especially like the guided imagery (p. 214) recording on depression produced by psychologist Belleruth Naparstek. Listen to it before going to sleep, or after breast-feeding, and bring its wisdom into your world.

- **T'AI CHI OR YOGA** The gentle movements of t'ai chi (p. 228) and yoga (p. 230) can be powerful allies in overcoming depression. Yoga classes for new moms (and dads too) are available in some areas.

- **NUTRITION** Carbo timing (p. 263) is an essential part of keeping your serotonin levels high throughout the day. Just a small amount of high-quality carbohydrates at each meal and for snacks will lift your mood. Remember, too, that if you're breast-feeding you're eating for two, so make good choices for both of you.

Q & A: PREGNANCY

Q. I'm thirty-three and expecting my baby later this year. Is the Three-Week Cure safe for me to follow during pregnancy?

A. The Three-Week Cure is safe for use during pregnancy *without the herbs and progesterone cream.* You should not take any herbs, like chasteberry or St. John's wort, or use progesterone cream. Although there haven't been problems reported with these herbs, I generally take a cautious approach and urge my patients *not* to take supplements during pregnancy (that includes 5HTP, which is probably harmless, but we really don't know for sure), except for what your ob-gyn recommends. During pregnancy your estrogen rises, and along with it your serotonin, accounting for many of the positive emotions (or relief from chronic Triple Whammy disorders) many pregnant women feel. The remaining non-supplement steps in the Triple Whammy Cure can only benefit you and your baby. Blessings!

14

PREMENSTRUAL SYNDROME (PMS)

If you've read "The Whammies, Explained" (p. 5) you already understand the inextricable link between your hormones and the feel-good, stress-buffering brain chemical serotonin. You also know that all women have less serotonin than men. Women who have especially low levels of serotonin are more susceptible to PMS and, to make matters worse, serotonin usually drops even further right before your period.

Your serotonin and estrogen levels are linked like two cars on a roller coaster, estrogen the front car, pulling serotonin up (happy) and down (not so happy) depending on the particular day of your cycle. Let's do a quick review of your female hormones:

- Estrogen is the dominant hormone in the first half of your cycle, from the time your period stops until you ovulate about two weeks later. The estrogen roller-coaster car is high on the track, with serotonin right behind it, high (and happy) too.

- When you ovulate, your estrogen drops a bit, and your progesterone (another female hormone) rises, preparing your uterus to receive a fertilized egg. If fertilization doesn't occur, both progesterone and estrogen plummet. Levels of progesterone drop to signal the inside lining of your uterus to shed (your menstrual flow). And as estrogen drops, so does happiness-producing serotonin.

PMS SYMPTOMS: TRIPLE WHAMMY, EXTRA LOUD

As you read this list of symptoms, you might realize that despite all the definitions of PMS you've ever come across, the most inclusive definition is that PMS is the Triple Whammy with the volume turned up extra loud. In fact, there are about 150 different symptoms associated with PMS, many of which are a "PMS-worsening" of symptoms from a seemingly unrelated medical problem, which (you guessed it) reads like a list of Triple Whammy disorders.

For example, conditions such as fibromyalgia, migraine, herpes, irritable bowel, and even asthma or arthritis frequently escalate during PMS days. And if you sit down with a calendar and track your PMS symptoms, you might discover that a medical problem you'd been seeing a specialist for, such as hair loss, chronic hives, or sinusitis, has a major PMS component to it. I'm hoping you'll discover as you treat your PMS with the recommendations in this section that any symptom flare from other conditions calms down dramatically once your PMS symptoms are quelled.

PMS symptoms include breast tenderness, abdominal bloating, fatigue, muscle aches, headaches, fluid retention (hands, feet, face), food cravings (carbohydrates, chocolate, salt), irritable bowel (constipation, diarrhea), sleep disturbances, mood swings, depression, anxiety, and panic, irritability, unexpected anger and rage, poor concentration, reduced short-term memory, clumsiness, reduced sex drive, and crying spells.

Doctors generally agree that an imbalance between hormones causes one of the two aspects of PMS mischief. If, during the decline of both hormones that occurs just before your period, you have a little too much estrogen in proportion to progesterone, you can experience symptoms like headaches, breast tenderness, and fluid retention. The herb chasteberry is simply amazing for this; I believe it's the single most useful product available for PMS. Acting on your pituitary, chasteberry balances your hormones and relieves these estrogen-dominant PMS symptoms. There's nothing in conventional medicine that can work as well, with most women reporting dramatic relief after two to four monthly cycles. The dose for chasteberry is 175–225 mg, once a day, when you're not menstruating, before a meal to maximize absorption. Remember, though, that because chasteberry affects hormone levels, you shouldn't use it if you're taking hormone replacement therapy or birth control pills (it can lessen their effectiveness), or if you're pregnant or nursing.

The second aspect of PMS trouble is the mood swings, irritability, anger, and brain fog that can occur during the days before your period, when dropping levels of estrogen drag down serotonin. If your predominant symptoms are mainly related to mood, shore up your serotonin with the amino acid 5HTP (5 hydroxytryptophan), taking 100 mg before bedtime, and the herb St. John's wort, taking 450 mg twice a day with food. Use both during the two calendar weeks before your anticipated period.

You can see this estrogen-serotonin phenomenon in other aspects of your life: most of my patients are cheerier during the first half of their cycles, as estrogen and serotonin both rise. Most are also very happy during a (wanted) pregnancy, not only because there's a baby on the way but because estrogen levels peak during pregnancy and, in turn, serotonin levels are also at their highest. After delivery, estrogen and serotonin both go into a free fall, which is why postpartum depression (p. 146) can occur. If you have had PMS, be aware that after pregnancy you may be vulnerable to postpartum depression or baby blues.

For some women, PMS isn't confined to just a few days before menstrual flow; if you're in this group, you start noticing symptoms beginning midcycle (at ovulation) that steadily worsen until your period starts. Other women have what I call Twin Peaks PMS: a few days of PMS symptoms around ovulation (when estrogen and serotonin dip), then a week or so of relief, and then a return of symptoms just prior to their period. Still others have industrial-strength PMS. My patients with this version report only a few good days each month, usually the single week after their period ends. That means for three weeks of every month, month in and month out, they feel undeniably crappy.

MEDICALIZING PMS

With the knowledge that the emotional misery of PMS was linked with serotonin, the medical profession "medicalized" it. First it was renamed "late luteal premenstrual dysphoric disorder," or LLPMDD. (Renaming is an essential part of health care. Your health insurance will cover expensive therapies for "gastroesophageal reflux disorder," or GERD, but could balk if your doctor called it "heartburn.") Then a prescription drug magically appeared. The good folks at Eli Lilly and Co., perhaps unhappy that the patent had expired on their antidepressant Prozac, got permission from the Food and Drug Administration to market Prozac as "Sarafem, approved for LLPMDD." Now, most women aren't truly eager to take antidepressants, especially for a condition that may only exist a few days of every month. While I'm happy to prescribe antidepressants for women who truly need them, this isn't always the case if you have PMS.

I can't physically feel your misery, but believe me, I understand what causes it and also can offer you some very straightforward steps to resolving it. Let's see what the Triple Whammy Cure has to offer.

STEP 1: TREAT PMS ON YOUR OWN

You can probably manage most PMS problems on your own, using the steps you learned in Three-Week Cure (p. 45). Naturopathic and nutritionally oriented physicians may have been the first to figure out that unhealthy lifestyle choices contributed mightily to PMS. With that in mind, a few simple steps will go a long way. So rather than begin by covering conventional and alternative therapies, let's go right to what you can do for yourself.

CHANGE WHAT (AND HOW) YOU EAT

By and large, women with PMS have the eating habits of a country whose flag is emblazoned with a pair of interlocking doughnuts. It's a country of junky and highly processed food: refined carbohydrates and saturated fats, a "supersize me" land with too much fat, salt, sugar, alcohol, and caffeine. Also, a place where high-quality carbohydrates, including whole grains, fruits, and veggies, are on the endangered species list. Exiting this toxic land can work wonders on PMS symptoms.

- **READ THE TRIPLE WHAMMY FOOD PLAN** (p. 245) and start eating the Triple Whammy way. Your PMS symptoms will greatly diminish.

USE NUTRITIONAL SUPPLEMENTS AND HERBS

Yes, those look-alike bottles lining health food store shelves will work, if you know how to use them. Most physicians should learn something about them or listen to their patients about their results. Perfectly good clinical studies have been published in conventional medical journals about treating PMS with the following:

- **CHASTEBERRY (VITEX)** Chasteberry is by far the single most important health food store product for PMS. It will balance your sex hormones. Most women report dramatic relief of PMS after two or three monthly cycles. Nothing in all of conventional medicine has been found to work as well. If you're following the Three-Week Cure (and, yes, you should be) and you're already taking chasteberry, don't add any extra. Chasteberry takes time to work—two to four menstrual cycles—so stick with it. You shouldn't use chasteberry if you're taking hormone replacement therapy or birth control pills (it can lessen their effectiveness), or if you're pregnant or nursing. **DOSE:** 175–225 mg per day, before meals to maximize absorption, when not menstruating.

- **VITAMIN B$_6$ (PYRIDOXINE)** Prescribed for PMS since the 1940s, B$_6$ apparently works as a catalyst to increase the production of serotonin. **DOSE:** 100 mg per day. If you're following the Three-Week Cure you'll get this much B$_6$ in your daily B complex 100 tablet, you needn't take any extra.

- **ESSENTIAL FATTY ACIDS (EFAS)** These raise the body's level of a chemical called prostaglandin, which seems to be involved in PMS symptoms like breast tenderness, depression, bloating, and headaches. You need to increase your level of gamma-linoleic acid (GLA), one of the EFAs, and to do so the exquisitely named evening primrose oil works nicely. Borage oil and rapeseed oil, also GLAs, are more economical and produce the same result. Read the bottle carefully to calculate the number of capsules you need to take. **DOSE:** 1,000–1,300 mg of evening primrose oil three times a day (or two capsules in the morning and one in the evening) with meals to enhance absorption. This will supply 240–300 mg of gamma linoleic acid per day.

- **MAGNESIUM** For reasons that aren't clear, the amount of magnesium in the red blood cells of women with PMS is low, possibly a consequence of vegetable-free junk food eating. Taking magnesium (in addition to cleaning up your diet) reduces PMS symptoms for many women. Start taking it two weeks after your period ends and take it daily until your next period arrives. **DOSE:** Start with 400 mg per day, increasing to 800 mg per day after two months if you don't notice improvement. Higher doses may give you diarrhea.

- **CALCIUM** Calcium is important in PMS management, so you might look for a product that combines calcium with magnesium. The mechanism of action is not completely clear, but apparently adequate calcium is needed for hormone production and balance. **DOSE:** You need about 1,000 mg of calcium every day. You can get part of this in a product that combines calcium and magnesium and the rest from your diet (dairy, dark green leafy vegetables, canned salmon, sardines).

- **ST. JOHN'S WORT** Consider adding this herb if your PMS is characterized by mood swings, depression, and anxiety. This useful herb will raise your serotonin levels much like an antidepressant, but it's milder and virtually free of side effects. Read more about St. John's wort on page 20. **DOSE:** 450 mg St. John's wort twice a day with food to avoid stomach irritation. Use during the two calendar weeks before your anticipated period. If your PMS includes breast tenderness, bloating, and other physical symptoms along with mood symptoms, a combination of St. John's wort with chasteberry, B$_6$, calcium/magnesium, and evening primrose oil should cover everything. Give this at least three cycles before moving on to natural progesterone (see below).

- **5HTP** Try 5HTP for the same reasons described in St. John's wort, just above. **DOSE:** 100 mg before you go to sleep. Use during the two calendar weeks before your anticipated period.

- **GABA** The full name of this supplement is gamma-aminobutyric acid. It acts on the brain as a mild tranquilizer but won't make you drowsy and isn't habit forming. Take GABA on an as-needed basis when you feel a teeth-grinding tension or anxiety coursing through your body and you can't escape to meditate, do some breathing exercises, or practice your t'ai chi. **DOSE:** GABA 250–500 mg two or three times a day, as needed.

- **NATURAL PROGESTERONE CREAM** Read the St. John's wort description and dose information above before starting this cream. Because of the link between low levels of progesterone and PMS (see The Background on PMS, p. 160), using progesterone to alleviate PMS has become popular. It works for some women, and does absolutely nothing for others, but it's so safe that you can try it for a couple of months and see if your symptoms improve. The cream must contain actual progesterone—so-called bioidentical progesterone—and not just wild yam (read more about this on page 54). Despite advertising to the contrary, your body cannot convert wild yam to progesterone, so don't waste your money. **DOSE:** Look for a product containing about 400 mg per ounce of cream. Then try this schedule: start approximately ten days after your last day of flow, applying one-quarter teaspoon daily where your skin is naturally thinner, such as on your inner arm or inner thigh, and continue until your period starts. If your symptoms are especially severe, double the quantity during the seven days before your period.

BEGIN SELF-CARE REMEDIES

Remember, you're still on your own here. Just keep going and you'll soon be out of the PMS woods.

- **EXERCISE** Women who exercise regularly have far less PMS than women who don't. Start with the twenty-minute daily walk outdoors described on page 47, building up to thirty minutes a day after a couple weeks. Take your walk every day, rain or shine. Consider it your minimum daily requirement. If you do no other exercise you'll still have your walk; if you can work out more, so much the better.

- **STRESS REDUCTION** Surveys among PMS patients report that symptoms increase during periods of stress, Whammy #1. If, as you're reading this, you sense a connection between the stress in your life and your PMS, read Chapter 20 (p. 197) and follow the steps there. Maybe it's time to recheck the schedule for that yoga class you've been eyeing this past year.

STEP 2: TRY ALTERNATIVES

By now you know I like alternative therapies, but when it comes to PMS, please first try the recommendations in Step 1. If you're still having problems with PMS, consider:

- **NATUROPATHY** (p. 281) If your state licenses naturopaths, these are the folks to see. Some of the best clinical studies from around the world involve herbal and nutritional medicine, and naturopaths are the experts here.

- **ACUPUNCTURE** Practitioners of traditional Chinese medicine (TCM, p. 285) offer a combination of acupuncture and Chinese herbal formulas for PMS. Their success rate is very high and the results can be long-lasting.

- **HOMEOPATHY** Homeopathic treatment can provide long-lasting PMS relief. Read more about homeopathy on page 277.

STEP 3: SEE YOUR DOCTOR

It's probably time to see your doctor if your PMS simply isn't budging despite your best efforts with Steps 1 and 2. See her sooner if you're stuck with a symptom like depression that prevents you from getting started in the first place.

- **ANTIDEPRESSANTS** Sarafem and Zoloft are the only antidepressants with FDA approval specifically for PMS, though any of the others that raise serotonin will probably work just as well. My own preference lies with Lexapro, mainly because it seems to act faster and has fewer side effects. Since your PMS mood issues are only a few days a month, you can limit your antidepressant use from ovulation (two weeks after your period ends) to the start of your next period. **DOSE:** Because women with low serotonin are generally quite medication sensitive, ask your doctor if you can start with half a tablet (5 mg) of Lexapro rather than the standard 10 mg dose.

- **BIRTH CONTROL HORMONES** The hormones in oral contraceptives dominate your own hormonal shifts, masking them and, for many women, helping PMS symptoms considerably. To me, taking birth control pills as first-step therapy is pure doctor-think. I don't endorse taking powerful medications that have side

THE BACKGROUND ON PMS

An estimated 75 percent of women have some PMS, with about 10 percent having symptoms severe enough to be virtually disabling. As an internist, I think a lot more than 10 percent of women are having severe PMS problems. These surveys are usually conducted by gynecologists or psychiatrists, and the questions asked are strictly PMS-oriented (mood, bloating, breast tenderness, and the like). Read PMS Symptoms: Triple Whammy, Extra Loud (p. 154) and you'll see what I mean.

The attitude of the medical community toward PMS has improved over the past two decades, but most physicians are still a long way from winning major awards for compassion. The late gynecologist Katharina Dalton performed the first serious research into the possible causes of PMS, discovering that many women with PMS had lower-than-normal levels of progesterone during the second half of their cycles. As a result, many doctors, both conventional and alternative, prescribe various forms of this hormone to alleviate PMS. And while some women improve, many do not. Other doctors see a greater link between PMS and low levels of estrogen. According to this model, prescribing some form of estrogen during the second half of a woman's cycle will help a lot.

There are two problems with placing too much emphasis on one hormone or the other, however. First, when blood or saliva levels of women with significant PMS are measured, the results are inconsistent. Some women have low levels of estrogen, some of progesterone, and many women with PMS have perfectly normal levels of both hormones.

The other problem with emphasizing hormones as the wonder drugs for PMS is that most women I talk to really don't want to take them. Did you know, for example, that even before the Women's Health Study linking hormones to breast cancer was published, most women who had been prescribed Premarin had stopped it after about two years on their own, often not telling their doctor?

The bioidentical hormones recommended in this section are taken in extremely low doses when compared to those manufactured by the pharmaceutical industry; they're also, in my experience, remarkably free of side effects. I recommend the 1-2-3 steps in this PMS healing path. If nutritional supplements aren't helping after three months of use, my patients switch to progesterone cream. If the cream works, fine. If not, they can move on to natural progesterone (see Bioidentical Hormones, p. 160) and/or an SSRI antidepressant.

effects to manage a condition that most of you can treat successfully by your-selves. But if you've tried the self-care and alternative therapies and it feels as if you're getting nowhere, consider birth controll pills. They should contain both es-trogen and progesterone to duplicate the two hormones in your body. The brand Yasmin contains estrogen and drospirenone, a substance similar to natural pro-gesterone.

– **BIOIDENTICAL HORMONES** When dealing with PMS, nutritionally oriented physi-cians and naturopaths generally limit their hormone prescribing to natural proges-terone. It's natural not because the product comes from wild yam, but because the molecule is exactly the same as a woman's own progesterone. These bioidentical hormones are available from compounding pharmacies (p. 289), in a variety of forms (capsules, under-the-tongue pellets, creams, and even rectal suppositories), but they all require a prescription, unlike the lower-strength progesterone skin cream described on page 158. A typical prescription for "oral micronized natural progesterone" is for 300-mg capsules, taken once or twice a day from midcycle (two weeks before your period) to start of flow. Many conventional physicians are unfamiliar with these products and because of this won't write you the prescription. In this case, the compounding pharmacy itself will help: Contact one in your area, explain your situation, and the pharmacist will be happy to provide you with a list of doctors who will write the prescription in appropriate situations.

TRIPLE WHAMMY CASE STUDY

PMS

Here was the real Victoria speaking, not her illness.

I remember Victoria with special clarity because she scowled at me for our entire first hour together. Though my heart went out to her, my choicest puns and dazzling *bons mots* fell flat, and I had the terrible feeling that if I couldn't come up with a treatment plan, I'd end up like a male praying mantis, head neatly chewed off by the female.

Not that I hadn't been warned in advance. Victoria had scheduled an appoint-ment and canceled twice before she finally showed up. There was some ruckus at the front desk as she complained about "all this paperwork" and seemed to blame my staff because she had left her insurance card at home. Then, despite the no-cell-phone rule in our waiting room, she'd been calling various people at her job who apparently worked for her, making dire comments about their incompetence and threats about their job security.

I myself was running about fifteen minutes behind schedule and she let everyone know this, both my staff and other patients in the area. As Mary, my nurse, escorted her into the consulting room, she gave me the "Brace yourself, David. This one will be tough" look. Then she mouthed "lunch" and smiled, reminding me that no matter how the next hour might go, lunch followed. Even doctors need comfort food.

When confronted with a patient like Victoria, a teaching from medical school always flashes through my mind: "Remember, if a patient presents with any behavior that seems hostile, angry, or difficult, what you'll hear during your meeting is the illness speaking—not the patient. Get rid of the illness and most likely a pretty decent human being will be underneath."

Victoria had written "PMS!" "Terrible!" in large, dramatic letters across the front of her information form. She had just turned forty and responded to my birthday wishes with a snort. "Twenty years of PMS, and each year it's getting worse."

She was right about that. In her teens, Victoria's PMS was limited to a single "blue" day, followed by a few cramps and that was that. By the time she'd left college, she could anticipate her period a week in advance with fatigue, bloating, and breast tenderness. Her single blue day became three days during which she struggled to retain her patience and hold back surges of rage.

Her doctor's prescription for birth control pills made her breasts hurt and triggered premenstrual migraines, so she had given up on those after a couple of months. By the time she was in her mid-thirties, a successful but overworked executive, she had only ten days of every month when she felt remotely well: the last three days of her period, and the first week thereafter. Then the dark cloud of PMS crept across the sky and three weeks of every month were sheer misery. At midcycle, when she ovulated, she felt drained and cranky. Then, in the two weeks that followed, her personality swung from "on the verge of tears" at the least criticism of her work to snarling rage if one of her staff had failed an assignment. I was tempted to get the names of all the people who worked for her and send them our office brochure on stress reduction.

Victoria acknowledged a general neglect of her health. Her coffee-and-Krispy Kreme breakfast was followed by a desk lunch of order-in "whatever" or a sandwich in cellophane from the minimart in her building. Her concession to "good health" was a carton of fluffy whipped yogurt from the cafeteria a couple of times a week. Victoria told me defensively that she knew she'd been drinking too much red wine after work each evening to help calm her down. Chocolate, which she once simply enjoyed, had become a nightly tranquilizer for her.

I spent quite some time describing what was happening in her body. I drew her a chart of her hormones, indicating trouble spots with a bright red highlighter. Then I gave what my staff calls my serotonin spiel, detailing the relationship between her hormones and the stress-buffer serotonin, the highs and lows, the roller coaster effect.

Her only comment was a semisnarl: "Are you trying to put me on antidepressants—is that it? I'm not depressed, you know."

Bravely, I changed the subject. "I'm going to suggest a lot of things to get you back on track. Your hormones are out of balance, and we can use herbs like chasteberry and dong quai to help this. Your diet is contributing mightily to your misery and some new food choices can really do you a lot of good. You'll need to dust off your treadmill or reactivate your health club membership. And most important, you need to get your serotonin levels shored up. Victoria, you are a poster child for PMDD—premenstrual dysphoric disorder," I told her. "It might be easier to remember this as Industrial Strength PMS."

"How do I get my serotonin up?"

"Normally, I'd use an herb and nutritional supplement, but that might take six weeks or so to kick up your serotonin. Even then, there's no guarantee they'd work.

"What I suggest instead is a tiny dose—half a tablet"—and, taking a deep breath, I ventured the name of a medication. "Yes, Victoria, it is an antidepressant, but let's agree we're not treating you for depression—just trying to bolster your serotonin. If this family of medications were renamed serotonin modulators, you and a lot of other people might be more receptive to them."

I ended by giving her an article I had written on PMS, since I really wondered how much of our conversation she had absorbed. She left without a smile and didn't schedule a return visit. I figured I'd never see her again and went to a comforting lunch at the noodle place, feeling very drained myself.

Six weeks later, I was in my office and the phone rang. "Guess who's on the line?" my nurse, Mary, asked. I was clueless until she handed me the chart. I felt my muscles involuntarily tense.

Suddenly, over the phone, I heard Victoria, laughing. "Dr. Edelberg! It's gone! My PMS is totally gone. I haven't had time to schedule my next visit but now I'm set for Thursday. There was actually one single day—one day—when the antidepressant and the PMS herbs all decided to kick in and I felt my body relax, my bad mood vanish. Plus, I've been walking every day and lifting weights at the gym. Oh, and I'm eating better too. It was the most amazing experience [more laughter]. I just called to tell you and also to ask what kind of cookies your staff would like. They earned them."

And I thought again about that line from medical school: here was the real Victoria speaking, not her illness.

15.

SEASONAL AFFECTIVE DISORDER (SAD) AND WINTERTIME BLUES

Feeling gloomy during the winter months is incredibly common among women living in northern cities around the world. If you've got seasonal affective disorder (SAD) or the less-severe wintertime blues, your symptoms can range from a relatively mild case of the blues during the darker months to a seasonal period of major depression. In addition, you might notice you're sleeping a bit more than usual and craving carbohydrates, especially sweets. As a result, weight gain comes easily, which for many women only aggravates depression.

On the opposite extreme, a few months later, you might feel almost giddy come springtime. On the first bright Saturday of spring, I am convinced that the women of Chicago go a little bit crazy. It may be only 50 degrees, but out come the summer clothes. In any patch of city park sunlight, sunbathers spread their blankets and bask in the emerging light.

If you've read the background on the Triple Whammy, you know the cause of SAD is a big fat lack of serotonin, Whammy #2. In fact, SAD is a classic illustration of how essential your daily walk in the light is to maintaining your serotonin levels. It also explains why all those Chicago women are capturing rays when it's 50 degrees out.

When the first reports of what ultimately would be named SAD appeared some years ago, I began asking my patients with other Triple Whammy disorders: "So, what happens to your symptoms in winter—you know, when it gets darker outside?" The responses frequently were that they had a general worsening of everything.

All people, but women in particular, need sunlight. Unfortunately, as our society became more industrialized we moved indoors, away from the sun. A woman living in Manhattan in the winter will travel between her dimly lit apartment to her artificially lit office using the subway, spending the day almost completely out of natural light. Even women in the suburbs can live a house-to-car-to-school-to-shopping mall existence that keeps them out of the sun most of their days.

Since sunlight stimulates your brain to produce serotonin, the result of sunlight deprivation, predictably, is a drop in the level of serotonin in your brain. And, as you know if you've read Whammy #2: Serotonin, Powerful Stress Buffer (p. 12), the reason women have so much difficulty with SAD is that they start off life with less serotonin in their brains than men. Come the winter months, with dimmer daytime light and longer periods of darkness, the serotonin you shored up all summer goes into decline. To compensate, women with SAD crave carbohydrates, which are needed to produce serotonin in the brain (later we'll talk about how to use that to your advantage).

Also during the winter months, your levels of the sleep-inducing brain hormone melatonin increase in response to the dim days and lengthening darkness. Our brains are programmed to produce melatonin in response to the dark. It's the melatonin that helps us sleep when we're in any dark place, like our bedrooms at night or even in a darkened theater. But the wintertime rise in melatonin has no healthful effect except to make us feel like hibernating bears. Women with SAD respond by sleeping more hours, burning fewer calories.

WOMEN FROM THE NORTH COUNTRY

It's estimated that 10 to 15 percent of the world population is affected by SAD, and that 75 percent of those are women. If you add the milder wintertime blues version of SAD, these percentages increase significantly. As you'd expect, the numbers are higher in northern cities that receive fewer hours of daylight during the winter months. If you live in a bright place such as Phoenix, Key West, or sunny Spain, you're probably clueless about all this suffering. But woe to the susceptible among you who find yourselves moving north, especially in January. My practice is located in the Lincoln Park neighborhood, a popular spot for people transferring to Chicago. By March, virtually every sunbelt native is questioning the wisdom of her decision to move here.

TREATING SAD AND WINTERTIME BLUES

Like many Triple Whammy disorders, just knowing that your SAD and wintertime blues are real and the symptoms aren't imaginary will help you start treating it. Recognizing the biochemical underpinnings (low serotonin, high melatonin) can help you understand why you've just spooned out the last of your Ben and Jerry's and cried when you remembered the story of *The Pokey Little Puppy*. It's the same reason that although it's barely eight at night, you are s-o-o-o-o sleepy.

Strictly speaking, the diagnosis of SAD requires that your depression lift completely during sunnier months, but my patients tell me that it's really more a matter of degree. Many women with either a mild case of the winter blues or actual SAD, both of which may include wintertime sleepiness and overeating, usually don't feel just fine come summer. They may feel a lot better in sunlight, but in many cases their symptoms really don't completely resolve in June and July if their stress levels are high or their hormones are out of whack. All the summer sunlight manages to do is turn down the volume on other symptoms.

On the plus side, if life happens to be going especially well, then the summertime serotonin surge may bring about a burst of creative energy and the undeniably pleasant sense of total joy.

LIVE IN THE LIGHT

Since the whole SAD/wintertime blues condition is triggered by darkness, the answer is, of course, to live in the light. Getting sufficient exposure to sunlight, especially in the winter, can be quite challenging. Given the choice between taking an antidepressant or a one-hour walk when, sun or no sun, the wind-chill factor is stuck at twenty below zero, most people with SAD would shrug and head for the medicine cabinet. But there are alternatives to drugs.

PRACTICAL STEPS TO INCREASE LIGHT

First, since not every winter day is bitterly cold, just force yourself to spend some time outside during the day. Yes, even if it's chilly, as long as you see sunlight, try to get your face in it (your daily twenty-minute walk outside is a fine time to tip up your head). When you work out, exercise near a window in the direct sunlight. If you're joining a health club, look for one with floor-to-ceiling windows. In your home, keep your curtains pulled open wide. Trim the trees around your house to let in more sun. Rearrange your furniture so you sit in the light. Before renting or buying a place to live, consider the windows and their exposure: southern and western exposures provide the most light. Paint your walls light colors. If you're planning some major home improvements, scratch the idea of a finished (dark) basement and add some skylights instead. If you have a car with a sunroof let the light shine in on you through the glass in the winter months. Plan vacations in sunlit climates. Increase the wattage on all your light bulbs, your best bet being subcompact fluorescent bulbs, which are a little more expensive but seem to last forever (mine are into their eighth year). The technology of fluorescent lighting has improved a lot during the past few years. The newer models no longer have the hum, flicker, and unpleasant light characteristic of the old tubular ones. They also use only one fourth the energy of a standard bulb.

Both tubular and subcompact fluorescent light bulbs provide full-spectrum light, but whereas the tube bulbs require special fixtures, you can use the subcompacts in most ceiling fixtures and table lamps. Your goal is to surround yourself with between 5,000 and 10,000 lux (units of light)—much brighter than the typical light emitted from standard light bulbs. If you are serious about lighting up your home and workplace, you can buy a lux meter at most camera stores or online for about $50.

LIGHT BOXES

I think lifestyle changes are a lot more sensible than the light boxes being sold for SAD. Sitting in front of a light box is undeniably helpful, but there are really no good studies that show a dramatic difference between using a light box and making the sensible environmental changes suggested above. The light source in boxes comes from the subcompact fluorescent bulbs described above, with most boxes providing anywhere between 5,000 and 10,000 lux. The big problem with a light box is that you need to sit in front of the thing for at least an hour each day. If you know you'll make the commitment to do this, light boxes are a fine (if expensive) way to increase your exposure. But light boxes often end up as frequently used as that treadmill now doubling as your clothes rack (although if you're already on the Three-Week Cure, you're using that treadmill again).

Another light source being touted for SAD is the light visor, which you wear on your head. They're expensive, though practical because you can move around while getting your light, but again you need to find the time to wear one for an hour a day.

TRIPLE WHAMMY APPROACH

Unless you're suffering from a truly incapacitating seasonal depression, before turning to antidepressants I suggest you next try the following, with complete commitment, for a few weeks. Ideally, you'll already be in full swing with the Three-Week Cure before autumn arrives with its darkening days. So, in addition to lighting up your life, address:

WHAMMY #1: STRESS Examine the terrain and see if stressful events are contributing to your winter symptoms. You might realize that last winter's SAD symptoms were especially severe because you hadn't quite figured out how to solve certain problems in your life, such as job pressure or your daughter's problems at school. If you intuitively sense that stress is a part of your SAD, turn to Chapter 20 (p. 197) and follow the steps there.

WHAMMY #2: LOW SEROTONIN At the heart of SAD is low serotonin. The three natural ways to increase serotonin—walking outside every day for twenty minutes in the daytime, taking B complex 100 and fish oil, and carbo timing—are described in detail in the Three-Week Cure. If after three weeks of trying these steps (faithfully!), your symptoms haven't improved, review the healing path on Depression (p. 78) and consider adding St. John's wort or 5HTP, both of which are involved in maintaining healthy levels of serotonin.

WHAMMY #3: HORMONES Track your emotions along with your period through a couple of calendar months. If you notice an overall worsening in the week or so before your period, your hormones are taking your serotonin on a roller-coaster ride (for more on how estrogen and serotonin conspire to be less than a carnival, see page 17). Premenstrual aggravation of SAD is common. If you're aware of a hormonal shift in symptoms, read and follow the PMS healing path (p. 153).

ALTERNATIVE THERAPIES

These are most effective when used in conjunction with the Three-Week Cure lifestyle changes to increase serotonin.

- **TRADITIONAL CHINESE MEDICINE** (TCM, p. 285) TCM has a seasonal component that makes it effective for SAD. Practitioners of TCM acknowledge a seasonal orientation to their selection of herbal remedies, as if thousands of years ago the physicians of ancient China anticipated what we call SAD today. Acupuncture and Chinese herbal remedies can help your mild-to-moderate seasonal depression.

– **HOMEOPATHY** (p. 277) An experienced homeopath would select a remedy that takes into account your physical and emotional symptoms, with special emphasis on the seasonal nature of SAD.

– **FLOWER ESSENCE THERAPY** (p. 220) A flower essence therapist may select such remedies as honeysuckle, gorse, mustard, or sweet chestnut, all of which have energizing and antidepressant qualities.

– **BODYWORK THERAPIES** Massage (p. 236), Reiki (p. 239), and reflexology (p. 223) can be very helpful. By relaxing your tense muscles and allowing your *chi* to flow freely through your body, you'll feel substantially better after each session. You'll notice a cumulative effect if you visit the practitioner weekly.

– **AROMATHERAPY** (p. 210) Bergamot, jasmine, and melissa are the three oils most commonly selected for their ability to alleviate a dark mood. Add a few drops to a warm bath, or place them in a diffuser.

ANTIDEPRESSANTS AND SAD

Although there's a place for drug therapy, my sense is that most doctors reach for the prescription pad too quickly, recommending antidepressants as a first line of treatment. My hope is that you'll try the other suggestions in this healing path initially, but if you've decided that you need an antidepressant to resolve your SAD symptoms, I recommend trying a small dose of one of the selective serotonin reuptake inhibitors (SSRIs) like Lexapro or Zoloft, keeping in mind that many women are able to discontinue their antidepressant once the days get longer.

Lexapro has the distinct advantage of working fairly quickly, usually within a week or two, as opposed to others, which may take as long as a month. The standard starting dose—10 mg—is too high for many women because it triggers side effects, like headache and wooziness. Most pharmacies stock 5-mg tablets, which can be cut in half to produce 2.5-mg doses. Your doctor will probably give you a thumbs-up to starting low and gradually increasing to the standard 10-mg dose (if you need it) during the following few weeks. Because doctors only receive samples of the 10-mg size, many are unaware that the smaller size even exists. Lexapro recently received FDA approval for generalized anxiety disorder, so if there's an anxiety component to your symptoms, this may be an excellent choice for you.

Zoloft, too, is an excellent antidepressant. The smallest tablet, 25 mg, can be cut in half to start and then slowly increased if needed. Both Zoloft and Lexapro will also nicely treat any premenstrual mood swings.

16.

SLEEP PROBLEMS

If you've ever been up around 3 a.m., staring blankly at an infomercial while those you live with lie deeply asleep, it may have crossed your foggy mind that women have a harder time with insomnia than men. Maybe you're the sort of insomniac who just can't fall asleep. Or you awaken too early or you're such a light sleeper that you jolt awake at the slightest sound. Maybe the culprit is a menopausal night sweat. Whatever the cause, your lack of sleep makes you start your day feeling tired, maybe a bit depressed, mentally sluggish, and struggling to hold back the snarkiness.

The list of factors that can interfere with your sleep is long, but for women, leading the list are the three whammies themselves: stress, low serotonin, and hormone fluctuations. When I ask my patients with other Triple Whammy disorders about their sleep, they almost always respond with a variation of the word "terrible."

Of course, men are not immune to insomnia. They'll lie awake with the stress of job insecurities, their cholesterol levels, or the well-being of their kids, just like women. Other factors can interfere with refreshing sleep for both men and women: too much alcohol, certain medications, jet lag, changing job shifts, or illness such as heart or lung disease.

WHAMMY #1, THE LEADING CAUSE OF INSOMNIA

Stress because of low serotonin is by far the leading cause of insomnia. Many stress triggers are temporary events, and the insomnia disappears when the stress is resolved. Let's face it, eventually you did stop lying awake worrying about your wedding plans, your son's SAT scores, your late period.

If you've been a sound sleeper and your insomnia is caused by something temporary, you probably don't need medication. However, do consider starting a stress-reduction technique to cope with whatever's causing your stress. Read Chapter 20 on stress (p. 197). Also keep in mind that insomnia does have a nasty way of becoming a self-fulfilling prophecy. When you start worrying less about what's stressing you and more about whether or not you're going to fall asleep, you might be ready for some additional help.

SLEEP CHANGES IN PERIMENOPAUSE AND MENOPAUSE

Shifting sex hormones during perimenopause and menopause make uninterrupted sleep a remote memory for many women. It's one unpleasant stew: waves of hot flashes, drenching night sweats, and anger at the repeated interruption of a peaceful night's sleep. Some women going through the menopause transition (p. 120) experience interrupted sleep for just a few weeks, while for others it goes on for years. As one of my patients told me: "Night sweats interrupted my sleep like some sort of horror movie, coming back again and again. Every time I'd get back to sleep I'd come awake with that incredible heat washing over me." Keep reading for ideas that can help.

LONG-STANDING SLEEP PROBLEMS

Most of my patients who have longstanding problems with sleep have an underlying Triple Whammy condition, most often depression, anxiety, fibromyalgia, chronic fatigue syndrome, or menopause. Many psychiatrists say that virtually everyone suffering frequent insomnia has some component of depression or an anxiety disorder.

For treatment to be successful, you need to address both problems—not only your insomnia but the underlying condition triggering it. You might be telling your doctor about your difficulties with sleep and find her asking questions about depression. Minutes later, as you weepily describe your marriage problems, your unemployment, or your sick mom, your doctor might remark, "Sounds like you're depressed" and give you instead of a prescription for a few sleeping pills the phone number of a psychotherapist. This is good medicine. Talking to a therapist is very helpful if stress, anxiety, depression, or other issues are at the root of your insomnia. In fact, in the Stress-Relief Menu (p. 204), you'll see that we've included counseling as one of your stress-relief options. It's smart to talk through what ails you.

Some doctors prescribe an antidepressant or antianxiety medication rather than a sleeping pill, especially when they diagnose an underlying mood disorder causing insomnia. They'll recommend an antidepressant with a side effect of drowsiness, like Elavil or Trazodone, or an antianxiety medicine such as Klonopin or Xanax, thereby treating two conditions with one medication.

THE TRIPLE WHAMMY APPROACH TO A BLISSFUL NIGHT OF SLEEP

You can make some significant lifestyle changes, including your work on the three whammies, that will improve your sleep very quickly. Jump right now to page 176 and read about sleeping pill options—a good choice if you have one of the underlying Triple Whammy disorders and need to regain the balance of a restful night's sleep—but *first* I'd like you to explore the steps that follow. Many women with sleep problems end up at sleep clinics, and I have no issue with them, but if you're honest about starting and staying with these simple changes, you probably won't need an evaluation at a sleep clinic.

LIFESTYLE CHANGES

– **CAFFEINE** Eliminate as much caffeine as possible. Some people metabolize caffeine more slowly than others, with the result that a Starbucks or diet cola at noon can interfere with sleep ten hours later. Some over-the-counter medicines contain ingredients that can keep you awake. Painkillers designed for migraine frequently contain a dollop of caffeine, and cold medications contain the decongestant pseudoephedrine. Taken during the day, these meds are fine, but if you take either after 4 p.m. or so, you might be staring at the ceiling at two in the morning and wondering why. Read labels to check for these less-obvious sources.

- **ALCOHOL** Some people are sleep-sensitive to alcohol, which may relax you at first but ultimately reduces the quality of your sleep.

- **FOODS THAT RAISE BLOOD SUGAR** Eating refined carbohydrates, including bakery goods, white bread, and sugary foods, in the evening may awaken you at 1 a.m. with hypoglycemia (low blood sugar). Read about high-quality carbohydrates on page 266.

- **TOBACCO** If you smoke, a few hours after your last cigarette you'll pass through the nervous irritation of nicotine withdrawal. And this can awaken you. The solution isn't to get up and smoke in the middle of the night, but rather to quit. For help with that, read the healing path on page 177.

- **GET MOVING** Sedentary people don't sleep as well as active people. Regular exercise will boost your serotonin levels, relieve stress, and help you fall asleep at night. Start with the twenty-minute brisk daily walk outside described on page 47. Do it every day even if that's all you do, but seriously consider doing another type of exercise three or more days of the week. Exercise is the original side-effect-free sleeping aid.

- **SCHEDULE** Go to bed and wake up at the same time every day. If your job requires frequent shift changes, which can devastate sleep patterns in some people, get a note from your doctor requesting a regular schedule. If you can't get your shift changed, some studies have shown that melatonin, the sleep aid available in health food stores, can speed the ability of your body to adjust to time changes. See dose suggestions on page 174.

- **DON'T LOLL AROUND IN BED** Use your bed only for sleep and sex.

- **IF YOU AWAKEN** No matter what time of night it happens to be, if you wake up and don't feel sleepy, don't lie there and suffer. Get up, go to another room, and read something relaxing (not a newspaper!) or listen to some soft music until you feel sleepy again. Guided imagery (see p. 214) can also be helpful in getting you back to a relaxed state for sleep.

- **DAYTIME NAPPING** If you can schedule a daytime nap, it may provide you with an energy boost for evening activities. Be aware, though, that napping will likely reduce the number of hours you'll sleep at night. This is okay, because what's important is the total number of hours you sleep. The "correct" number of hours is the number you need to awaken easily, ideally without an alarm clock, and feel reasonably refreshed. Some people need only five or six hours; others need ten. Sleep specialists tell us to sleep at least seven hours in a twenty-four-hour period.

WHAMMY #1: REDUCE STRESS Remember, stress is the most common reason for sleep problems. Read Chapter 20, "Stress Less" (p. 197), and start identifying and coping with the inevitable stress in your life.

WHAMMY #2: BOOST SEROTONIN The natural methods of raising serotonin described in the Three-Week Cure will help improve your sleep because serotonin itself is the major chemical regulator of sleep in the brain. In the normal metabolic pathway, some of the serotonin not used as a neurotransmitter converts to melatonin, the sleep hormone. Once you're in a darkened room, the brain releases its store of melatonin and you fall asleep. However, if you don't have enough serotonin, you won't have enough melatonin.

WHAMMY #3: BALANCE HORMONES The two Triple Whammy disorders most closely tied to hormone imbalance are PMS and the menopause transition, and both can lead to impaired sleep. Balancing your hormones with a focus on preventing significant shifts in estrogen can help restore sound sleep.

NUTRITIONAL SUPPLEMENTS

I recommend that my patients try nutritional supplements *before* resorting to prescription sleep medications. Interestingly, although every one of these is extremely safe and not habit forming, each acts on the brain much like a prescription medication, only milder. If you're new to using something for sleep, you'll likely be sensitive to even the most mild of sedatives. Why go for knockout drops when something gentle will work just as well? Try one, or another, or use them in pairs.

- **5HTP (5-HYDROXYTRYPTOPHAN)** 5HTP converts to serotonin in the brain and is quite effective as a sleep aid without any trace of a morning hangover. However, *don't* take 5HTP if you're already using an SSRI antidepressant because you actually might make an excessive amount of serotonin, which, curiously enough, can then keep you awake. **DOSE:** 100–150 mg about 30 to 60 minutes before bedtime.

- **VALERIAN** The ancient Greeks referred to this herb as "pfui" because of its unpleasant odor. Valerian has been in continuous use for thousands of years as an effective treatment for sleep disorders and more than two hundred scientific studies attest to its value. **DOSE:** 800–900 mg at bedtime.

- **MELATONIN** The melatonin you can buy at health food stores is a pharmaceutical copy of the sleep hormone produced by the pineal gland, located deep within your brain. Melatonin is released in response to darkness, so taking it at bedtime will not only make you sleepy but will improve your "sleep architecture" and help you sleep soundly through the night as well. **DOSE:** 1–3 mg at bedtime.

ALTERNATIVE MEDICINE FOR BETTER SLEEP

A number of alternative therapies have worked well for my patients with troubled sleep. Over the years, though, I've been most impressed with traditional Chinese medicine and homeopathy, but others, like Reiki and reflexology, often work just as well. These are all completely safe, so there's no downside to seeing if they'll work for you.

- **TRADITIONAL CHINESE MEDICINE** (TCM, p. 285) Under the guidance of an experienced practitioner, you can obtain effective acupuncture and Chinese herbal formulations to treat chronic sleep disorders.

- **HOMEOPATHY** Long-standing sleep problems require an individualized constitutional remedy from an experienced homeopath. However, for temporary periods of insomnia, you can try the following remedies yourself: coffea, when you feel your mind is overactive and you feel restless; nux vomica, if you awaken between 2 and 4 a.m. and have problems returning to sleep; or pulsatilla, if you can't get comfortable under your blankets or because you're excessively sensitive to the temperature in your bedroom. You may be puzzled that "coffea" (which sounds suspiciously like coffee) is a remedy for insomia. If you turn to Homeopathy (p. 277) you'll learn that in homeopathic theory, substances that trigger symptoms will, when highly diluted, actually relieve those same symptoms. Try the remedies individually or in a good homeopathic combination remedy. If you're working with individual remedies, use 30C strength (a homeopathic term describing the degree to which the substance has been diluted) about one hour before going to bed.

SELF-CARE

You can use these self-care techniques with any of the other approaches to sleeplessness—alternative medicine, nutritional supplements, lifestyle changes, and prescription drugs.

- **AROMATHERAPY** Make a relaxing bedtime bath (p. 211) by adding a few drops of Roman chamomile, geranium, lavender, marjoram, or ylang-ylang. You can use a single oil or a combination.

- **FLOWER ESSENCE THERAPY** Read about flower essence therapy (p. 220) and try white chestnut if you have difficulty suppressing unwanted thoughts; scleranthus for indecision; or vervain to address emotional stress and an inability to relax.

- **GUIDED IMAGERY** The audio tapes "Perfect Sleep" (Deepak Chopra, M.D.) and "Healthful Sleep" (Belleruth Naparstek) are excellent. Read more about guided imagery (p. 214) and use your tape in bed with the lights off. Make sure you have a tape player that will turn off automatically, as you'll be too deeply asleep to do it yourself.

- **REFLEXOLOGY** Using a reflexology (p. 223) foot chart, work on the diaphragm, ovary, thyroid, and adrenal glands, the foot points associated with improving sleep.

SLEEPING PILLS

Sleep is so important for women that I readily recommend prescription sleeping medications after lifestyle changes, nutritional supplements, and self-care haven't helped. Medicines to help you get a decent night's sleep carry a bad reputation they no longer deserve. The older pills caused all sorts of problems that have now been eliminated. Gone are the next-day hangover feeling, addiction, and need for an ever-increasing dose to remain effective. Thankfully gone as well is the news-paper phrase "fatal overdose of sleeping pills." The new medications work quickly, effectively, and are extremely safe and rarely habit forming. Here's how to use them:

- **IF YOU HAVE DIFFICULTY FALLING ASLEEP,** try Ambien (zolpidem) 10 mg or Restoril (temazepam) 7.5 mg about thirty minutes before going to bed.

- **IF YOU AWAKEN IN THE MIDDLE OF THE NIGHT,** have a glass of water and one 10-mg Sonata (zaleplon) capsule on your bedside table. Sonata is quickly deacti-vated and cleared from your body by your hardworking liver so that if you take it at 3 a.m., you'll often awake on your own and refreshed at 7 a.m. without any hang-over effect.

Most people rarely need sleeping aids for longer than a few nights during a month, but if you have a chronic sleep problem that isn't helped by addressing the underlying cause, such as the Triple Whammy disorders mentioned earlier, you need some extra help. Although the FDA tries to discourage doctors from pre-scribing sleep medications for longer than three weeks, this thinking is based on the older, dangerous sleeping pills that aren't even available anymore. Studies from Europe have shown that people can use medications like Ambien, Restoril, or Sonata for up to two or three years without it losing effect and without the need for an increased dose.

- **FOR CHRONIC SLEEP PROBLEMS,** ask your doctor to prescribe Ambien 10 mg or Restoril 7.5 mg. Take the drug thirty minutes before going to bed for about one week or until you've restored a pattern of restful night sleeping.

AVOIDING REBOUND INSOMNIA

When you decide to stop using one of these medications after having taken them for weeks or months continuously, the usual effect is a night or two of what's called rebound insomnia, with some definite problems falling asleep. To avoid it, after stopping your prescription medication begin taking 800–900 mg of valerian at bedtime. Then taper off your valerian dose by 400 mg over the next few nights and, if you wish, stop the valerian completely.

17.

SMOKING

It shouldn't surprise you that addiction to cigarettes is one of the Triple Whammy disorders. After all, women who smoke aren't stupid. They're aware of the health dangers, yet they continue to light up because smoking relieves Whammy #1—stress—and its sister, anxiety.

Smoking is also related to Whammy #2, low serotonin. Smoking cigarettes calms you by quickly raising levels in your brain of feel-good neurotransmitters, including serotonin and dopamine. How quickly? Probably within three or four puffs. Of course, it's not the serotonin that gets you addicted, but the nicotine. This nasty chemical, as addictive as heroin, stimulates a part of the brain called the addiction center. Once activated, turning off this center becomes quite a challenge.

How challenging? I myself started smoking in medical school (we were actually allowed to smoke during hospital rounds, occasionally sharing cigarettes with our patients). I stopped smoking during my residency when I was in charge of a ward of emphysema patients, more than thirty years ago. As I write this, I'm asking myself, "Could I go for a smoke right now?" And the answer, which won't come as news to any ex-smoker, is "Absolutely." I can still remember the exact sensation of the first deep puff, thirty years later. Now *that's* a powerful effect on the brain.

I've not read any studies to confirm this observation, but women who smoke tell me they smoke more during their PMS days, when Whammy #3, hormones, comes into play. You would expect this: declining levels of estrogen and, as a consequence, declining serotonin need support during this time, and smoking delivers it. (Read more about the relationship between serotonin and estrogen on page 17.)

Because women start out with lower levels of serotonin than men, it's more difficult for women to give up cigarettes. It's been reported that the primary fear of women smokers is that they'll gain weight after quitting, and admittedly this is common. However, the weight gain is not caused simply by overeating to quell the need for something oral (if that were the case, you'd be delighted with celery sticks), but rather a craving for carbohydrates to shore up the now unsupported (and falling) levels of serotonin and other neurotransmitters.

MOTIVATION AND A PLAN TO QUIT

Doctors advise their patients never to stop taking antidepressant medications cold turkey because the brain has gotten used to the higher levels of neurotransmitters that these drugs deliver. Precisely the same logic applies to cigarette smoking. (You might reasonably ask: if your brain gets addicted to tobacco, does it get addicted to antidepressants? The answer is no, because antidepressants don't contain nicotine.) If you're motivated to stop smoking, you can do so in about thirty days, with some help from the Triple Whammy Cure. It's best to plan ahead, rather than impulsively throw your pack away, declaring as you do, "That's it, I'm stopping" (although if this works for you I'm all for it).

Talk to your doctor, your family, and a circle of friends about your intentions. Choose a calendar month and dedicate it to the end of your addiction. There's a heavy psychological component to smoking and you need to prepare yourself. Now's an excellent time to start following the Three-Week Cure (p. 45) if you haven't already begun. More on that below.

Based on what you've been reading so far about cigarette addiction, the plan is to:

- shore up and maintain the neurotransmitters, including serotonin, in your brain

- gradually reduce your daily intake of nicotine

- use a nicotine source other than cigarettes in order to appease the addiction center

Don't stop smoking during a period of stress. You'll only provide yourself with a ready justification for why you failed. On the other hand, don't use some pathetic stress like "the dry cleaning was late" as a reason to keep smoking. Tell everybody you're quitting and ask for their help. Support groups to help smokers quit are available in every community, often through hospitals. These groups can provide enormous personal support by bringing smokers together to discuss strategies and plan quit dates. They're also vital for many people during the follow-through period, when you may need to talk to another ex-smoker who fully recognizes the challenge of quitting. The groups also teach you how to manage powerful psychological cues—your morning coffee, cocktail hour, or missing your friends in the smoking lounge—that can set you back.

QUITTING

To begin, ask your doctor and pharmacist for two drugs that will ease your entry into nonsmoking:

1. **ZYBAN,** another name for the serotonin-boosting prescription antidepressant Wellbutrin, is the first. You'll start Zyban for about two weeks before you quit smoking and stay on it for about two months.

2. **YOUR REPLACEMENT NICOTINE SOURCE,** such as a nicotine patch, inhaler, nasal spray, or gum, will help reduce your cravings by providing a constant source of nicotine in your bloodstream so you don't feel withdrawal as dramatically as stopping nicotine altogether. Many nicotine replacements are available without a prescription. *Never* smoke while using a nicotine replacement.

If you're a heavy smoker (one and a half to two packs per day), consider using both the Zyban and the highest-potency nicotine replacement patch. Begin with the Zyban for two to three weeks with the goal of cutting back your number of daily cigarettes by at least half. Then, add the nicotine replacement source and at the same time stop smoking completely. Then, over the next month taper off your nicotine replacement source, and after two to three months stop taking Zyban as well. If you smoke less than that, start the Zyban and sometime during the second week quit smoking and use a lower-potency nicotine replacement if you need it.

Next, get yourself shored up on three important fronts by following the Three-Week Cure:

– **REDUCE STRESS** by closely following each of the stress-relief steps in the Three-Week Cure. Add some vigorous exercise to further offset the stress of quitting cigarettes.

– **RAISE SEROTONIN** using all the strategies. This is not the time to experiment with a low-carb diet. In fact you should be timing your intake of carbs (p. 263) throughout the day to keep serotonin elevated.

- **BALANCE YOUR HORMONES** if you're aware of a hormonal component to your smoking patterns.

ALTERNATIVE APPROACHES

If you can't afford Zyban, have side effects from it (rare, but possible), or simply want to try a nonprescription alternative:

- **ST. JOHN'S WORT** (450 mg twice a day) and **5HTP** (100–150 mg at bedtime) can be taken in combination—meaning I want you to take both every day. They act slowly on serotonin levels, so start them at least two weeks before quitting. And please don't combine St. John's wort and 5HTP with Wellbutrin/Zyban. Doing so can actually create too much serotonin in your brain, making you feel headachy, lightheaded, or "wired."

Next, add one of the following mild, natural, and nonsedating tranquilizers, available at health food stores or online. You can safely use either of these with Wellbutrin/Zyban and nicotine replacement:

- **VALERIAN** had its first recorded use in ancient Greece. This herb may act by increasing levels of GABA (see below). Safe and effective as a daytime tranquilizer, 400 mg once or twice during the day can relieve any anxiety from quitting. By adding an additional 400 mg at bedtime, valerian becomes a very effective sleep aid.

- **GABA** (gamma aminobutyric acid) is an amino acid in your body that functions to protect your brain from overreacting to anxiety-related signals. Called the body's natural tranquilizer, GABA promotes relaxation. This is probably why many antianxiety drugs (including Valium) target GABA receptors in the brain. Unlike prescription tranquilizers, GABA is not habit forming and won't make you drowsy. Take 250–500 mg two or three times a day to relieve the anxiety of nicotine withdrawal.

Finally, consider:

- **ACUPUNCTURE** (p. 285), shown unequivocally to reduce cravings that come with addictions, including addiction to smoking and to other drugs such as cocaine and heroin. If you have an acupuncturist in your community, make her part of your team.

18.

TEMPOROMANDIBULAR JOINT DISORDER (TMJ)

What does TMJ have in common with migraine headache, PMS, or any of the other Triple Whammy disorders? Quite honestly, whenever there's a condition linked to the phrases, "We don't know what causes it" and "It seems related to stress," my curiosity antennae perk up.

Let's get the anatomy out of the way first. If you reach up, grab your chin, and open and close your mouth, you are holding your jaw bone, or mandible. It's attached to either side of your skull, just in front of your ears, in an area called the temporal region (hence temporo + mandible = temporomandibular). If you place your finger on this spot in front of your ear, and open and close your mouth, you can feel the joint move.

When you've got TMJ, the joint in front of your ear becomes inflamed and painful. Often you wake up in the morning with pain right over the joint, although sometimes the pain also radiates to your ears, neck, and upper back. Chewing becomes uncomfortable, yawning even worse. The muscles of your jaw involved in chewing are called the masseters and, for their size, are among the strongest in your body. Using strong masseters, circus performers dangle in the air by their teeth and college students open bottles of beer.

For most people, TMJ is a consequence of using the powerful masseters to grind their teeth in their asleep. (The medical term for this is bruxism, and after all these years being a doctor I can't understand why the simple act of tooth grinding deserves its own word, especially one that sounds more like a political movement or an obscure religion.) Since they're asleep while they're grinding away, most bruxists learn of their problem through the annoyed comments of their bed mates: "You're grinding woke me up again." Dentists can spot evidence of grinding on the tooth enamel surface during a checkup.

After a night of teeth grinding, you awaken with an achy jaw, the joint itself tender when you push it with your finger or when you wag your chin back and forth. Most TMJ flare-ups are temporary, the grinding having triggered some in-flammation in your jaw joint. In rare cases, TMJ is caused by faulty posture, like holding the phone between your ear and neck for hours at a time. Dentists look for malocclusion—an uneven bite in your jaw when you clamp down, caused by a protruding tooth—as a source of TMJ.

MOST COMMON CAUSE OF TMJ

The most common reason for grinding at night is Whammy #1, stress. Just as many of my women patients will tell me they hold their stress in their neck, people with TMJ are essentially holding their stress a bit forward from the neck in the masseter muscles. And, yes, far more women than men suffer from TMJ. For many, flare-ups occur during PMS days, revealing a hormonal component (Whammy #3) as well.

But why the jaw muscles in particular? Why do we grind at night? Let's look at the stress/muscle spasm problem symbolically by asking, "What does this *mean*?" If you picture a person holding stress in her neck and upper back, you can see that this is the posture you'd unconsciously assume when anticipating some sort of blow. When you tense up in preparation for a conflict (you hear the door open downstairs as your alcoholic husband comes home), your neck and upper back tighten.

The psychological associations with jaw grinding are different, but not all that much. Women with bruxism and TMJ problems often acknowledge an emotional conflict in which they have a very strong opinion about something but are reluctant to release it. During sleep (when everyone's guard is down), the conflict surfaces and almost gets released, but then the woman with TMJ silences herself, holding back her anger or resentment by clamping shut her mouth. Al-cohol, which lowers inhibitions even further, is known to make grinding worse, perhaps because conflicts and resentments are permitted to surface a bit more with alcohol, though they're still blocked from being released by the jaw.

TRIPLE WHAMMY APPROACH TO TMJ

If you have TMJ, there are numerous steps you can take before considering the surgery that is commonly offered (and seldom worthwhile). Many are practical steps, while others delve a little more deeply into the possible underlying reasons for your TMJ. Read through the healing path that follows and see what your intuition tells you about where to start.

LIFESTYLE CHANGES

- **TAKE AN ANTI-INFLAMMATORY** medication like aspirin or ibuprofen to reduce the painful swelling at your jaw joint.

- **SELECT SOFT FOODS** that require minimal chewing: thick soups, cooked veggies and fruits, yogurt, eggs.

- **APPLY A WARM MOIST COMPRESS** to your jaw joint area, followed by a few minutes of fingertip massage, right over the joint. This will hurt a little at first but improves blood flow to the joint, and this will wash away the chemicals released during inflammation.

- **DON'T CHEW UNNECESSARILY:** avoid gum, your fingernails, and tasty pencils.

- **TRY NOT TO YAWN.**

Next, work on your whammies . . .

WHAMMY #1: STRESS Get a handle on what's triggering the TMJ. If this is a constant or recurring problem, check with your dentist first to make sure you don't actually have an uneven bite—the malocclusion mentioned earlier. If your bite is uneven, your dentist can take care of it. If not and she suggests you wear a mouth guard at night, that's okay but it sort of misses the point. If you came to see me explaining that you had a headache as a consequence of banging your head against a wall, I would suggest we explore why you feel compelled to bang your head and look at options to help you stop. I would not suggest nailing up foam padding to soften the blows. To me, this is what a mouth guard basically accomplishes. You almost certainly will benefit from reading Chapter 20 on stress (p. 197), and applying the techniques to manage stress. Yoga (p. 230) is a good stress-reducing choice for those with TMJ, and self-exploration with a therapist is always helpful. Read about counseling on page 232 and consider some short-term psychotherapy to explore areas of conflict in your life that you're keeping locked up inside.

WHAMMY #2: LOW SEROTONIN Raising your brain levels of serotonin—your factory-installed buffer against stress—can help. Begin with the natural ways to increase serotonin, outlined in the Three-Week Cure and in Nutritional Supplements below. Most people don't need prescription antidepressants for TMJ, but very small doses—from 10 to 25 mg—of the older antidepressant amitriptyline (Elavil) can provide multiple benefits: deepening sleep, relieving muscle tightness, and raising serotonin.

WHAMMY #3: HORMONES If you're menstruating, use a calendar to track your TMJ symptoms against your periods to see if there's a premenstrual trigger involved. If there is, you'll need to address both problems—the TMJ and the PMS—if you want to make progress. To get started, read and follow the PMS healing path (p. 153). If your TMJ surfaced during perimenopause, read the Menopause Transition healing path (p. 120) and begin the conservative measures like exercise, dietary changes, black cohosh, and soy products.

NUTRITIONAL SUPPLEMENTS

The goal of using nutritional supplements is to build up your serotonin stress buffer, improve the depth of your sleep, and reduce the inflammation within your temporomandibular joint. These objectives can be accomplished with safe natural products from your health food store.

- **5HTP,** 50–150 mg at bedtime, will deepen your sleep and raise levels of serotonin.

- **ST. JOHN'S WORT** acts as a mild antidepressant and along with 5HTP will raise serotonin levels over the course of several weeks. Take 450 mg twice a day, with food.

- **VALERIAN** is an effective sleep aid. Take 800–900 mg about an hour before bedtime. You can also use this herb as a mild daytime tranquilizer in a smaller dose, usually in the range of 200–400 mg once or twice a day.

- **GLUCOSAMINE SULFATE,** used as a supplement for arthritis, can act as a natural antiinflammatory and provide the building blocks for healthy joint repair, including your temporomandibular joint. Glucosamine usually comes in 500 mg capsules; you'll need 1,500 mg per day. I recommend two capsules in the morning and one in the evening since everyone (including me) manages to miss the midday dose.

ALTERNATIVE MEDICINE FOR TMJ

I've been very impressed with the results of alternative therapies for TMJ. Also (and this is a profound insight into the obvious): most people feel much less anxious anticipating a visit to a chiropractor, acupuncturist, or Reiki therapist than to a dentist or an oral surgeon. You'll also feel a whole lot better after you leave.

- **CHIROPRACTIC** (p. 275) People whose TMJ is caused by a misaligned spine or a repetitive injury, such as gripping the telephone between face and shoulder, may find chiropratic adjustment very helpful.

- **TRADITIONAL CHINESE MEDICINE (TCM)** Several sessions of acupuncture (p. 285) can dramatically reduce the pain and inflammation of TMJ.

- **REIKI** (p. 239) Therapists skilled in balancing subtle energies see TMJ as a block-age of energy at the level of your neck and throat (the throat chakra, one of seven such energy centers in the body). Safe and gentle techniques that allow energy, *chi,* to flow freely may allow you to experience a dramatic release of tension. You might actually start articulating aloud for the first time those conflicts you'd been uncon-sciously suppressing.

SELF-CARE

All of these methods can be used in conjunction with any of the other treatments for TMJ:

- **ACUPRESSURE** (p. 207) The points that relax your jaw muscles are located about one inch above the angle of your lower jaw under your ear. Press these points with your fingertip for one full minute three or four times a day.

- **AROMATHERAPY** (p. 210) Select the oils commonly used for relaxation: lavender, marjoram, or ylang-ylang. Treat yourself to a relaxing bath (p. 211) just before bed.

- **FLOWER ESSENCE THERAPY** (p. 220) A trained therapist can be valuable in se-lecting a remedy specific to your emotional needs. She may select scleranthus (for indecision and uncertainty), agrimony (hiding worries), or white chestnut (persistent worries, mental arguments).

CONVENTIONAL THERAPIES

Most dentists looking for the cause of TMJ will check for malocclusion (uneven bite) and then prescribe a mouth guard. There's a new mouth guard available, called an NTI device, that is placed on the two front teeth only. It's a lot more comfortable than the bulkier full-mouth version but, as discussed earlier, try some of the other measures first.

Some dentists suggest a variety of procedures, such as orthodontic braces, attaching crowns, or even sanding down perfectly good teeth in order to balance your bite. These are generally useless and expensive procedures. If your dentist recommends surgery for TMJ, get a second or third opinion on it. The thought of someone grinding down my teeth makes my toes curl, so I would try every-thing in this chapter before considering surgery.

TRIPLE WHAMMY CASE STUDY

TMJ

"I was out apartment hunting with my fiancé . . ."

Caroline made an appointment with me to consider, as she put it, "something alternative" before moving ahead with what her dentist was planning for her TMJ.

"He said that I was in pain not just because I was grinding my teeth, but it looked as if I was doing it unevenly. He thought if he could shift a couple of my back teeth with braces, then sand down some uneven ridges, I'd still be grinding, but doing it more evenly and maybe the pain would go away."

Remembering my own discomfort with braces as a child, and shuddering at the thought of sanding down perfectly good teeth, I agreed with Caroline that she should explore other options for her TMJ. I asked when her grinding had started.

"You know," she answered, "I almost remember the day, because it was the first time in my life I ever woke up with pain in my jaw. I was barely able to open my mouth, and wondered what was going on. The day before, I'd been out apartment hunting with my fiancé. We're getting married in a few months and thought it would be nice to get a place together early. We found a beautiful apartment and we're sitting down with the landlady, looking at the lease, when Bill's cell phone rings. It was his mother.

"Bill told her about the apartment, and then all of a sudden says into the phone, 'Okay, Mom.' Do you know what he agreed to? That we wouldn't take the apartment, even after we were married, but would move in with her out in the suburbs. She's a widow, with plenty of space in her house. She said Bill and I could have the big bedroom and that she'd sleep in Bill's old room."

"And that's when you woke up with the pain/started grinding your teeth?"

"Yep. I knew I was mad, but I didn't say anything. I figured I'd just get over it. He's a really good guy, and his mother's house is very nice. It's just that I wanted something to be ours."

"And Bill?"

"Oh, I think he's really happy with it. You know, two women taking care of him . . ."

I told Caroline that some psychologists believe TMJ can begin when a person is experiencing an internal conflict: an intense urge to speak up but an equally strong sense to clam up. Rather than trying to sort this out with a counselor, I suggested she work with our Reiki therapist to see if together they could free up energy around her throat. After a couple of Reiki sessions, Caroline didn't come in for a few weeks. No one on my staff heard from her and I wondered if she was being fitted for her braces or her teeth were being sandpapered.

She then suddenly appeared for a follow-up visit, starting off our conversation by saying that her TMJ was history, and that her very first Reiki session had opened up her mind in ways both clear and subtle to what was happening in her life. The TMJ had gone, as had her fiancé and his mother, and the house in the suburbs. Caroline said, "It was like I saw my future during that ride home. I knew if I didn't break it off, I'd be grinding my teeth till death do us part. And that the death would probably be mine."

19.

WEIGHT LOSS AGONIES

Far and away the most common Triple Whammy disorder concerns the uniquely female preoccupation with losing weight. At any given moment, it is estimated that about 120 million Americans, mainly women, are on some sort of diet. Because we live in a culture that places an absurd emphasis on being thin, many women spend much of their lives feeling terrible about their bodies. Many weight-loss nutritional supplements have turned out to be quite dangerous. The ever-helpful pharmaceutical industry has stepped in over the years with highly addicting amphetamines and their cousins, heart-damaging fen-phen, along with the "fat blocking" Xenical, whose users were horrified to discover oil dripping out of their rear ends, staining their leotards. Most recently, there is Meridia, a Prozac-like drug whose side effects of appetite suppression, dry mouth, and persistent metallic taste were put to good economic use by savvy marketing as a weight-loss pill. Intestinal bypass surgery, liquid protein diets, jaw wiring, and high doses of thyroid hormone have also been used. We've also added other potentially dangerous surgical procedures, banding our stomachs and liposuctioning our love handles.

You need to know that virtually nothing ever works. Weight that you lose on a diet or with the above methods is almost always regained. Women feel emotionally miserable when they're dieting, and even worse when they see the pounds coming back. Who needs this? If I could have one wish fulfilled about women's emotional and physical well-being, it would be that you would never again think about your weight, instead unequivocally accepting that you're just fine as you are and that you enjoy what you eat and unconditionally love your body and yourself in the process.

DOCTORS SHOULD LEAVE WOMEN ALONE ABOUT THEIR WEIGHT

Of course it would help considerably if the medical profession would leave women alone about weight. Several years ago, the Surgeon General of the United States joined a long line of previous surgeons general by intoning that America's greatest health danger was obesity. Personally, I would think that our greatest health problem is that 45 million of us can't afford health care, but apparently he thinks otherwise.

The Surgeon General is quite wrong about this and it's wrong of him to be an alarmist. Being overweight is vastly overrated as a health risk. I wouldn't argue that the 5 percent of overweight people in the morbidly obese range (300 pounds and over) are at a greater risk for diabetes, high blood pressure, heart disease, and arthritis. I agree that being overweight and sedentary does place you at greater risk for a variety of chronic illnesses. But if you're moderately overweight, you don't have to spend your life trying to reduce poundage to reduce your health risks. All epidemiologic data show that overweight people *who are physically active* will remain as healthy as those who are "normal" weight and physically active. In addition, overweight physically active people of both sexes will, in the long run, remain healthier than their underweight, sedentary counterparts.

The patients in my medical practice are about 85 percent female, between twenty and sixty-five years old. Homemakers, legal assistants, corporate workers, teachers, business owners, white, black, Asian, and Latina—a representative cross-section of urban women, as far as I can tell. I would take as their weights something in the range of 140 to 175 pounds. Many of the younger women are fairly svelte, but after a few years of married life and a couple of kids, most gain some weight (a normal state of affairs).

Some of my patients are pushing 200 pounds, a few even higher. By the Surgeon General's standards, almost all are overweight. Yet those who exercise are extraordinarily healthy. A few, both thin and heavy, have high blood pressure, diabetes, or high cholesterol, but not a lot. What's really unfortunate is that despite their good health, virtually all are unhappy with their current weight, dislike their bodies, and think about their weight almost every time they sit down to

eat. Most have tried dieting, and failed, and tried again and failed again, throughout their lives.

So, if almost half the population of the United States (mainly women and
now, horrifically, young girls) endlessly thinks about food, diet, and weight, and
yet continues to overeat and gain more weight, I think it can fairly be said that
the problem is not an obesity epidemic, but rather an epidemic of eating disorders triggered by a society that places a bizarrely high value on being thin and
young, and little value on simply being who you are. The whole mess is fueled
by the health care industry misreading research evidence and profiting in the
process.

A real factor in all this is that we're surrounded by food. Good things to eat are
cheap and available everywhere. We eat out more and restaurants serve enormous
portions. We're endlessly snacking as we stroll through shopping malls or drive.
And then we sit down to dinner, where everyone is encouraged to have seconds.

HOW IS AGONIZING ABOUT MY WEIGHT
A TRIPLE WHAMMY DISORDER?

First, regarding Whammy #1, the source of stress is self-evident. If you're thinking about your weight endlessly, or dislike your body or how your clothes fit,
then you're clearly experiencing stress (quite aside from the everyday stress a majority of women face keeping family together, working, and caring for children
and/or aging parents). If everything you eat is accompanied by an approach-
avoidance conflict—"I'd love the potato. I can't eat the potato. I want the potato.
I'm fat. I'm hungry. I'm starving. I'm fat. I'm unattractive"—then you're under
stress throughout the day. Day? Many women live like this for years.

Enter Whammy #2, low serotonin. Remember that this feel-good neurotransmitter, in sufficient levels, acts as a buffer against stress. Men, with plenty of
serotonin on board, are less susceptible to the ravages of stress, and also have a
more lenient cultural norm to live up to. But women, with low levels of serotonin, can be tortured by this. So what's available to calm you down and raise
your serotonin? That's right, food, and often in the form of not-so-high-quality
carbs—comfort foods like chips and candy—and frequently at the expense of
nutrient-packed whole foods. By the way, this is why I beg women not to start
low-carb programs. Without carbs (and by this I mean high-quality carbs—see
page 266 for more), serotonin drops and emotional vulnerability escalates. Men
do better on low-carb diets. After all, men don't really regard a steak, salad, and

martini as dieting. Women, on the other hand, can experience a real snarkiness born of carbohydrate restriction.

And Whammy #3, monthly hormone shifts, definitely don't help you here. During those few days before your period starts, as estrogen falls, it drags serotonin down with it. To shore up serotonin, many women start craving carbs before their periods.

How many men do you know who crave certain foods? Men may like chocolate, but if a typical guy were told "You can never have a piece of chocolate again in your life" (something that would devastate many women), most would shrug and ask, "What about caramel?"

TRIPLE WHAMMY APPROACH TO WEIGHT AGONIES

What I present here is frequently met with a look that implies, "If you knew what it was like to be ten (or fifteen or twenty-five or fifty) pounds overweight, with your stomach bloated and your clothes too tight, then you'd understand." Have you ever wondered why men's clothes aren't "too tight"? Maybe it's because men don't think about this stuff, and buy looser pants. If you follow these suggestions, casting aside doubt and moving forward with confidence, concerns about your weight will play an ever-diminishing role in your life.

WHAMMY #1: STRESS An excellent start to relieving the stress of failed diets and the way you look is to accept yourself unconditionally. In our world we're surrounded by love that's dependent on conditions—good grades, more money, clear skin, better housekeeping, and (need I even say it) being thin. What I'm asking is that you bite the bullet, ignore all the nonsense of the youth culture, accept that you will never look like a sixteen-year-old waif, and love yourself. This may require some stress-relieving measures, among them counseling (p. 232). Please also read through the entire stress chapter (p. 197) and begin to cope with your stress.

WHAMMY #2: LOW SEROTONIN Although conventional physicians might suggest Meridia or a prescription antidepressant to raise your serotonin, I'd like you to follow the natural serotonin-boosting steps in the Three-Week Cure instead, including the supplements and light exposure. Exercise is a winning bet, because it will bring you cardiovascular fitness while raising your serotonin (and it reduces stress in the process). High-quality carbs are your friends because your brain needs them to make serotonin. Learn more about carbo timing on page 263.

WHAMMY #3: HORMONES Track your menstrual cycle for a month or two to determine if there's a hormonal component to your eating. Read the PMS healing path on page 153 for ways to bring your hormones into balance.

- **IF YOU DON'T WANT TO GAIN WEIGHT,** eat what you enjoy but eat a small portion of it. Multicultural America has a vast variety of wonderful things to eat. Enjoy them all in moderation—carbs, fats, proteins, everything—and keep your in-between-meal snacking to fruits and veggies. With that said, let me just add that a substantial number of people are grazers, eating fewer smaller meals and snacks throughout the day. This is just fine, though meal eaters and grazers alike need to keep an eye on their portions. Follow the Triple Whammy Food plan and you'll be fine. And if one morning you wake up thinking, "I'd kill for a Ho-Ho," just have it. You won't explode. (I have a friend who treats herself to one full-fat, giant-sized just-like-mom-used-to-make-it chocolate malt per year. She enjoys just anticipating it every summer.)

- **THROW AWAY YOUR DIET BOOKS AND WEIGHT-LOSS SUPPLEMENTS AND NEVER BUY ANOTHER AGAIN.** No matter what they promise, diet books are misleading you. Everything in a health food store marked "for weight loss" is lying. Every infomercial you see on TV for weight loss is lying. If you took all the money you've spent on diet books, special foods to eat on diet programs, and any other diet-related expenditures, how much would you have? Enough to take a few weeks' worth of yoga courses? Enough to go to a spa for a few days? Enough to walk with a friend for an hour and then have a nice lunch and conversation? Any of these latter ideas is a far more productive use of your money and time.

- **MORE THAN ANYTHING ELSE, WATCH YOUR PORTIONS.** The French, a decidedly thin nation, truly enjoy good food, including high-fat everything, as long as they can have a glass of wine with it, and rarely skip dessert. When I was much younger (and fatter), visiting Paris for the first time, I was outraged that the meal portions were so small. Now I'm smarter and understand that they eat all foods—a vast variety of them—in moderation, don't eat between meals, and don't eat fast food and snack foods (or at least most don't). The other thing to keep in mind about the French is that they really appreciate the sexuality and beauty of older women, the cultural opposite of the United States.

- **HOW EXERCISE FITS IN.** It's been established beyond doubt that people of any weight who achieve cardiovascular fitness have a lower risk of death from all causes than do sedentary so-called normal-weight people. Please reread that sentence aloud. It's an essential piece of information. Don't even think about using exercise just to lose weight; it doesn't work and you'll be disappointed. Starting tomorrow, your purpose for exercising regularly is to stay healthy or become healthier. To build muscle and keep flexible. To challenge your heart. Honestly, people of every weight who exercise have it written all over their bodies—their skin glows, their posture is exceptional because of their muscle strength, and their eyes sparkle. Maybe it's the serotonin, too, and the other feel-good neurotransmitters that exercise kicks up, even as it damps down stress.

- **DON'T ALLOW ANYONE TO CRITICIZE YOU.** Your weight-loss friends may be scandalized that you aren't suffering with them anymore. Find a new shared enthusiasm, such as tutoring some kids or joining a book club.

- **IF YOU SMOKE BECAUSE YOU THINK YOU'RE GOING TO GAIN WEIGHT IF YOU STOP SMOKING, STOP SMOKING ANYWAY.** Yes, you might actually gain some weight, but you will have eliminated from your life a very real health risk, infinitely more dangerous than a few extra pounds in a person who works out. See the healing path on page 177 for some help.

WHAT ALTERNATIVE MEDICINE OFFERS

If alternative medicine could solve America's obsession with weight, alternative practitioners would be mainstream. There are a few good options, however. As with other Triple Whammy disorders, three supplements used for serotonin and hormone imbalance can sometimes help with sugar and carbohydrate cravings. If there's a hormonal component to your overeating, start all three at once.

- **5HTP** 100 mg at bedtime will raise serotonin and reduce cravings for sweets and carbohydrates.

- **ST. JOHN'S WORT** 450 mg twice a day will work together with 5HTP to raise serotonin and suppress carb urges.

- **CHASTEBERRY** Take 175–225 mg twice a day when not menstruating to balance your sex hormones and help reduce PMS sugar and chocolate cravings. Because chasteberry affects hormone levels, you shouldn't use it if you're taking hormone replacement therapy or birth control pills (it can lessen their effectiveness), or if you're pregnant or nursing.

MY WIFE AND HER WEIGHT

I have to close by letting you know something about how my wife, Ann, has maintained her weight for our thirty-odd years of marriage. First, she eats whatever she wants. She loves Mexican food, thick Chicago-style pizza, and never says no to a glass of wine or a good dessert. Second, she simply stops eating whenever her hunger is sated, no matter how much food is left on the plate. Third, she never eats anything other than an apple between meals. Fourth, she exercises three or four times a week, not all that vigorously (in my opinion), but consistently. When she was pregnant with our boys, she gained weight, which is normal. Within a year or two, without any dieting, she was back to her original weight. Of course, some of this is genetic, but mostly it's portion control. She simply will not eat junk food, fast food, or between meals. Maybe she's French and I never noticed it.

CONVENTIONAL MEDICINE
AND WEIGHT ISSUES

Don't let anyone "helpfully" calculate your BMI (body mass index). This is one of the poorest means of deciding who is overweight and who isn't because it places every person, regardless of their fitness level, into the same mathematical formula. Everyone with a BMI over 25 is automatically labeled overweight and allegedly "at risk," even if that person is crossing the finish line of a triathlon without a drop of sweat on her brow.

Nothing conventional medicine can offer will help with long-term weight loss—drugs, surgery, diet, or otherwise. (If exercise is suggested, that's fine, but remember it's to improve your fitness level.) Prescription medicines for weight control don't work, are expensive, aren't paid for by most insurance companies, and have potentially dangerous side effects. Find a doctor who will leave you alone about your weight. Tell her upfront that you don't wish to discuss weight and if she nags you on the subject, you'll find another doctor. Remember, she has nothing—absolutely nothing—to offer except incorrect medical information about the so-called dangers of being overweight. (If your insurance company paid for membership in a health club, now that would be something to offer.)

To begin with, she incorrectly assumes that being fat places you at risk for heart disease, but if your cholesterol level is normal, and your blood pressure is normal (which is a result of your working out, not your weight), statistical evidence has shown you are at no greater risk than someone whose weight falls beneath the sacred BMI of 25. Or conversely, even though there are more overweight people than ever before, our rate of heart disease, especially sudden deaths from heart attacks, has, during the past ten years, steadily dropped. She will then wag a finger about diabetes because overweight people are more prone to developing diabetes than those of normal weight. But do we really have the much-touted "epidemic" of diabetes? Doctors are seeing more patients with diabetes because we screen for it more frequently than we did a generation ago, not because there are more overweight people. In this respect, it's like the "epidemic" of high cholesterol. If you start testing the cholesterol levels of virtually everyone who breathes and, at the same time, lower the definition of high cholesterol from 220 to 200, it's going to look like we're in the middle of an epidemic.

The evidence associating being overweight with increased cancer risks is even (pardon the pun) thinner, with studies even showing that being overweight has a protective advantage. So if you can't visit your doctor without tensing up for her inevitable weight loss lecture, or you feel on the verge of tears when you're wrapped in a paper gown and the nurse moves that slider thing on the doctor's scale toward higher and higher numbers, just find another doctor.

PART IV

TRIPLE WHAMMY
RESOURCES

20.

STRESS LESS

LIFETIME LESSONS:
LEARNING TO LIMIT STRESS

Stress is the trigger, the catalyst, for your whole Triple Whammy problem. You might want to review "Whammy #1: The Chemistry of Stress" on page 5 in conjunction with reading this section to fully understand the implications of unchecked stress for your health. To limit, manage, or eliminate stress altogether you first must uncover those factors in your life that are relentlessly pushing your buttons. This can be daunting, with stressors popping up like those "Whack-A-Mole" games you see at carnivals. You also need to explore why certain things do in fact push your buttons. Limiting stress is a process, and self-awareness can be a painful part of it, but it's also a major step in controlling bursts of resentment, moodiness, and tension that bollix up the simple pleasures of your day. Once you've pegged your stressors, you've got to teach your body to control its stress response. The three lessons that follow are deceptively simple. Like learning meditation, getting these lessons right requires perseverance and regular practice.

LESSON ONE

STRESS JOURNAL

Once you understand where stress is coming from and how it's affecting you emotionally and physically, you can use the other tools in this chapter to curb its impact. What is stressing you out is probably no secret to you: finances, relationships, work, time pressures. We develop reactions to stress in situations where something prevents us from being in full control of our lives, whether it's a terrible boss or a traffic jam, a mountain of unwashed laundry or a boyfriend who won't make a long-term commitment. Survey your life for a few weeks and see where stress may be chipping away at your sense of self and happiness. Once you recognize the extent and effects of stress, you can improve your coping skills or even take a deep breath and exit the scene altogether.

KEEPING A STRESS JOURNAL

TOOLS Purchase a nice, wide-ruled spiral notebook. Get a pen.

COMMITMENT Make a contract with yourself to devote fifteen minutes at the end of each day to complete that day's entry.

ON PAGE ONE Make a Stress Symptom Survey. This is your personal master list of how stress affects you. Divide this page into two columns, one headed "Mental/Emotional," the other "Physical." Then, working from the following lists, write down as many of these symptoms as regularly appear in your life:

Mental/Emotional: Anger; anxiety; burnout; crying spells; depression; fearfulness; frustration; guilt; irritability; loss of sense of humor; mind racing; nervous habits (hair pulling, nail biting, mindless eating); pessimism; poor concentration and memory; powerlessness; resentment; short temper

Physical: Chest tightness; exhaustion/fatigue; frequent colds; headache; heart pounding; insomnia; teeth grinding; irritable bowel syndrome; muscle aches or tightness; sudden dry mouth or bad taste; intuitive physical sensation of "something not right"

ORGANIZATION Plan the rest of your journal in the following format: Devote each page to a single day in your life. Divide the top two-thirds of the page into two equal columns, which you'll head (1) The Stressful Event and (2) Emotional/Physical Symptoms. Include in the event column direct quotes from anyone who is a source of stress in your life: boss, husband, roommate. You'll leave the area in the bottom third of the page open for your own thoughts, such as what you learned about yourself, how you might have responded differently, and what changes you can make in the future. It might also be helpful to track your menstrual cycle in this diary, just to see if your stress shifts up during the days, or even weeks, before your period.

Carry your journal with you during the day, to record those moments when you're experiencing symptoms. You can fill in the details later. In a few short days, you'll likely see patterns emerging. You may learn how those tense muscles in the back of your neck throb after your agonizing commute to work. How the recurring thoughts that interfere with sleep are mainly about your problems with your husband. Or how the sentence "I think we should just keep living together and not get married" tightens a knot in your stomach (gut feelings represent the very best of your female intuitive skills). You may discover it's time to consider a job closer to home or to get into therapy with your husband or boyfriend.

The physical act of writing and recording, and then reading what you've written, is powerful. It's one thing to say to your doctor, "Stress triggers my migraines" as she refills your pain medication and then forget you said it by the time you reach your car. It's quite another to realize that you've had ten migraines in the previous month, most of them on days when, for example, your boss had been unpleasant and demanding. "Gosh, look at this," you might say aloud, flipping through your diary pages. "Oh, my!" And with that "Oh, my!" it's time to start one of the stress-relieving activities found in Lesson Two (p. 200).

SYMPTOMS AS MESSAGES

A doctor practicing holistic medicine takes care of the whole person and, as part of this process, is keenly interested in knowing the story of your life and how you *became* ill. To me, the single most interesting principle of holistic medicine is that symptoms, both physical and emotional, are frequently messages from the body asking its owner to make changes. Since symptoms-as-messages are only trying to help, they require a good listener (you and, with luck, your doctor) in order to be understood. In this light, symptoms of stress, whether anxiety or headaches, anger or fatigue, are all, in a peculiar way, gifts. A typical holistic approach asks "What is this headache trying to tell you? What is your body trying to say by giving you this headache?" Part of the process of dealing with stress (or any symptom) is to learn to listen to your body.

And while we're on this topic of symptoms as messages, here's a good general rule: try to avoid taking medicines for a condition you can cure by making lifestyle changes. The real help for a smoker's cough is not cough syrup but quitting cigarettes. The real solution to heartburn is not the purple pill, but to stop stuffing yourself with lasagna before bedtime. And, yes, the real treatments for stress-induced anxiety or depression are not tranquilizers or antidepressants, but rather to see clearly your sources of stress and learn to cope with them—or walk away from them.

LESSON TWO

USING YOUR BODY TO CALM DOWN YOUR MIND

Your first project of Lesson Two is to start practicing one stress-reducing technique every day. You can choose from among yoga, t'ai chi, guided imagery, meditation, acupuncture, massage—any of the techniques described in the Stress-Relief Menu on page 204. Of course, if you discover you don't like your first choice (and it stresses you out), try something different. Some new patients react with surprise when I prescribe stress-reducing techniques as a part of their care. They tell me it's the first time a physician has suggested such a thing, much less considered it a medical necessity. Some people view acupuncture, massage, or self-hypnosis as self-indulgent, or a little "woo-woo"—interesting to try but not necessarily beneficial or worth the time.

My view is precisely the opposite. Your health *depends* on taking this time for yourself, and every one of the stress reducers on the menu can be remarkably effective. Doctors in Europe routinely send their patients off to spas. It's a real point of pride with me that every year I send far more patients to health spas than I do to hospitals.

PUT WORRY BEHIND YOU

Your second project will be learning to overcome worry. You know what I mean here. Worrying is that utterly useless endeavor in which you relentlessly work over a problem (or two, or more) like a dog worrying an old bone. Worry is a major source of stress. Sometimes worry drives us to find a solution in response to pressures at work or home or concerns about family, relationships, or money. But other times (and all too often) we collapse into a bundle of nerves and engage in mental hand-wringing and perseveration. If you've made worry a daytime activity or it's keeping you awake at night, you're certainly enjoying life a lot less while you're worrying. And since you're agonizing about events that may never occur, you're also engaged in an ultimate waste of time. Here are a few practical steps to help you conquer worry (or at least learn to deal with it better):

- **CONSIDER THE WORST-CASE SCENARIO.** A tried-and-true formula for overcoming worry is to analyze the situation carefully, listing all the possibilities you're obsessing about. Then select the worst eventuality of all and "live it." Actually imagine how this awful possibility has occurred ("I've been fired!") and accept it emotionally. "Oh, dear," you can say to yourself, "It's happened. Just what I was worried about." Now devote your energy to figuring out what you're going to do next. List the steps you'll have to take. Write them down so you have them to refer to should it happen. When you start intelligently and objectively solving what once so terrified you, you break down that huge ball of worry into conquerable chunks.

- **FIGURE THE ODDS.** Try to be as objective as possible. Ask yourself, "Really, what are the chances that the worst scenario I'm afraid of will actually happen?" Fortunately, our worst fears rarely do come to pass. Few planes crash; most people won't get the West Nile virus.

- **CREATE A "WORRY TIME."** Make a conscious choice to delay your thinking about a problem until a specific time every day—say between 8 and 8:30 p.m., or any other time that works for you. Then, during that half hour, concentrate on your problems all at once instead of letting bits of anxiety undermine your whole day. This does require some mental discipline. Whenever a "worry" thought drifts up (especially in the middle of the night), simply tell yourself "I will think about that during worry time tomorrow." And then put it in a mental box and force your mind to move elsewhere.

- **RENAME AND MOVE FORWARD.** Some worries do have a basis in reality. However, if you sit around wringing your hands in helpless despair, you'll never get anywhere. Review the real sources of your trouble, and rename them "challenges." Simply renaming your worries will place them within your power. Now go ahead and tackle each challenge.

- **ACCEPT THE INEVITABLE.** When the company you work for is doing badly, you just might get laid off. (Have hope: I can't tell you how many of my patients were sick—literally—of their jobs but became well and even optimistic after losing them.) Public transportation will generally make you late. The IRS will find something during its audit that will cost you money. "God grant me the serenity to accept things I cannot change . . ." can be a very helpful motto.

- **FIND PROPER PERSPECTIVE.** One fast way to gain perspective is to find someone who needs your help—a sick friend, an elderly acquaintance, a child who needs tutoring—and do something for that person. Ask just about anybody who volunteers even a little bit of her time and she'll tell you that she receives much more than she gives, and that volunteering provides a helpful perspective.

- **MOVE FORWARD.** You can't change the past, no matter how hard you try. Better not to waste a whole lot of time worrying about what you could have (or should have) done. Sorry, but once you've turned in your final exam, you can't go back and change the answers. Accept that whatever occurred is now over, apologize if you hurt someone, and call it a lesson in learning from your mistakes.

- **GET HELP.** If, after trying these suggestions, you simply can't stop worrying, consider professional help. Obsessing endlessly about the same issues to the point where you can't get on with your life may require some counseling (p. 232) or a support group to help you develop different perspectives. Life's too precious to bring it to a halt with worry.

LESSON THREE

CULTIVATE A POSITIVE ATTITUDE

Your first project of Lesson Three is quite pleasant, and an essential component in learning to limit stress. Using the same notebook in which you've been keeping your Stress Journal, you'll now stop your daily recording of stressful events and create instead a Cultivate a Positive Attitude list. Tag a page about halfway through your notebook so you can flip to it easily (reserve a few pages in the stress section so you can jot down any special-occasion stressors). Title the page something pleasantly hokey like "The Good in My Day." And, starting today, you'll focus on cultivating the positive. You don't need any gardening tools to tend this patch, just a keen eye for the optimistic. Starting now, record something each day, no matter how small, for which you feel a sense of wonder, thanks, or optimism. This may be an act of kindness someone did for you or you did for someone else, some flowers you saw during lunch, or the way your cat rubbed against your leg. Once you begin, you'll actually find yourself looking for—or better yet, creating—the day's sweet spot so that you can record it later. And remember that helping others generates measurably higher levels of serotonin. As the weeks progress, you'll discover that the entries on your positive attitude list will fill page after page, while the Stress Journal you started weeks ago will become an interesting but dated reference to your old way of thinking.

MANAGING ANGER: HUMOR IT, PICTURE IT,
OR HEAD FOR THE GYM

Chronically stressed people are more prone to anger, which often represents a climax of accumulated stress. If you recognize in yourself a tendency to easy anger or periods of smoldering resentment, put the brakes on an episode of anger and thoughtfully analyze it. What may surprise you is the complex path you took to arrive at your present state. Exploring just how your button got pushed can give you some real insight into yourself.

Anger can be triggered by a specific person (partner, boss, best friend) or an event (delayed flight, neighbor's yappy dog, car alarm keeping you awake). Consider the anger at your boss; she's done you some sort of an injustice, but since she's still your boss and does control your paycheck, you feel helpless and nurse a brooding resentment. Or say your son comes home with a second nose ring. Your anger (if you pause to think) comes less from his looking like an idiot than from the realization that you can't control him the way you could when he was three.

Your body's response to anger and stress are very similar, and as you'd expect, it ain't healthy. Chronically angry people have high blood pressure, strokes, heart attacks, and actually die younger. And of course chronic anger equals chronic stress, Whammy #1. While you'll never be able to rid your world of people or incidents that can enrage you, you can learn to control your reactions to them. The next time your blood pressure (and temper) start to rise, put one or two of the ideas in this section into practice. You'll be well on your way to stopping anger in its tracks—or at least keeping it at bay.

- **THINK BEFORE YOU SPEAK.** When you feel yourself getting angry, pause. Counting to ten does this nicely and, of course, if you're really angry make it one hundred. Think carefully of the consequences of your angry outburst before, not after, your explosion. The regret you might feel at making a fool of yourself may be painful indeed. No matter how you reframe "hotheaded loudmouth," you can't make it into an admirable characteristic. An angry outburst can adversely affect reasonable relationships forever.

- **TRY HUMOR.** When the situation seems to call for an angry outburst, stop and tell yourself, "The universe is testing my sense of calm. I will get an A in peaceful resolution." Wallow in your new sense of goodness. Crack a joke. Practice irony. "Angry about my computer crashing and losing the report? Me? I've got nothing but time." Take comfort in the knowledge that people who burst into angry rages are not the brightest of our planetary citizens.

- **WHAT IF YOU COULDN'T APOLOGIZE?** Imagine how you'd feel if the person who received your explosion of anger were actually to die during the next twenty-four hours. There's a bit of a jolt for you. No opportunity to apologize; no chance ever to make amends. And over something so silly.

- **CHANGE YOUR TIMING.** This is a good one if anger erupts in your household with predictable regularity. If you and your partner tend to fight when you get home from work because you're exhausted and hungry, avoid discussing important issues then. Remember, though, that changing the time doesn't change the issues. If you're at each other's throats frequently, something is amiss in the relationship and you may want to see a counselor (p. 232).

– **GIVE YOURSELF A BREAK.** Make sure you have some personal "downtime" scheduled for periods you know are particularly stressful. If you're a mom who flares up when the kids leap on you as you walk through the door at 5:30, make a rule that nobody talks to mom for fifteen minutes after she gets home. Your kids may not like it at first, but they'll soon realize that you do adore them and you're not blowing up at them quite as often as before. One of my patients who works at home takes a hot aromatherapy bath (p. 211) to mark the break in her day from working to not working. She reads, relaxes, and everybody knows not to bother her before she emerges.

– **PICTURE YOURSELF AT YOUR ANGRIEST.** Nothing is as effective as anger when it comes to an unsightly distortion of what you thought were your good looks. Few people ever look gorgeous during an outburst of fury. As a bonus, if you're angry often enough, you'll etch deep frown wrinkles into your face permanently (remember what your mother said: "Your face can get stuck there forever!"). That vision alone may calm you down and help you get a grip.

– **GET SOME EXERCISE.** Working out your stress through exercise is a medically sanctioned means of processing your anger. If you've read the Three-Week Cure, you know that a daily twenty-minute brisk walk in sunlight increases the flow of blood to your brain and elevates your levels of feel-good endorphins, including serotonin. That vigorous walk outside can work magic as you breathe, sweat, and adjust your mind-set.

STRESS-RELIEF MENU

So here's the situation: you're being buffeted by the Triple Whammy, you've read about how the whammies interact to make you feel crummy, and you've started the Three-Week Cure. Good. You're already into Week 1 and you've noticed that the twenty minutes of brisk walking each day is making a real difference in how you feel. Maybe you're browsing this section, or perhaps you've landed here because this is part of the Week 2 assignment. Whatever the reason, you might be thinking to yourself, "Uh-oh, this is the part where I add my stress reliever and I don't think I have the time—isn't my twenty-minute walk enough?" I can confirm that you're entering that section of the book where you need to step up and really get involved. I also ask that you choose one or more of the stress-relievers in this section and start doing it every day—yes, in addition to your walk.

But please: stay optimistic and stay with me here. The menu of relaxation techniques that follows is luxurious, vigorous, and fun. Starting this project should definitely not stress you out. Addressing Whammies #2 and #3 is important, but addressing Whammy #1, Stress, is essential. Your good health depends on it.

PRESCRIPTION FOR STRESS RELIEF

Remember, I'm the doctor who sends more patients to health spas than to hospitals, and I consider this a badge of honor. If you need to justify to yourself or anyone else taking time each day to release stress, consider this book my handwritten, personalized prescription to do just that. This section isn't meant to be a comprehensive list of choices. If you're crazy about Pilates (a superb workout), stay with it and choose one or more other methods of stress relief for your days off Pilates. My aim here is for you to reach a state of happy relaxation that you've felt before, perhaps when you took a week off work and just puttered, or maybe when you went on a cruise or spent a day in nature. Read Guided Imagery (p. 214) and learn how to bring back all the sensations of your most relaxing memories.

Vital to all of this is learning what sets off your stress response and, more important, avoiding those stressors or adjusting your reaction to them. For help with that, please also read Lifetime Lessons: Learning to Limit Stress (p. 197).

CATHY'S COMMUTER ANXIETY

Keep in mind that stress is different for everyone. Oh sure, certain things get to all of us, but mostly I find it's pretty specific to the individual. I had a patient named Cathy whose daily dose of stress was primarily getting to work. Cathy was punctual and it was essential to her job that she arrive on time, and yet she lived at the mercy of the uncertain daily schedules of her commuter train and then a bus. The daily stomach-churning she endured—Cathy called it commuter anxiety—finally triggered what ultimately cured her: she moved from the suburbs to the city, where she could walk to work and combine her daily exercise with her commute. Even before she had settled into her new apartment, she realized that she now had two hours every day that were hers instead of belonging to the vagaries of mass transit. This came to five hundred hours a year—almost three solid weeks—that she "got back." That's a solution that might not work for everybody, but it made a remarkable difference in Cathy's life. The lion's share of her stress melted away like April snow and she was far better equipped to handle the daily work stresses, which of course continued to present themselves.

HEALTH SPAS

Consider a week at a health spa. Daily yoga classes are part of virtually every spa routine, as are healthy food, massages, and scenic walks. The absence of phones doesn't hurt either. Before you say something like "I can't spend all that money just for myself," bear in mind that spa prices vary considerably. A few minutes on www.spafinder.com may surprise you. For women facing any Triple Whammy disorder, a week at a spa can be life altering. There you'll realize how well you can feel by eliminating the stress that triggers your whammies.

YOUR CALL: BY YOURSELF, IN A GROUP, WITH A THERAPIST

This section is organized into three groups: working alone, with a group, and with a therapist. I have no shortage of patients for whom problems with time management play a significant role in the source of their stress and tension. I recognize many women need to get up early to start an exhausting, tension-filled day and roll their eyes or shake their heads in disbelief when I suggest a morning t'ai chi class or a yoga session a couple of times a week, muttering to themselves, "He's got to be kidding. With my schedule?" Others dislike group activities of any kind and anticipate something like a yoga class with the same enthusiasm as a root canal repair. You can do many of the techniques presented here alone; others you can learn from a therapist and then use regularly on yourself at home, so be sure to read through all the sections. You can easily learn techniques such as self-hypnosis, guided imagery, and reflexology, which are portable, always ready to be used at home, at work, on an airplane, or even in the dentist's chair. The descriptions in this section are brief. Lots more information is available at your health food store or library, and on the Internet. Read through this section using your intuition to see what intrigues you, and follow through from there.

Q & A: STRESS RELIEF ON A BUDGET

Q. My husband got laid off last year and my hours were just reduced. Needless to say, stress is a big factor at our house (and in my Triple Whammy symptoms!). Because money's so tight, I wonder if you could suggest a few no-cost stress relievers.

A. Many of the stress relievers described in the section starting on page 204 cost nothing, including breathing meditation, self-hypnosis, the relaxing bath, and guided imagery. Start one or more immediately free of charge. Then get a notebook and pen and create the stress and blessing journals described in Weeks 1 and 3 of the Three-Week Cure. Especially important will be your ability to recognize stress triggers and learn new ways of coping with them. Because it sounds like stress has taken over your home, I would calm down the house itself by making a small shrine in your living room honoring the blessings your family has experienced over the years. Treasured photos, of course, but also little *tchotchkes,* like somebody's graduation ribbon, baby's rubber ducky, and a recipe from grandmother. Visit your shrine daily to be reminded of all you have and to give thanks.

Finally, find yourself a private spot outside your home, ideally in a place of nature. A park bench can do nicely, adjacent to some grass or flowers. Make this place "yours" in your heart. Care for it; plant a few seeds. If the weather is dry, water it. Try to visit your nature place at least daily and when you're there, practice the breathing exercise described on page 217. You might consider using your twenty-minute brisk walk to get to your nature place, receiving the benefits of stress-protective serotonin along the way.

WORKING ALONE

ACUPRESSURE AND SHIATSU

It's pitch dark in your living room. You bang your shin hard against the edge of a coffee table, and for a moment you actually see stars. Then you reach down and rub the sore spot; within seconds you actually feel a little better. Although you may not think you've just entered a field of alternative medicine, you're performing acupressure.

Touch heals, even when it's your own. You press your fingers against your temples when you feel a headache surge, you hold both hands over your lower abdomen for menstrual cramps, you instinctively rub the back of your neck when you feel tense. And here's the best part of acupressure: you don't have to pay anyone to do this. It's self-care *par excellence.*

The idea that finger and hand pressure could actually accomplish something predates acupuncture by 2,500 years. Doctors in ancient China introduced needles to enhance acupressure's fingertip pressure. Because of this, the rules of traditional Chinese medicine (p. 285) apply to acupressure. The body's vital energy, or *chi,* flows through channels called meridians. When the channels go out of kilter, the energy flow slows down or excessively speeds up. In a system like this, the goal of maintaining good health, as well as healing symptoms, is to balance the flow of *chi.* If you're totally healthy, say doctors of Chinese medicine, your *chi* flows freely, like water through pipes.

Along the fourteen meridian paths are 365 individual points that open the meridian when pressure is applied or an acupuncturist inserts a needle. Each point is named according to its channel and by a number.

Most of the acupressure in China is done for acute illnesses and as first aid for injuries. Acupuncture generally is reserved for more chronic medical problems. In the United States, many people use acupressure for stress reduction, pain relief, and improvement of overall well-being. By and large, acupressure is a self-administered therapy. Since the points are identical to those in acupuncture, practitioners of Chinese medicine can perform it, but generally limit it to patients who become excessively anxious at the sight of a needle. For this reason, you don't find a lot of practitioners who specialize in acupressure. If you search for an acupressurist on the Internet, for example, you'll usually locate a Shiatsu practitioner instead (see p. 210).

DO IT YOURSELF

There's a right way to press on a point and here's how: you'll be using your thumb, finger, palm, or knuckle. If finger, choose the middle one, as it's the strongest. You have to push firmly; don't wimp out, but don't be a masochist either. It's supposed to be a "good" hurt, but if you don't press fairly hard, nothing is going to happen.

Your first press should be for a slow count of twenty; release gently and repeat, adding twenty until your final push holds for about a minute and a half. This translates to four separate pushes, each successive one a count of twenty longer than the one preceding it (20–40–60–80). Acupressure points follow a left-right symmetry, so upon completing a spot on one side, repeat on the other.

Two other techniques are important. If you're treating points in large muscles, like your calf or thigh, firmly massage the area first with the heel of your hand. This will loosen the muscle and allow you better access to the acupressure point. If a point is located just beneath your skin, such as a scalp or facial point, tap the area quickly with two fingers before applying fingertip or thumb pressure.

You can learn acupressure techniques for stress reduction, anxiety control, energy enhancement, and overall good health from a variety of acupressure do-it-yourself books. There'll be diagrams of the meridians, with labeled dots indicating acupressure points. If you have some misgivings about exactly where your points are located, visit a licensed acupuncturist and have her perform a full traditional Chinese medicine evaluation. She'll ask you about your medical history, check your pulses and tongue for further diagnostic information, and give you an acupuncture treatment. At the end of the session, ask what points you yourself might use for acupressure self-treatment. She can dot them with a skin marker and show you what kind of pressure is needed.

A self-treatment from an acupressure text would read something like this: "For stress reduction, press and hold P-6 with your thumb, take a few deep breaths, and release. Repeat three times, increasing the length of pressure each time. Follow this by firm pressure at the spot between your eyebrows." You'd discover that P-6 is on the underside of your wrist, about an inch below the palm of your hand. Some other commonly used points:

- **FOR STRESS,** B-38, between your shoulder blades at the level of your heart (you needn't contort yourself, just lie on a pair of tennis balls).

- **FOR TENSION HEADACHE** and to induce sleepiness, work GB-20, beneath the back of your skull, two inches outward from the midline.

- **FOR FRONTAL HEADACHES,** go for LI-4, treated by pinching the webbing between your forefinger and thumb.

Now before you roll your eyes and snort in disbelief, believe me, I've tried acupressure personally and it's extremely effective.

SHIATSU

Shiatsu is a Japanese form of acupressure. All the Shiatsu practitioners I've met wear a nifty white robe with a black belt that definitely enhances the drama of your treatment session. You'll be fully clothed and lie on the floor on a mat. Beginning with your abdomen, the practitioner will touch certain areas of your body to determine where most of your tension lies. The treatment will focus on these areas, releasing blocked energy and restoring energy flow. As the Shiatsu treatment continues, you may experience some strange but not unpleasant sensations in your body, like a loud gurgle in your stomach or a quiver through some muscles as you release tension. Sometimes, if the practitioner releases tension caused by an emotional trauma from the past, you may suddenly and unexpectedly start crying. This is all part of your healing process and a good Shiatsu practitioner will be compassionate and support you through it.

At the end of your Shiatsu session, you may feel very relaxed and want to drift off to sleep. The sense of well-being that follows your treatment may last as long as a week.

AROMATHERAPY

You've probably seen one of those aromatherapy displays in health food stores and thought, "One of these days, I'm going to learn something about aromatherapy." I must admit that being confronted with the forty-odd different oils put me off aromatherapy for a long time. Here we're going to keep it simple and quickly eliminate thirty-five of the forty oils—not that they don't serve good purposes. If after trying the first five you decide to take up aromatherapy seriously, you can always explore the other scents. But good oils cost about ten dollars a bottle, so you want to be informed when buying. The five oils that alleviate stress, tension, and frazzled nerves are lavender, geranium, melissa, clary sage, and ylang-ylang. Breathe a little bit of each and see if one calls out to you. If you need some direction and you're going to try a single oil for relaxation, start with lavender.

While you're still in the store, get a small bottle of unscented carrier oil, like sweet almond oil (you'll need it later) and a simple diffuser. The easiest diffuser is a device that positions a shallow dish above a candle. A few drops of the oil placed in the dish and heated will fill a room with the oil's aroma.

AT HOME WITH YOUR SCENTS

Home with a few bottles of essential oils, you can:

- Simply open the bottle and inhale the scent, or shake a drop or two into a hand-kerchief and carry it with you, breathing deeply from it when tension knocks. For a less intense effect, use your candle-operated diffuser.

- Make an aromatherapy massage oil by adding just a few drops to a small amount of the carrier oil. Gently rub it into your tense muscles, like your neck and upper back. Then lie down and listen to some soft music. If you're planning a visit to a massage therapist (p. 236), take your personalized massage oil with you.

- Add the oils to your bath. Adding eight to fifteen drops of an essential oil to your bath after the water has finished running creates a relaxing atmosphere and allows the oil to seep into your skin. It's best not to use soap in an aromatherapy bath, be-cause it may interfere with the absorption of the oil.

RECIPE FOR A RELAXING BATH

In showers, we wash up and exit. In baths, we can luxuriate. Baths have an unde-niable ritual aspect about them. You may never be Cleopatra, who luxuriated in baths of hot milk, or lie back in heated wine, like Mary, Queen of Scots, but a slow warm soak can make bath time the most peaceful part of your day, an es-cape from noise, worry, and tension. Your muscles relax and your mind wanders.

- **PLAN AHEAD.** This is your time. Turn off your phone, get a sitter for the kids, tell your partner to take a hike. Don't rush through your bath because dinner needs to be prepared or you've got theater tickets.

ACUPRESSURE AND THE TRIPLE WHAMMY

In addition to acupressure's ability to relieve stress, it can be extremely effective as part of the treatment for any of the Triple Whammy Disorders. For example, the painful trigger points of fibromyalgia or the jaw tightness of TMJ can melt away with regular acupressure. Anytime I recommend using traditional Chinese medi-cine for a Triple Whammy disorder, you can take this to mean that acupressure can also help. Get your specific points from a reference book or an acupuncturist. Then perform your acupressure ritual daily for at least two weeks, then every other day for two weeks, and, finally, as often as needed.

- **GET THE BATHROOM READY.** You want everything as comfy as possible before you slide into the tub. Have plenty of fluffy towels at hand. Make sure you haven't left your robe somewhere else in the house. Light a candle. Have a soft eye mask ready. Put on a CD (not near the water!). A glass of wine might complete the ritual.

- **TEST THE WATER TEMPERATURE.** Use your foot, not your hand. Your foot is much more sensitive to temperature.

- **USE A DRAIN BLOCK AND A BACK PILLOW.** Buy these two very useful items from a bath and bed store. You'll be able to fill the tub to the very brim and lean back with something soft to support your neck.

- **WITH THE TUB FULL, ADD YOUR ESSENTIAL OILS.** The hot water and the warm, steamy room will yield the richest effect from just a few drops added to your bath. As you soak, the oils will soften your skin while the scented air calms your mind. Try one oil alone, or combine two or more of them. Close your eyes, inhale, and empty your mind. Combine your bath with guided imagery (p. 214) or meditation (p. 215) for an extraordinary escape from your hectic life.

AROMATHERAPY AND THE TRIPLE WHAMMY

Many women with Triple Whammy disorders are more chemically sensitive than others and frequently experience side effects from medicines unless the dose is reduced to pediatric levels. Your sense of smell is especially acute. Maybe you feel nausea from the odor of cigarette smoke, newsprint, or nail polish and you regularly toss out the perfumed pages found in magazines. This sensitivity can work to your advantage if you learn the fundamentals of aromatherapy and use them to dramatically reduce daily tension and stress.

BIOFEEDBACK, GUIDED IMAGERY, AND MEDITATION

Each of these techniques, when done regularly, has been proven unequivocally to have a calming effect on both mind and body. Each is also very portable—once you've learned how to enter a relaxed state you can do it on the bus heading for work, in your gynecologist's stirrups, in an airplane at 35,000 feet, or just before you're called in for your job interview.

BIOFEEDBACK

For many years, scientists thought that many functions inside the body were beyond voluntary control. Although it's certainly possible to slow down your breathing or relax your muscles at will, researchers thought it quite another matter to lower your blood pressure, slow your heart rate, or change the temperature on the surface of your skin. The invention of biofeedback devices almost forty years ago disproved this thinking forever.

A biofeedback device measures some of the functions of your body that change during states of stress. Some examples: when you're anxious, your skin temperature cools and your heart rate speeds up. When you calm down your skin warms, your heart rate slows. Articles in conventional medical journals that reported that biofeedback successfully reduced migraine severity began appearing more than ten years ago and now some health insurers cover treatments.

Now, let's say you're holding in your cold, stressed hand a skin temperature sensor, attached to a small biofeedback device that reflects your temperature by a series of colored lights, ranging in color from red to green. (The device is really no larger than a cell phone.) Your cold hand causes the red to light up. You breathe deeply, relax, calm your thoughts, the red goes out, and an orange light appears. During real relaxation, you "reach the green" and hold it there for a few minutes. And then it will dawn on you. You are indeed feeling calmer and more relaxed, your muscles less tense, your mind clearer.

To me, the best part of biofeedback is that when you get reasonably adept with the device, you can dispense with it altogether and reach that state of relaxation on your own. Then, at various times throughout your day, if you can find a quiet place for only a few minutes, you can achieve that sense of peace and release the internal tension you drearily carry with you like some backpack filled with rock samples.

Like early computers, biofeedback devices were once large, expensive affairs and a requisite computer nerd (or "biofeedback practitioner") had to sit next to you to incessantly adjust a dial or tighten your headband. Today you can find excellent biofeedback devices with simple instruction manuals on the Internet for less than $100. Type "biofeedback" into your search engine and brace yourself for an onslaught of hype. Just get one that looks easy to use because they're all pretty similar. Two excellent units are ThoughtStream and GSR2, both available online. Work with the device until you feel confident you can achieve and hold the relaxed state on your own. Then use throughout your day as needed.

GUIDED IMAGERY

The first studies using guided imagery appeared about the same time as biofeed-back, when researchers were exploring the powers of the mind and how it acted on the physical body. With guided imagery, you deliberately and consciously use the power of your imagination to create positive images (called healing visual-izations) that will trigger healthful changes within. The whole concept of guided imagery works because whether your brain pictures something or actually expe-riences it, the physiological effects are very similar.

Let's pretend that last year you took a Caribbean vacation and remember the total bliss and relaxation you felt in the warm sun, lying on the beach, sipping your piña colada just served by that delectable waiter. Now if you go into a quiet and darkened room, and get into a very comfortable chair, you can actually transport your mind to that beach. Brush aside all other thoughts, turn off the phone, and think carefully and completely how you felt that very day. In a few minutes, you might even recall the taste of the piña colada, the smell of the sun block slathered on your skin, the warmth of the sun on your body. If you're head-ing in the right direction, you have recreated what your mind and body felt that lovely day one long year ago.

Psychotherapists are now routinely using guided imagery during patient ses-sions with excellent results, but you can easily do this on your own. My own pa-tients have done best using audio tapes or CDs that are now available for just about every illness and human frailty imaginable. Unlike biofeedback, where some effort is required, guided imagery is passive. You simply allocate some time in a private place, pop in a tape or CD, and lie back. You'll hear soothing music, and then a very relaxing voice guiding your imagination to a place of healing and wellness. You may even fall asleep, so NEVER listen to a guided imagery tape while driving.

And again, like biofeedback, you'll soon be able to reach that relaxed state without the tape and without the comfortable chair in your quiet room.

Among the numerous guided imagery tapes available, I do have two recom-mendations. My patients have been using two series, one recorded by Belleruth Naparstek, the other by Alexandra Dickerman, for many years. Belleruth's cata-log is online at www.healthjourneys.com and includes "General Wellness," "Re-duce Anxiety," and even "Fibromyalgia and Chronic Fatigue." Alexandra, at www.soulvoices.org, lists CDs for deep relaxation, preparation for surgery, and weight loss. There are many other excellent guided imagery recordings available, but these are the ones we've used most frequently, and with excellent results.

MEDITATION

Requiring no devices, meditation is the simplest of the relaxation techniques to explain, and by far the hardest to master. Like acupuncture, yoga, sushi bars, and Thai restaurants, meditation comes to us from the East, via religious practices that required quiet contemplation in order to induce a state of tranquility. The three most popular meditation techniques are breath meditation, mindfulness meditation, and transcendental meditation (TM).

- **BREATH MEDITATION** asks you to sit quietly, empty your mind, and focus only on the act of breathing in and breathing out in order to clear the mind. It sounds pretty simple, but like any discipline it takes practice. Breath meditation requires that you sit comfortably in a chair, eyes closed, breathing in and out, focusing only on your inhalations and exhalations. Breathe from your belly, placing a hand there to feel its rise and fall with each breath. Keeping your mind empty of thoughts can be the greatest challenge, and if your mind wanders, don't berate yourself; just return your attention to your breathing. Many of us are so overcommitted that our minds wander to our "to do" list—the laundry, the birthday gift that needs buying, the report that needs to be finished. Remind yourself before you start that all those obligations will be waiting for you after your meditation is completed.

- **MINDFULNESS MEDITATION,** as developed by Jon Kabat-Zinn, director of the Stress Reduction Clinic at the University of Massachusetts, involves intensely focusing on the present moment, acknowledging thoughts as they appear, and observing the thoughts without judgment. The goal with mindfulness meditation is to become increasingly aware of events within your body. The technique may include a "body scan" in which you focus on each body part, starting from your head and working downward. As you release images associated with each body part, you release associated tension.

- **IN TRANSCENDENTAL MEDITATION (TM),** introduced by the Beatles' guru, Maharishi Mahesh Yogi, in the 1960s, you repeat to yourself a single word or sound (called a mantra) throughout the meditation. This allows you to focus your thinking and achieve a state of calm.

These days, meditation is embraced by conventional medicine as a perfectly acceptable means of lowering blood pressure, reducing pain, helping to alleviate migraines, remedying menstrual cramps, and, most important, reducing stress and anxiety. Not surprisingly, people who engage in regular meditation go through life in a calmer state, live longer, develop fewer chronic illnesses, are hospitalized less often, and take fewer prescription medications.

You can learn meditation through an assortment of books, tapes, or in groups at colleges, community centers, and hospitals. A typical tape guides you through a thirty-minute meditation. Ultimately it's recommended that you meditate twice daily, in two twenty-minute sessions, once before breakfast and once at bedtime.

BIOFEEDBACK, GUIDED IMAGERY, MEDITATION, AND THE TRIPLE WHAMMY

When using creative imaging to heal yourself, use your imagination. For example, picture your painful fibromyalgia trigger points as red hot circles on your body and as you relax, imagine them changing from red to orange to a cool and soothing blue. If you're depressed, picture yourself in a bleak gray day and visualize the clouds parting, sun beaming through, and flowers appearing around you.

EXERCISE

Without a doubt, one of the best ways to handle stress on a day-to-day basis is through exercise. Of course, eating, smoking, drinking diet soda, and watching TV seem so much easier. But one of the reasons women outlive men is because they're more aware of the importance of exercise and act accordingly. Because of the effect of exercise on serotonin, many women are also aware of the good feeling and de-stressing they feel after an exercise session. If you're already exercising regularly, read the rest of this Stress-Relief Menu and choose something new to try—Reiki, massage, t'ai chi—in addition to your workout.

Basic truth, like it or not: we all need regular exercise. I don't think there's anyone remaining in the United States who doesn't know this. But for anyone just emerging from a cave, here's a quick list of the benefits of exercise: overall your health will improve pretty dramatically (especially your heart, lungs, muscle strength, blood pressure, and cholesterol), as will your sense of well-being, the quality of your sleep, and your energy level. If you're exercising regularly, you might recall the moment you made a commitment to change things. You might also remember the event that triggered the gasping, "Boy, am I out of shape!"

THE WRONG WAY, THE RIGHT WAY

If you're just getting started, there are two ways to go about it. I'll begin by telling you my own path as an example of the wrong way. When I joined my local health club in my thirties, the last time I had actually done anything physically challenging may have been in fourth grade. So not without some trepidation, I signed up for Beginning Aerobics, and in my spanking new sweat suit found myself in the midst of thirty or so women, most of whom in my opinion looked pretty fit already. That I was the sole male didn't bother me as much as it should have because I distinctly remembering thinking something about "we guys have more endurance and more muscle mass anyway."

This was my last coherent thought.

No more than ten minutes into a routine that had me bouncing around like a Rockette, I was drenched with sweat, gasping for air, and had turned the color of my gray sweat suit. The instructor took me aside and asked, "You've never done this before, have you?" before leading me into a corner to do some pathetic, wimpy stretches.

Here's the right way to start an exercise program: if you're under thirty-five and your health is good, you should feel free to start an exercise program with-

BREATHING OUT STRESS

This breathing out stress exercise can be done when you're all alone with eyes closed in a quiet place or when chaos seems to surround you (rush hour traffic), but with your eyes open and hands on the wheel, please. Sit quietly in a straight backed chair with your eyes closed, palms down on your thighs. Now breathe in slowly, through your nose, filling your lungs from the bottom to the top. Focus on your belly, letting it relax and expand outward as you breathe in. Then, slowly exhale through your mouth. Repeat ten times.

out a medical check-up. Everyone else should have a quick exam beforehand, and enjoy the congratulations you'll receive from your doctor for starting. Realize of course that from this visit on, every time she sees you she'll be asking, "So how's the exercise program going?"

Then start slowly. Your physical fitness program will start producing four significant returns almost from the day you start:

- **WITH IMPROVED HEART AND LUNG ENDURANCE,** you'll no longer gasp at climbing a flight of stairs or walking your golden retriever.

- **BETTER MUSCLE STRENGTH** improves your posture as the core muscles in your torso strengthen, lifting and lengthening your midsection.

- **BUILDING MUSCULAR ENDURANCE** will allow you to participate in some really enjoyable sports like bicycling, kayaking, and kickboxing, and will give you a brilliant form during t'ai chi (p. 228). Remember, everything physical doesn't happen at a health club.

- **AND LAST, IMPROVED FLEXIBILITY** will allow you to tie your shoes even after you've grown old.

There's a fifth and utterly important payoff in that you get better body composition. A fitness program will slow down and even reverse that otherwise inexorable shift of your body composition from muscle to fat. I always have hated thinking about that, waking up each morning with just a little more fat and a little less muscle. And with more muscle, you burn more calories at rest, producing more energy and feeling more energetic.

Keeping in mind these four basic goals of a fitness program, if you consciously plan to include some of each of the following each week, you'll cover everything you need. And remember that you can do your daily twenty-minute walk outside in conjunction with these other recommendations. Patients frequently ask me what I would consider a reasonable exercise program. Physician members of the American Holistic Medical Association really try to live up to their own recommendations, so what follows is pretty much what I do myself, three times a week at my local health club:

- **WARM YOURSELF UP.** Begin with a ten-minute warm-up. Stretch your body in every direction, which encourages flexibility, rolling your neck toward each shoulder and to the front and back. Walk a little, twirl your arms about, do some knee lifts. This alerts the rest of your body that it will be busy during the next hour or so.

- **STRENGTHEN YOUR MUSCLES.** Follow your warm-up with twenty minutes of muscle strengthening. Your best bet here is to use free weights, available in many sizes, from one pound on up. Just make sure all muscle groups are covered. On days you aren't up to muscle strengthening, try instead to . . .

- **INCREASE YOUR MUSCULAR ENDURANCE.** Again, you want a twenty-minute session aimed at endurance. Use the exercise machines. You want to perform three sets of eight repetitions each, again covering all the major muscle groups, each week steadily increasing the resistance.

- **IMPROVE YOUR CARDIAC FITNESS.** The all-important cardiorespiratory endurance, thirty minutes, three times a week, strengthens your heart and lungs. A variety of activities satisfies this requirement: jogging, alternating walking and running, elliptical training, stairmaster, NordicTrack, treadmill, exercise bicycle, aerobic class, swimming, racquetball, tennis, and dancing.

- **COOL DOWN.** At the end of a workout, cool down for about five minutes by just walking around and stretching some more.

What this comes to takes a little more than one hour. It's pretty standard stuff, what a personal fitness trainer might suggest. You can vary this quite a bit, like during the summer skipping a session to go on a ninety-minute bike ride or out for a jog. Remember that sticking with a single activity, like jogging, is not a good idea because you need to vary the challenges to your muscles.

It actually doesn't make a whole lot of difference what time of day you exercise. Surveys show most people exercise after work, apparently to de-stress and unwind, but many of my patients exercise first thing in the morning to rev up their engines. In addition, try to add a few hidden exercises throughout your day, every day. Each of these is a great calorie burner:

- Park your car far from your destination and walk. Better yet, get rid of your car altogether and walk, bike, or take public transportation everywhere. If you do take public transportation, exit early and walk in.

- Take the stairs instead of the elevator—every day

- Get away from your desk and do stretches several times a day

- Walk faster

- Carry your own packages

- Do all your own gardening and lawn care

- Plan vacations that involve physical activity, like biking, camping, or kayaking

The real key to success with physical fitness is to keep going, making your exercise program into a habit. Don't give up if you miss a day or two; just get back on track the next day. Vary your program, both inside and outdoors, never allowing bad weather to prevent you from doing something, even if it means shoveling snow (a great exercise!).

And finally, be patient. If you're out of shape it's going to take a few weeks to regain what years of TV watching have cost you. It took me about eight weeks to finally survive one complete aerobics class. But at the end of those two months, an exercise habit kicked in that's remained with me for many years, mostly because it makes me feel so good.

EXERCISE AND THE TRIPLE WHAMMY

Because exercise generates feel-good endorphins—including serotonin—doing it regularly relieves stress and eases depression, improves the quality of your sleep, increases mental sharpness, and bolsters your ability to cope with difficult situations. I suspect that women feel the effects of the serotonin boost more dramatically than men simply based on what I see at virtually every health club I've visited. Namely, on the machines that require real work, like the treadmills and the ellipticals, 90 percent of users seem to be women. Meanwhile, over in the corner, the men hang around talking about the Cubs. Then, every once in a while, one of them will lift some weights, dry himself off, and go watch the TV.

FLOWER ESSENCE THERAPY

I first encountered flower remedies some years back when visiting a couple who had recently lost a long-awaited infant by miscarriage. Although their home was very much a place of mourning, they bore their grief with fortitude. At one point during the conversation, they brought out a small bottle, placed a few drops under each other's tongues, and continued with the conversation. I had to ask.

They were using Bach's Rescue Remedy, they answered, a combination of several of Bach's homeopathic flower remedies. Handing me the bottle to inspect, they added that Rescue Remedy should be in everyone's medicine chest. Just as the name implied, I was told how the contents of the little bottle could calm the spirit and restore the soul during times of greatest distress. After a little research into this, I learned that Rescue Remedy works the way everything else seems to work in alternative medicine: by stabilizing the body's vital energies (*chi* in Chinese medicine). With energies balanced, peace is restored to the soul.

Conventional medicine would have given the young couple some tranquilizers, which we doctors shove down people's throats by the ton. Of course, tranquilizers (the preferred term is now antianxiety agents) make you feel tranquil to the point of fogginess. But restoratives to the soul? Nothing like that figures anywhere in the *Physicians' Desk Reference,* not even as a side effect.

Bach Flower remedies are available in health food stores in a neat little display of identical tiny bottles bearing lovely names like Sweet Chestnut, Clematis, Rock Rose, and Star of Bethlehem: thirty-eight plants from the British Isles, plus the combination Rescue Remedy. Modern day spin-offs from the original Bach Remedies have been extracted from other plant species and even from rocks and gems. You can work with a Bach Flower practitioner if you like but, really, if you're willing to ponder the emotional issues in your life and you're open to alternative therapies, you can use Bach remedies on your own.

Edward Bach was a British homeopathic physician during the early part of the twentieth century. The homeopathic approach evaluates a patient's symptoms and cures them by administering a minuscule amount of something that could induce the same symptom if given in large amounts to a healthy person ("Like cures like"). Bach added to this the principle that emotional turmoil can result in disease. The key to both preventing and treating illness, Bach felt, should begin on the emotional level. He wisely perceived that emotional states such as chronic grief, loneliness, hypersensitivity, and lack of confidence could be underlying reasons for chronic health disorders. Bach would agree with what I call the "whammy of stress" as a source of ill health, but would go a step further and ask, "Yes, but why are you so stressed? Is it unresolved grief, or endlessly being hurried, or simply feeling overwhelmed with life?" If you want to make progress on your personal healing path, these unhealthful psychological traits need to be addressed.

But just how do you go about treating greed, jealousy, and boredom with life? Bach set about this by homeopathic "provings." He experimented on himself, placing under his tongue the dew from a variety of English plants, and then entering an almost meditative state to determine what physical and emotion sensations were surfacing.

Almost every plant yielded up a variety of physical and emotional sensations, but only thirty-eight plants produced emotional symptoms alone. These thirty-eight became the basis of Bach Flower remedies, designed for healing emotional issues only, never for physical ones. Since the 1970s, hundreds of other provings by practitioners around the world have yielded a veritable library of flower essence remedies, now used for both physical and emotional problems.

For your personal use, staying with Bach's original thirty-eight remedies is quite sufficient. If you like the results, you may later want to work with a certified flower essence therapist, who'll spend a lot of time exploring your physical and emotional symptoms and then put together a personalized combination from the hundreds of essences currently available. For example, if you take a concentrated form of the flower gentian, you might feel a sense of pessimism and apathy. But if you take a highly diluted solution of gentian, opposite emotions like faith, self-confidence, and optimism would begin to emerge.

Not surprisingly, conventional physicians soundly ostracized Bach for his views. He was removed from the British medical register five years after his books were published and later he voluntarily abandoned his license to practice medicine. Now, seventy years later, flower essence therapies are used worldwide. People use them for self-treatment and an increasing number of holistically oriented psychotherapists and counselors are including them in their practices.

HOW DO I CHOOSE MY REMEDIES?

The Bach Center has prepared a self-help questionnaire to guide you through the remedy selection process. The questionnaire is usually tucked next to the remedy display at health food stores, but you can find it online by searching for "Bach questionnaire." When you work through the questionnaire, you'll need to acknowledge your emotional shortcomings. Although the phrase "I'm self-centered, unfeeling, and generally lazy" does not actually appear in those words anywhere on the questionnaire, you'll be compelled to face your dark side with honesty and candor if you want the remedies to be successful. Anyway, nobody's looking over your shoulder.

Once you've completed the questionnaire, you'll be able to determine the remedies best suited for your emotional state. Most people discover they'll need anywhere from two to six separate essence remedies, reasonably priced at about $8 apiece. The remedies are in a highly concentrated form, and if used correctly, a bottle will last about six months. (By contrast, a month's supply of a typical prescription tranquilizer is almost $100.) While you're at the store, remember to buy an empty dosage bottle. You'll need it to prepare your own remedies.

When you get home, place a few drops of each remedy into your dosage bottle and fill it with distilled water. Remember, in homeopathy, diluting a remedy increases its strength. Then, at least twice a day, place a few drops from your dosage bottle into a small amount of water and sip it slowly. Or, easier still, place a few drops directly under your tongue.

Don't expect a quick fix. Homeopathic remedies work from within, and it may take from two to ten weeks before you begin to perceive changes. Conventionally prescribed tranquilizers work fast but wear off quickly. The action of flower therapies is subtle, but you will perceive a shift from within as negative emotions begin to fade away.

If you've got the courage to confront a few of your stress-causing demons, bring up the questionnaire on your computer and see what remedies are right for you.

FLOWER ESSENCE THERAPY AND THE TRIPLE WHAMMY

Women whose serotonin is very low and who take an antidepressant frequently ask me this: "I really don't want to go off my antidepressant. Can I use flower essence therapies, too?" Flower essence therapies can be combined with your conventional medication and any counseling you may be having.

REFLEXOLOGY

I personally postponed trying reflexology myself because of extreme ticklishness. Just the thought of something other than a floor or a pair of socks touching the soles of my feet sent shivers up and down my spine. But the soles of the feet are connected to the meridians of Chinese medicine, so I bit the bullet and located a certified reflexologist. I clambered into his chair, chatted as he worked on my feet, but was also aware that every muscle in my body was becoming more and more relaxed. Unlike my acupuncture experience, where I actually fell deeply asleep, with reflexology I simply felt all physical stress vanish from my body.

A SHORT HISTORY OF REFLEXOLOGY

Let's face it. It feels good when someone's rubbing your feet. You can trace foot massage as therapy back to ancient Egypt and China. Despite conventional medicine's scorn of reflexology as a therapy for anything, I'm pleased to tell you it was an American ear-nose-throat specialist, William Fitzgerald, MD, who discovered that if you applied pressure to the fingers and toes, you could relieve pain in areas like the neck, face, and mouth. After discovering the effect of applying pressure, Fitzgerald then divided the body into ten zones—five on each side of the body—each zone terminating in a single finger and toe. He named what he had discovered "Zone Therapy."

Fitzgerald was little appreciated by his conventional colleagues, who tried to take away his medical license. Later, a massage therapist, Eunice Ingham, mapped areas of the hands and feet that she felt "connected" with internal organs. She then developed techniques of foot and hand massage that could selectively treat affected areas. Ingham termed the various points on the hands and feet "reflexes," and massaging these points sent energy flow up through Fitzgerald's zones. She also renamed zone therapy "reflexology."

In traditional Chinese medicine (p. 285), the zones would correspond to meridians. In fact, the idea that the body can be mapped out on the hands and feet has its roots in Chinese medicine. Reflexologists believe that stimulating certain points (reflexes) will allow the body's natural energies (*chi*) to flow freely and trigger natural healing processes. These practitioners don't diagnose or treat any specific illness. Rather, when they perform an initial evaluation to the hands and feet, they are literally feeling for blockages to the natural energy flow, which they describe as "lumpy" or "gritty" sensations to their own fingertips.

Seeing a picture of the hand and foot with its reflexes mapped out helps show all this better than my description. You can view a reflexology map online by just typing "reflexology map" into your search engine. Health food stores offer wallet-sized reflexology cards.

There are several schools for reflexology and quite a few people have become certified reflexologists. Many are massage therapists who've wanted to expand their areas of expertise. A typical introductory session with a reflexologist will include a discussion about your health issues and concerns, and then a slow and careful examination called a "thumb walk," which you can actually learn to do yourself.

With a thumb walk, you use the outside edge of your thumb to take little steps, or bites, up and down the sole and sides of the feet, repeating the process on the palms of your hands. This allows you to place pressure on individual points. According to practitioners, when you get good at it, you'll actually feel areas of blockage and dysfunction during the thumb walk. The reflex areas are small, so the "bites" must be small as well.

An actual treatment session will focus on those newly revealed blocked zones, using a variety of techniques, including rubbing the zone with a hard object like a golf ball. The key is to apply sufficient pressure, and that means you might actually feel a little (but not a lot of) pain. It's a "good" hurt, though, as it releases blockages.

Reflexology lends itself well to self-treatment and there are many instruction manuals on how to care for yourself or family members. Reflexologists encourage preventive maintenance, and a treatment session may end with instructions on how to do a little work on your feet every day. If you go to a health club or day spa, you might inquire if the massage therapist is trained in reflexology; many of them are. Otherwise, self-care reflexology is worth exploring. A few minutes every day can really make a difference in your life.

REFLEXOLOGY AND THE TRIPLE WHAMMY

Reflexology lends itself well as part of self-care for a Triple Whammy disorder because a reflexology chart allows you to focus on specific areas of your body. For example, for PMS, you'd treat the brain (pituitary gland), breasts, uterus, and ovary areas. For irritable bowel syndrome, again your brain, but this time also your large and small intestines. The easiest way to give yourself a regular treatment is to use an indelible skin marker, drawing the anatomical correlations on the sole of each foot. Then, whenever you have a moment of privacy, give yourself a five- or ten-minute treatment.

SELF-HYPNOSIS

The power of suggestion surrounds us constantly, and as a general rule doesn't instigate healthy behavior. Advertisers endlessly remind us that we need to buy objects we don't need and eat large portions of unhealthy food, but many years ago, psychologists learned that through hypnosis, the deliberately induced power of suggestion, they could reverse unhealthy habits. Using hypnotherapy, smokers are able to toss out their cigarettes and anxious people relax. Self-hypnosis is a lot like guided imagery (p. 214) at a deeper level. You can purchase dozens of excellent self-hypnosis tapes and CDs on the Internet. Or you can record one yourself.

Your tape will be approximately twenty to thirty minutes long. Lying down comfortably in a quiet room, where you can remain undisturbed for a half hour, you'll record something like the following. (By the way, the three paragraphs that follow are not original. I found them written on a yellowed piece of paper in an alternative medicine book I acquired at a garage sale several years ago. Luckier people at garage sales have uncovered copies of the Declaration of Independence in the backs of framed pictures, but I think this script is very good and credit whoever wrote it with a heartfelt thanks.)

"Breathe slowly and deeply through your nostrils. Allow your mind to travel throughout your body and start relaxing yourself from your head downward. Relax the top of your head, your eyebrows, eyelids, and face. Especially relax that tension spot between your eyebrows.

"Relax your jaw, neck, shoulders, arms, hands, and fingers. Exhale and inhale slowly five times, permitting your tummy to rise and fall.

"Relax your chest, stomach, abdomen, lower back, hips, thighs, calves, ankles, feet, and toes. Feel your inhalations and exhalations coursing through your entire body, like a cleansing breeze. Concentrate only on your breathing, as every muscle in your body remains in a totally relaxed state. Expel from your body all tension, anxieties, and worries, and continue to breathe slowly and deeply."

From there, your voice on the tape can begin to count slowly backward from 100. This is called a "deepening," wherein you begin to tap into your unconscious. When you reach the number one, your voice will read the suggestion or suggestions you wish to instill in your mind. People write their own scripts for de-stressing, stopping cigarettes, eating less. Here's an example:

"In the past, I have always been a tense and anxious person. This has been caused by my fears of the unknown. But I really am a courageous person, and I can survive . . . and thrive. My anxieties and fears have chipped away at my courage and have prevented me from making my best decisions. Worries and anxieties have kept me from my dreams and goals. From this time forward, I will not allow myself to be afraid. I will face all crises with calm and good judgment. Each day, I will spend a few minutes in quiet calm and focus, and when I feel a surge of anxiety, I'll say aloud, 'This is not me. This is not who I am. I am a calm and wise person, and will exercise good and careful judgment. And when I awaken, stress and anxiety will be banished from my life. I will not allow fear-based emotions to dominate my life again.'"

Now it will be time to awaken yourself. You can do this quite easily by recording:

"It is now time to wake up. At 'one,' you feel yourself slowly emerging from your deep sleep. ONE. At 'two,' you'll feel energy coursing through your body. TWO. And at 'three,' you'll wake up completely, feeling alert, refreshed, and energetic. You will remember the lessons you have taught yourself. THREE. You are awake."

You might want to lie quietly for a minute or two before you get up. I don't recommend going to sleep afterward, as you'll then associate self-hypnosis with sleep and you'll end up putting yourself to sleep each time, rather than accomplishing anything. Self-hypnosis is a lovely low-tech way to merge the force of positive suggestion with deep relaxation.

SELF-HYPNOSIS AND THE TRIPLE WHAMMY

For decades, doctors have known that suggestion can help in the healing process. One "right" phrase from any healer, conventional or alternative, can work wonders. Consider how you felt when you heard, "You're going to get better." Sufferers of Triple Whammy disorders are familiar with phrases such as, "You'll have to learn to live with it." But for a doctor to say this only reflects a reluctance to make a commitment to deal with a complex health problem. Call this therapy whatever you like—self-hypnosis, self-suggestion, power of mind—you yourself can bring hope, optimism, and courage (three definitely useful traits) into your healing path, and you don't need "permission" from your doctor to do so.

WORKING WITH A GROUP

T'AI CHI

Chi is the invisible life energy flowing through all living things. *Chi* travels down paths called meridians, and the flow can be directed by stimulating certain points on the body, either using fingertip pressure (acupressure, Shiatsu) or needles (acupuncture). This life energy is believed to originate from the sun, which explains why in China t'ai chi is performed outdoors at dawn. It's also connected to breathing and affected by emotions. It can be controlled by the mind, communicated from one person to another, and conducted through inanimate objects. It is for this last reason that t'ai chi classes are often held in city parks, allowing participants to absorb the energy given off by the trees.

THE CRANE AND THE SNAKE

Originally, t'ai chi was developed as a noncombative martial art and, in fact, the full name *t'ai chi chuan* translates to "the supreme way of the fist." My favorite of the several legends about the development of t'ai chi tells of a thirteenth century Taoist monk and martial arts expert, Chang San Feng, who saw from his window a battle between a crane and a snake. The swooping attacks from the crane and the wily, elusive movements of the much smaller snake inspired him to integrate the movements into his martial arts. During the past twenty years, t'ai chi has spread throughout the world, making the liquid, slow, ballet-like movements the most popular form of exercise on the planet.

The basis of t'ai chi is learning what is called "the form." A form is a set of slow and deliberate graceful exercises performed in a definite pattern. The movements of the forms are basically martial arts, and have names like "Kick with the right heel," or "Punch with a concealed fist." There are long forms, which can take anywhere from twenty to sixty minutes to perform, and short forms, rarely taking more than five or ten minutes to complete.

The health benefits from regular practice of t'ai chi have been studied by physicians both in the Orient and the West. It's universally agreed that those who have made t'ai chi a part of their lives are calmer, physically stronger, and more optimistic about life. T'ai chi limbers joints, lowers blood pressure, slows the pulse, improves balance, and speeds recovery from illness. And perhaps most important, engaging in any regular physical activity, such as t'ai chi, usually triggers a person to start paying a bit more attention to other aspects of her health.

Although the movements look easy, they require concentration, patience, and practice. Your reward will be a sense of peaceful calm and harmony as the *chi* moves smoothly throughout your body, reducing stress and anxiety. As an aerobic exercise, t'ai chi is also extremely beneficial, increasing muscle strength, enhancing balance, and improving flexibility.

GETTING STARTED

To get started on this health-enhancing, stress-busting, strength-developing project, you'll need to find a class. Numerous tapes and DVDs are available, but you need an instructor to help you see what you are doing right and wrong. I've tried the tapes myself, but I got quite anxious trying to see exactly what the man on the screen was doing, and then trying to do the movements myself. My living room, with the cats and the kids and the phone and the neighbors, was not exactly conducive to slow graceful meditative movements.

To locate a class, inquire at local health clubs, colleges, city recreation departments, YMCAs, health food stores, or even hospitals. If your town has a martial arts school, check there too—many martial arts students begin their class with several minutes of t'ai chi. One of my patients from a small Illinois town told me she got her class started by talking to the owner of a local Chinese restaurant. It turned out that his elderly father had taught t'ai chi in China and was practicing every morning in the family back yard. Yes, he would be delighted to teach a class!

Perfecting the art of t'ai chi requires patience, focus, and a unity of mind, body, and spirit. Practice is essential. Try to do your t'ai chi at the same time every day: either make it an invigorating start to your morning or practice it after work, to ease the tension from your hectic day. Some people with extra cash choose to learn their t'ai chi in private lessons from a t'ai chi master. I guess this is okay, but there's something about the group energy from a class that is almost palpable. A typical class lasts anywhere between sixty and ninety minutes, and usually begins with fifteen minutes of basic warm-up exercises before you learn the components of a form. Keep in mind that forms are made up of different movements, and that learning a specific form is not easy. A long form can require more than one hundred subtle movements and can take a year or two to learn properly. You can always do some extra practice on your form in the privacy of your home.

Like meditation and yoga, you can learn the very basic principles of t'ai chi in about an hour, and then spend the rest of your incarnation getting them right.

T'AI CHI AND THE TRIPLE WHAMMY

Remember that the natural ways to raise serotonin include exercise and sunlight. A t'ai chi class outdoors, surrounded by nature, breathing fresh, clean air, will boost your feel-good brain chemicals and reduce stress simultaneously. Even people with devastating Triple Whammy disorders such as chronic fatigue syndrome or fibromyalgia can tolerate (and benefit from) a few minutes of t'ai chi daily. Then, each week, add a few more minutes. After three or four months of steady increase, you'll be in charge of your life again.

YOGA

If you want to take a major step in reversing whatever Triple Whammy problem ails you, sign up for a yoga class and stick with it. There are now classes in virtually every town and community large enough to have paved roads. The people who teach and attend yoga classes are some of the nicest people on our planet, and sometimes good health (and other good things) comes about by being around nice people.

There's very little about yoga not to like. It's inexpensive, safe, and there are no pills to swallow. You won't have to deal with health insurance and most people don't need a referral from their doctor (though people who've had a joint replacement should ask their doctors if yoga is permitted). You'll need no special equipment except your body in some loose comfortable clothing and a "sticky mat." This is exactly what it sounds like, and keeps your hands and feet from sliding all over the place. The very best part of yoga is that within a few weeks, your friends will remark on how good you're looking. And so calm and peaceful.

Yoga has been around as long as acupuncture—at least six thousand years—arriving in the United States a little more than one hundred years ago. The word yoga itself means "yoke" or "union" in the ancient language of Sanskrit, and the ultimate goal of yoga is to achieve a state of harmony—a union—among mind, body, and spirit. It's not a cult or religion, but rather a way of looking at life in a more spiritual and meditative way. Whatever your religious beliefs, they'll likely be enhanced by a yoga perspective.

FORMS OF YOGA

Most yoga classes teach Hatha yoga, a system of postures, and the instructor will guide you through some postures (asanas) in each session. Astonishingly, there are over one thousand asanas, ranging from simple quiet sitting to positions that seem impossibly contorted. In addition to Hatha yoga, there are now more than a dozen twentieth century Hatha-based forms of yoga available in larger cities. Iyengar yoga adds some nifty props, like chairs, blocks, and belts. Kripalu yoga emphasizes breath and meditation. Astanga, or power yoga, is a strength and muscle builder. Viniyoga, the precursor of Iyengar and Astanga, is tailored toward a person's body type, and stresses a sense of harmonious healing. And not for the faint of heart or underhydrated, Bikram yoga practices its twenty-six asanas in a room heated to 105 degrees. If you're not in such great shape, think twice about Astanga or Bikram yoga, as these are physically very challenging.

Clinical studies from around the world have shown that students of yoga are healthier than the rest of the population. They have more energy, better strength, muscle, and joint flexibility, are more relaxed, have lower blood pressures, slower pulses, stronger hearts, better sleep, improved digestion, and more positive outlooks on life. Emotionally, yoga students have increased self-awareness, better coping skills, and a more relaxed approach to any stress, whether on the job or in a family crisis. This may be partially due to a slew of the feel-good endorphins, including serotonin, released during yoga postures.

In-person yoga classes are far superior to videotape instruction. You will need some guidance as you learn the postures, and then you'll be able to move along at your own pace. Yoga instructors are not health care professionals and do not have to have formal licenses to teach. It's probably a good idea to ask about an instructor's formal training, certification, and the number of years she's been teaching. Be sure to let your instructor know of any health issues that might require you to vary how you follow the routine she teaches. Some people like a morning session to energize them throughout the day. Others like an evening session for improved sleep. Whatever time you select, arrive with an empty stomach and don't plan to eat for a couple of hours afterward. All classes end with a few minutes of deep relaxation, a roomful of students sprawled comfortably and blissfully across the floor.

Plan on two or three sessions a week and you'll learn some techniques for daily practice as well. Yoga classes are usually about an hour long, and your daily at-home practice can be about twenty to thirty minutes. If you're uncertain which form of yoga is for you, try a few and see which is most appealing. You'll be more inclined to stick with a class that is geographically convenient and fits into your schedule. And like everything else in life, if you go to class regularly for about three weeks, it becomes a habit.

YOGA AND THE TRIPLE WHAMMY

Whatever form of yoga you choose, you'll start feeling relief from Triple Whammy problems after your very first session. The integration of mind and body that results from the postures will allow you to feel a real sense of calm and peacefulness. Stress begins to melt away and you feel yourself becoming centered. Muscle tension disappears and every joint feels more limber and flexible.

WORKING WITH A THERAPIST

COUNSELING

I'm a major proponent of psychological counseling. Let's put it this way: you know you're a pretty complicated person. You've been living with yourself all these years, creating the story of your life. If you ever sat down with a tape recorder with the goal of recording everything you remembered (like the life-assessing character in Samuel Beckett's play *Krapp's Last Tape*), you'd go on for days. If you're willing to acknowledge your complexity, then you know there's simply no way to separate what happens in your body from what goes on in your mind. In fact, lots of my patients can look back on their lives and make a connection between the start of their Triple Whammy symptoms and a significantly stressful period, such as feeling pressured as a youngster at school, going through the divorce of parents or a death in the family, or going away to college. The section Looking for Clues in Your Life Story on page 33 is a good place to start thinking about these things; counseling can help you sort it out and make real strides in getting healthy.

Conventional medicine has been very remiss by not encouraging patients to spend time reflecting on their lives and how reactions to life events might be responsible for health problems. On those occasions when a patient reveals emotional distress, too many doctors feel discomfort and are impatient, trying for a quick psychiatric diagnosis instead, usually choosing either depression or anxiety, and reaching for the latest drug samples. Referrals to psychotherapists, though not overtly discouraged, are rarely chosen as a first option.

So, let's consider that first Whammy again, stress. When you start to list stressors in situations where outside forces apparently control your life, the list can get long: the schoolyard bully when you were a child, lacking a date for the prom, anticipating job interviews, being unhappy with your weight, getting into a toxic relationship, working at a suffocating job. This definition of stress leaves something out, however. Psychotherapy explores the often unasked question, "Why do I keep doing this?"

BEFORE COUNSELING . . . AND AFTER

Here's an image of you before counseling: you're sitting in front of a bookcase endlessly rearranging the volumes, each titled with a variation of "My Perspectives on Life." Same titles, day after day, year after year, pulling a volume out, then squeezing it back in. That's an image of you being stuck. You don't necessarily enjoy titles like *My Physical Symptoms* or *My Inability to Say No*, but there you are. Psychotherapy gives you the tools to get rid of some of the old titles and add some new, positive ones.

What is the relationship between being stuck in some behavior pattern and an actual definable emotional illness, such as clinical depression or panic disorder? To a large extent, it's a matter of degree, of severity of symptoms. If you keep getting involved with abusive men, you need some insight into your behavior patterns—you need some new book titles. But if you're involved with such a man *and* you're having major panic attacks on the way home from work, you need both insight therapy and medication to shore up your fragile neurotransmitters, like serotonin.

When personal insights start surfacing, and you experience a few "Aha!" moments, then your psychotherapy gets extremely interesting. You may even learn that you make choices, no matter how bad they seem on the surface, deliberately to protect you from something else. Maybe you choose abusive men just because these are the only ones you feel comfortable dealing with. And even though the price of your decision may be emotional turmoil like depression or even physical symptoms like fibromyalgia, in the whole system that is you, the choices made sense given your lack of awareness of other options. Those choices were a defense against something you really didn't want to face.

I don't send everyone off for counseling, but remember that many women with chronic Triple Whammy disorders have a life story that contributes significantly to their poor health. There are many stresses in our lives, historical and current, and counseling can be a remarkably effective way to understand all the "books" on your shelf and get you some new titles.

FINDING A THERAPIST

Right up front, don't start with a psychiatrist. Look for a psychologist (PhD), psychotherapist (PsyD), or Licensed Clinical Social Worker (LCSW). Psychiatrists are medical doctors whose major training is now geared toward medication rather than counseling. Because psychologists (as well as clinical social workers and other psychotherapists) can't write prescriptions, they call on psychiatrists mainly when they think their patient needs medication. Second, check credentials and licensing. Anyone, licensed or not, can call herself a counselor. Your family doctor may know a good therapist; support groups are also a good source.

The Internet is a superb resource, with therapists listed along with their areas of expertise. A truly excellent website to learn about counseling is www.about psychotherapy.com. The site's recommendations for finding a psychotherapist, including asking individuals you respect for suggestions, are very good. To find a list of therapists in your area, you can also type "psychotherapy" and the name of your town into your Internet search engine.

Another way to find a therapist is by looking in *Psychology Today,* which has a free directory called "Find a Therapist" that was specifically created so you can locate a therapist in your area and review credentials, philosophy, and even price before you commit. It's at www.psychologytoday.com.

Don't be overwhelmed by the jargon of different therapies. Different terms, although very faddish, will make little difference. The goal of psychotherapy is insight. If you're buffeted by one Triple Whammy disorder or another, just know that, figuratively speaking, it's possible you made a bad left turn and headed down the wrong road. Psychotherapy gives you an opportunity to backtrack, and head down a better one. It really can be quite an adventure.

COMMON OBJECTIONS TO COUNSELING

- **DO I REALLY WANT TO DO THIS?** The phrase "know thyself" endlessly surfaces throughout the history of Western civilization. Even when what you find out might not be the best news, you're better off knowing why you behave the way you do. For example, one of my patients said she had always felt she was stupid. She felt humiliated as long as she could remember, and was endlessly being reminded that she was capable of doing more. Her relationships were spotty, her job history worse. When, after a single session, a psychologist diagnosed her with attention deficit disorder, she burst into tears of relief.

- **I CAN'T AFFORD IT.** There's a good chance you can. If you have health insurance, read the Mental Health Benefits section in your policy carefully. Most people have better coverage than they realize. You may have a deductible and some out-of-pocket expenses, but for heaven's sake, this is your life we're talking about. If you have no health insurance, many therapists offer a fee adjustment that is based on what you're able to pay. Just ask.

- **THERAPY LASTS FOREVER.** It doesn't have to. Major insights can surface in relatively few sessions—something on the order of a few weeks or months. Some people need just a few sessions to help clarify what they've known all along and set a new course.

- **I COME FROM A FAMILY THAT DOESN'T ACKNOWLEDGE EMOTIONAL PROBLEMS AND BELIEVES SEEING A THERAPIST IS FOR WIMPS.** For many people, this is a real part of the problem. Recognize that you are your own person who makes her own decisions; then try a couple sessions with a therapist. You don't have to tell anyone you're seeing a counselor if you choose not to.

- **I TRIED IT ONCE. I DIDN'T LIKE THE THERAPIST.** The "good fit" between people and counselors sometimes requires more than one try. Give it a second chance.

- **WILL IT MAKE ME HAPPIER?** I was hoping you wouldn't ask that. Freud himself said that psychoanalysis wasn't going to make you any happier but at least you'd learn why you are unhappy. At a minimum, every week you get to relate the soap opera that is your life to someone who is interested in what you're saying. And at best, I myself think that if you get that far, you have a chance to change things.

COUNSELING AND THE TRIPLE WHAMMY

If you've got a Triple Whammy disorder, by now you're understanding that simply "taking something" to relieve your symptoms will be a singularly unproductive maneuver in the overall path to getting completely well. Like it or not, you need to dig deeply and uncover the why and how of your illness. If counseling brings up something that's especially painful and you can let go of it after all these years, it's one fibromyalgia muscle knot, or one intestinal cramp, or one migraine headache you've released as well.

MASSAGE AND OTHER BODYWORK THERAPIES

I'm endlessly mystified about the excuses I hear for why my patients don't enjoy an occasional massage. Generally, they boil down to variations on the "I don't deserve such self-indulgent luxury" theme. I especially bristle when a patient reveals that her significant other has just bought his second snowmobile or is heading off on a week-long fishing trip with the boys.

Even physicians from ancient times knew that massage ranks highly as an effective treatment. Ponder this the next time your health insurer denies massage coverage as "medically unnecessary" or your HMO primary care physician refuses to write a referral because she "doubts if it will help anything."

There are more than one hundred different forms of massage and various bodywork therapies. The majority of massage therapists perform a combination of traditional European massage and contemporary Western massage, which are based on Western concepts of anatomy and physiology.

Let's briefly review other bodywork therapies, which fall into two broad categories:

- **THE STRUCTURAL REALIGNMENT AND MOVEMENT INTEGRATION GROUP.** These methods work to integrate the body in relation to gravity, through both manipulations and correction of poor movement patterns, and include Alexander Technique, Feldenkrais Method, and Rolfing.

- **THE "ENERGY" GROUP.** In all of these, the therapist is manipulating invisible energies, like *chi* or *prana,* which follow energy flow patterns (meridians or chakras). Some are from the Orient, like Shiatsu, Tui-Na, or Reiki (p. 239). Others are energy medicine that has been westernized, like Therapeutic Touch (p. 242) and Polarity Therapy.

THE POWER OF TOUCH

To me, by far the most important aspect of massage and other forms of body-work therapy is the healing power of one human being touching another. Physicians have all but forgotten this, or have become so paranoid about malpractice suits that physical contact is limited to a handshake. Alternative practitioners, on the other hand, have no such agonies and virtually all of them will give you a friendly or sympathetic hug when it looks like you need one. In plainest language, touch conveys a sense of caring. It is a form of communication, and within the human body this caring touch will relax your muscles, reduce your output of the stress hormones adrenalin and cortisol, and increase your feel-good endorphins, including the endlessly important serotonin.

The various massage techniques relax tense, stressed, and overworked muscles, improve circulation of both blood and lymphatic fluid to the muscles, and flush out waste products like lactic acid. No shortage of medical research studies has confirmed the health benefits of massage, which to me are "great insights into the obvious." For instance, one was titled "People with Muscle Pain Report More Relief After Massage than People Not Receiving Massage." The most annoying study was recently conducted in a hospice, where people were dying from terminal illness. Researchers proudly reported that people receiving regular daily massages experienced less depression than people who weren't touched at all. Just mulling over a study in which dying people were deliberately deprived of massage makes me want these researchers breaded and deep-fried.

Probably the best way to find a massage therapist is by word of mouth, getting information from someone you trust. Your chiropractor may know a good therapist; you can also look for business cards on the bulletin boards at health food stores and health clubs, check ads in local papers, or go online and enter "massage" and the name of your town into your search engine. Look for a massage therapist who has completed a formal training program and is certified. The American Massage Therapy Association's website (www.amtamassage.org) has an effective "find a massage therapist" search engine. But beyond skills and credentials, you yourself need to feel a healing connection with your therapist. If not, find another.

WHAT YOU CAN EXPECT FROM A MASSAGE SESSION

On your first visit, your therapist will ask what you'd like from massage. You may want stress reduction, pain relief, or just about anything else. She'll inquire into any medical conditions, and ask about your lifestyle and stress levels. Her therapy room itself is usually warm, inviting, and softly lit. She'll play soft music if you wish, or burn a candle for a pleasant scent. She'll ask if you want her to use massage oil, and if she knows some aromatherapy (which many do), she'll discuss her selection.

You'll be asked to disrobe partially or completely, but only to a point where you feel comfortable and not anxious. You'll be given a sheet to drape over areas of your body not being massaged. You'll lie down on a softly padded, sheet-covered table, usually with a special face rest that allows you to lie face-down without turning your head. A typical session lasts anywhere from thirty to sixty minutes.

After the massage, you'll likely feel extremely relaxed and calm, refreshed and restored. Sometimes, previously tense muscles feel a bit achy after a particularly vigorous massage, but this clears up after a day or two. It's helpful to drink a lot of water after a massage to help your body clear away the muscle toxins and waste products that have been released.

Although health insurance companies don't relish paying for something that might give you some actual pleasure, there are some perfectly legal methods to get them to pay for your health-giving massage sessions. Ask your doctor to write a prescription for physical therapy that specifies massage. Your doctor will need to give you a diagnosis, which will be legitimate because somewhere in your body your muscles are tight. On the prescription, the physician will need to write the number of sessions and the number of weeks. Usually, four weekly treatments are prescribed.

You'll have to pay the therapist, but take the paid receipt and submit it for reimbursement, attaching a copy of the prescription. This may or may not work, but it certainly doesn't hurt to try. Insurance companies process tens of thousands of claims daily, and your little claim might slip through. If you're in an HMO, it's harder to get a referral for massage, but nagging your doctor until she wants you out of her sight can be a very effective strategy.

MASSAGE, OTHER BODYWORK THERAPIES, AND THE TRIPLE WHAMMY

For women with Triple Whammy symptoms, regular massage, along with healthful eating and exercise, is a wonderful avenue to health and longevity. Because the effects of massage and bodywork are so positive for both your mind and body, you certainly don't have to wait for something to go wrong before considering massage. Many people budget time and money for regular massages as a means to keep stress from chipping away at the quality of their lives.

REIKI

I've referred patients to Reiki (pronounced "ray-kee") therapists for many years and regard their insights as extremely valuable. If this section seems to carry on a bit much about Reiki, it's because of the good work the therapists have done for so many of my patients. I myself have had several Reiki sessions with different practitioners, the most recent during the very week I wrote this piece. Like all my encounters with Reiki, when the session was over I sat up and said, "That was nothing short of amazing. I'll never be able to explain this to another doctor." But I'll try to explain it to you.

I first heard about Reiki in (of all places) a hospital cafeteria when I was pulled to a quiet corner by a physician who knew I was involved with alternative medicine. She was clearly uneasy with what she was about to tell me. "It's like nothing you've ever experienced," she began. "You actually feel the energy pouring through her hands, and you feel newly strengthened, like a power surge." Then she paused, unsure whether or not her next revelation might permanently damage her career: "I believe this woman can heal."

Physicians frequently ask me if I actually believe all the claims of alternative medicine. "Of course not," I answer, "any more than I believe the claims of the pharmaceutical industry." But too much skepticism can keep some real eye-openers from entering your life.

Reiki is so completely relaxing that I couldn't help dozing off during my own first treatment, which I'd decided to try for a stubbornly aching hip. Then, half-awake, I felt a tingling sensation, like a tiny series of electric shocks, around the painful area and thought to myself, "Oh, she's using an electrical stimulation unit," a piece of equipment used regularly by professional physical therapists. I thought, "Well, it feels good enough, but is it Reiki?" Then I opened my eyes and lifted my head up to see what she was doing. She was sitting next to me, eyes closed, in deep concentration. And her hands were a full inch above my hip. No equipment. Nothing but her hands.

The "rei" of Reiki means "universal" while "ki" is the Japanese form of the word *chi*, the invisible energy coursing through our bodies. As taught in traditional Chinese medicine, acupressure, or t'ai chi, when you're healthy, this energy passes smoothly throughout your entire body, but during any form of ill health there are imbalances, blockages, and depletions that need to be balanced and restored.

Reiki—literally the "universal life-force energy"—connects with the energy of the universe, directs it through your body, balances the flow, and releases the blockages and stresses within both your body and your mind. I have always liked the image of the Reiki practitioner as sort of a human lightning rod who, after entering her own meditative state, directs the life-force "lightning" through her client to awaken a self-healing process.

Reiki was discovered during the nineteenth century by the Japanese Christian minister Mikao Usui, who also studied Buddhism. After a solitary fast and meditation, he felt he had discovered a healing technique that could easily be passed on to others. Usui felt that anyone at all could learn Reiki and, by the year 2000, Reiki students numbered well into the hundreds of thousands.

Although most people who take Reiki training use it for self-care, many are so amazed with the results that they take advanced training and move on to become practitioners themselves. A form of energy healing similar to Reiki called Therapeutic Touch (p. 242) has become very popular among holistically oriented nurses. If you live in almost any urban area, you'll be able to find classes in Reiki and practitioners. I suggest that you schedule a couple of sessions and experience Reiki yourself. After a first session, my patients regularly say, "I've never felt so totally relaxed in my life," "I really felt energy shifting within me," and "It was like a release—I started crying and I didn't know where the tears were coming from. Then all of a sudden, I knew what I had to do with my life."

After a visit to a conventional internist, no patient in the history of medicine has ever said, "I never felt so totally relaxed in my life." Mainly as an internist, I've been trained to give people pills that make them feel nauseated.

YOUR FIRST REIKI SESSION

Just so you don't become anxious at the thought of getting into something "woo-woo," here's what generally happens during a Reiki session. You'll remain fully clothed and enter a dimly lit room where some soft music may be playing. You'll climb on to a padded massage table, lie back, and get as comfortable as possible. The therapist will then place her hands very gently on you in a series of pre-scribed positions, starting at your head, and will remain in each position for as long as five minutes (her hands are never placed on your breasts or near your genitals). The pressure is very light, passive, and still, without any massage.

About halfway through the session, you'll roll over face-down, and she'll be-gin again. You'll feel the heat of the *chi* energy from her hands, a pleasant sensa-tion like an electric heating pad or hot water bottle. Some therapists "scan" your entire body with their hands before the actual treatment begins, moving their hands slowly above your entire body, trying to sense specific areas of energy blockage or depletion. If she finds something, like a sense of heat or cold, the therapist may inquire about problems in the area, something physical, like an ill-ness or injury in the past, or some emotional issue.

During the session, you may fall asleep or enter a deep meditation-like re-laxation. After the session is over, you might feel as if you've been in a dream-like state, and now have awakened from a refreshingly deep sleep. The Reiki therapist may ask you questions about what you felt and how you might interpret these sensations.

Regular Reiki sessions, though undeniably beneficial, can begin to get ex-pensive, as they're not covered by insurance. Asking your HMO primary physi-cian for a Reiki referral will get you a stony silence, and a claim for Reiki will likely be rejected.

You might consider learning Reiki yourself. There are three traditional levels of Reiki. First-degree Reiki is designed for personal use; you'll learn how to tap into the universal energy that defines Reiki and master several hand positions for self-healing. Second and third degree levels are designed for those who wish to become Reiki practitioners. Most classes are taught in all-day sessions over two or three weekends.

Finding a Reiki practitioner is pretty simple. Type "Reiki" and your town's name into your Internet search engine. I tried this for a small town in Illinois, where I have a cabin for weekend retreats. I located one practitioner affiliated

with the local community hospital and another in a nearby town. I can't describe
how delighted I was. When a local hospital in a small town in Illinois has a Reiki
therapist on its staff, the future is actually a bit brighter for good patient care.

REIKI AND THE TRIPLE WHAMMY

The combination of psychological counseling and an energy therapy like Reiki will
help you more quickly heal your Triple Whammy disorder. Manifestations of
trapped issues remain energetically in your body as knotted muscles, intestinal turmoil, and the throb of migraine. A Reiki therapist senses these areas of congestion
and blockage and releases them. Whether it's depression or fibromyalgia, panic
attacks, IBS, or PMS, Triple Whammy disorders are generally not well served by
conventional physicians, male or female. By telling you that getting well can be a
reality when you use therapies like Reiki, counseling, meditation, and herbs, I am
also saying that you need doctors a whole lot less than you think you do.

THERAPEUTIC TOUCH

A nurse's aide giving a soothing back rub to a patient in a hospital bed, a physical therapist's arm around the shoulder of a patient attempting his first step on a
new hip, a nurse taking a pulse, and as she does so, holding her patient's hand in
both of her own. These are all transfers of healing energy. This is how people actually recover from illness. The tens of thousands of TT practitioners are mainly
nurses working in hospitals, although an increasing number of doctors are being
trained as well. I've grown accustomed to my office nurse, Mary Nagle, heading
off to perform therapeutic touch for a patient in distress. She's very good at spot-
ting people suffering in silence, reluctant to talk about their physical or emotional pain. After a few minutes of treatment in a quiet, dimly lit room, our
patient emerges relaxed, a little more cheerful, and better prepared to deal with
issues that may be contributing to her ill health.

Therapeutic touch was developed in the 1970s through the joint efforts of a
nurse, Dolores Krieger, RN, who was also a professor at New York University, and
Dora Kunz, a self-taught hands-on healer. Like many of the other alternative
therapies we've discussed here, TT is based on the energy that surrounds us and

works within our bodies. The TT practitioner centers her own personal energy field and passes its healing forces to her client.

The word "touch" in therapeutic touch can be misleading because the practitioner need not touch her client at all. You remain fully clothed, as your practitioner moves through the four phases of healing:

- First, the practitioner focuses her mind on the conscious intent to heal another living being. This is a centering process that tunes out any distractions.

- Second, she'll use the natural sensitivity of her palm to assess your energy field. She'll hold her hands about three inches above your body. Then, starting at your head and still keeping her hands just above your body, she will "smooth" her hands over your face, the sides of your head and neck, torso, pelvis, and legs. She tries to sense differences in your energy flow, including left-right imbalances and peculiar sensations, such as temperature shifts or tingling.

- She then shifts those areas in your energy field that seem congested or sluggish, moving her hands in slow rhythmic strokes to smooth out areas of inappropriate accumulation or deficiency.

- Finally, she reassesses your energy field, verifying that her treatment was successful.

One of the best aspects of therapeutic touch is that you can learn it quickly for self-treatment or to treat your family and friends. Women seem much more aware of energy fields than men and quickly perceive positive and negative energies emanating from an individual, a group, or a place, while most men feel more comfortable with an instruction manual. Women can feel their personal space being invaded and can react quickly. By the same token, the female of any species is virtually hardwired as a healing and nurturing force. The concept of "touching with an intent to heal" is almost as natural to the feminine soul as breathing.

To try TT on yourself: sit in a backless chair and repeat steps one through four listed above. The centering process is basically you entering a meditative state, eyes closed, concentrating on each breath. Then pass your hands downward slowly, focusing on any irregularities in your energy field. Smooth these out, rest your hands on your lap, and return to your meditative state for a minute or two.

To find a TT practitioner, try the nursing office at your local hospital; ask your chiropractor, massage therapist, or at a local health food store. Experience TT on your own; then ask the practitioner about taking a course for yourself.

I heard this TT story from Barbara Dossey, RN, author of several excellent books on healing and holistic nursing: She tells of a hospital in Colorado where TT had become very popular among the nurses and patients alike. However, the hospital's administrators were very uncomfortable with the idea of nurses waving hands in the air above patients. So they posted a sign "There shall be no healing in this hospital" in the nurse's lounge. Barbara would conclude her talk on energy healing with a slide of this sign, reminding everyone of the challenges we all face within the modern health care system.

THERAPEUTIC TOUCH AND THE TRIPLE WHAMMY

Healing does seem like something we all should be doing naturally, voluntarily, without ever being asked, one caring, compassionate human being relieving the pain and suffering of another. There's an essential "rightness" to it. A real healer will heal with a few reassuring words, maybe a silent prayer, and then a summoning up and a transfer of her love and energies.

21

THE TRIPLE WHAMMY FOOD PLAN

Many people go through life seeing capable, committed doctors who never once mention that the quality of what we eat has a dramatic effect on our health and vitality. Obviously, these doctors need some reeducation, and their patients need different doctors.

Any eating program plan that includes the words "never" or "must" gives me the willies. You don't want to go overboard on the do's and don'ts of healthful eating. An occasional splurge, a guilty pleasure, these are fine by me. So let's clear the air right up front. If you're aching for some pâté or a slice of pecan pie, just enjoy yourself. An indulgence every once in a while won't move your efforts back to square one.

The Triple Whammy Food Plan is delicious and uncomplicated. It contains a wide variety of whole, health-giving foods. It's designed to balance the action of your hormones and keep your serotonin levels at a nice constant high by timing your intake of complex carbohydrates. And it boosts your overall resistance to disease by bolstering your immune system.

You'll dramatically reduce how much you eat of some foods—notably processed foods, which contain inordinate amounts of sugar, salt, and saturated fats—and increase your intake of colorful, nutrient-packed fruits and veggies, complex carbohydrates, and lean protein. You'll drink more water, too. Once you start following the food plan you'll feel and look so much better you'll wonder how you ever ate any other way.

As you explore the health benefits of eating well (far more than we have room to include here), check out this website that I refer my patients to: The World's Healthiest Foods (www.whfoods.com) contains reliable information on the value of nutrient-rich whole foods, plus delicious recipes. This chapter is divided into two easy steps. Let's get started.

STEP ONE: EAT THE TRIPLE WHAMMY WAY

Eating the Triple Whammy way means eating mostly whole foods—the ones you buy in their original form that haven't been processed at all or are only minimally processed, like a can of beans that have been cooked to make them edible. Our most stunning examples of whole foods are fresh fruits and vegetables, the colorful array of them, each with a distinct texture, flavor, and health-giving force. Nuts and seeds are also whole foods, as are eggs and whole grains. These foods contain all the nutrients nature endowed them with, unlike foods that have been highly processed or to which lots of artificial ingredients (color, preservatives, chemical enhancers, and the like) have been added. Meats and fish are also whole foods, but should be eaten sparingly because many do contain pollutants.

Eating the Triple Whammy way requires spending more time in the fresh produce section of your market, where you don't need to waste time reading labels. But if fruits and vegetables were labeled, you'd discover that in addition to providing vitamin C and lots of fiber, your apple also contains significant amounts of antioxidants—substances that protect us against conditions ranging from the sight-robbing macular degeneration to cholesterol problems and heart disease. The individual compounds that make up whole foods are less important than the way all the compounds interact. Thus, taking a vitamin C supplement won't provide anywhere near the range of benefits that eating a whole apple can.

Eating mostly whole foods will also balance your hormones and quell Triple Whammy symptoms. Surveys show that women eating a largely junk-food diet, with refined sugar and saturated fats, suffer more symptoms of PMS and perimenopause. Although carbs of any kind, from a bran muffin to a Twinkie, will give your serotonin a boost, the sugar-laden Twinkie will be followed quickly by a low blood sugar crash (and a craving for the Twinkie you left in the package).

Now, I *won't* be telling you *not* to have carbs. *Women need carbs.* But I want you to eat healthy carbs and I'll show you how.

EAT FOOD AS NOUNS, NOT ADJECTIVES

Choosing to eat a plant-based diet most of the time—vegetables, fruits, whole grains, and nuts—will unequivocally improve your health in a couple ways. First, these foods are nutrient-dense. When you choose an apple instead of an apple pastry, a slice of bread made from whole grains over a slice of bread made with refined white flour, you're eating the food itself instead of something made with a part of that food or a processed version of that food.

Here's an easy way to think about it: eat foods as nouns rather than adjectives. Noun: I'm eating blueberries. Adjective: I'm eating a refined white-flour blueberry muffin. Noun: I'm eating a sweet potato. Adjective: I'm eating sweet potato pie.

Move your thinking away from how much fat or how many calories you're taking in and focus instead on increasing the number of fruits and vegetables you eat every day, along with several servings of whole grains, nuts, and seeds. This can be daunting at first if you're not in the habit, but you're smart and you can stick with it for the payoff—you'll feel and look better. Fruits and veggies contain vitamins, minerals, healthy fats, and roughage in the form of fiber. They strengthen your bones and heart, keep your memory and eyesight sharp, help your blood vessels stay clear, and lower your risk of cancer.

They do this because they contain phytochemicals ("phyto" means "plant-based"), powerful substances that exist naturally in veggies and fruits as well as in nuts and whole grains. Phytochemicals prevent disease and boost your immune system. Scientists have identified hundreds of phytochemicals in whole foods, and they expect to find many more. Most fruits and vegetables appear to contain more than one kind; all-stars like kale and broccoli have five different types each. In fact, phytochemicals give fruits and vegetables their colors, and a good rule of thumb is to include as many colors as you can in your daily eating. Broccoli's great, but if you ate only broccoli you'd be missing the equally powerful—but different—phytochemicals in eggplant, radishes, and sweet potatoes.

Once you start reducing the foods on the Reduce list (p. 248), instead of taking in all manner of marginal fats and chemicals, you'll be able to add your own spices and beneficial fats (no chemicals!) to food, including wonderfully flavored cheeses, olive oils, and avocados. For example, a sweet potato baked and topped with a big dollop of low-fat sour cream and a sprinkle of cinnamon is a delicious, nutritionally powerful part of lunch or dinner—it's loaded with the phytochemical beta-carotene and also complex carbohydrates to keep your serotonin high (see page 263 for more on this).

An avocado (lusciously satisfying and bearing beneficial fats) sliced onto your favorite whole-grain bread with a slab of tomato, a handful of baby spinach, and a bit of sharp cheese provides enough complex carbs to keep your serotonin up, represents three servings of your daily fruits and vegetables, and makes a healthful breakfast, lunch, or dinner.

REDUCE, INCREASE, REPLACE

Follow these guidelines to start reshaping your food choices:

1. REDUCE

You've already gathered that I generally dislike eating plans that tell you what not to eat. Usually they list foods that we love and want to have at least occasionally. I'm not asking you to completely avoid foods like ice cream, dark chocolate, and butter. Nor am I asking you to quit eating all sugar or even most (heaven forbid) carbohydrates. But from the list below, there's one category I'd like you to start reducing and then consider giving up as much as you possibly can: the chemical swill of processed and prepared foods.

PROCESSED FOODS

HOW TO DO IT: Start today reducing or eliminating nearly all of the prepared and processed foods from your diet unless you know and feel comfortable with the source. Leading this category are most of the so-called meals that you find in the freezer compartment at your grocery. Back in the 1950s, we called them TV dinners. I think you know what I'm referring to here—the cuisines in a box that are "lean" only because they contain minuscule portions of actual food. The list of ingredients for your tiny (and expensive) dinner reads like a list of chemical additives. These processed meals are brought to you by agribusiness giants that create this junk and market it heavily to time-pressed, weight-conscious, and nutrient-starved women. If your body could speak aloud, it might say, "What are you trying to do to me with this stuff?" Instead, your body speaks to you in the language of symptoms: low energy, weight gain, unhealthy-looking skin and hair. When you start eating well, and you both look and feel better, your body is saying "Hey, girl, thanks for listening!"

Processed foods contain a lot of sugar, unhealthful fats like hydrogenated fats (p. 250), and salt, three of the main players on our Reduce list. The processing itself removes most of the nutrients from the food. Instead of steaming your own spinach, broccoli, or kale and adding a healthy couple of shots of olive oil and a crumbling of intensely flavored cheese, you're often consuming the ever-bad trans fats, a huge amount of sodium (salt), and sugar in the form of high-fructose corn sweetener. You could drown a bowl of steamed broccoli in cheese sauce and still come out ahead, because you'd be eating actual broccoli.

Cut back on eating processed foods unless you can recognize most of the ingredients on the label. Many organic frozen meals, including burritos, contain mostly actual food. Become a reader of labels and you'll see what I mean. My wife and I frequently get prepared meals from Whole Foods and Trader Joe's, but certainly not every community has these options or every family the money to purchase high-quality prepared food.

Read the labels on boxed prepared foods, too, including mixes to which you add hamburger or chicken. These products have more fake ingredients than real ones, and you can just as easily make the meal without the "helper" by adding rice, beans, or noodles, canned tomatoes, and a few spices to ground beef or turkey. To get started, see the delicious black bean soup recipe on page 272, which you can easily turn into black bean chili or, cooked down a bit and tucked into a tortilla, a burrito.

SUGARY DRINKS AND FOODS

HOW TO DO IT: Reduce your intake of all fruit juices (eat whole fruit instead), soft drinks including diet sodas, and "sports" drinks. Don't add sugar to food, and minimize how many sugar-containing foods you eat every day—though by this I certainly don't mean limit your fruits. They are champions at satisfying a sweet tooth. It's simply amazing the amount of sugar we're eating these days. Because sugar is being added to everything from boxed cereal to potato salad (and especially in the form of high-fructose corn syrup), we're eating about 150 pounds per year. That's close to a half pound of sugar a day!

FOODS HIGH IN SATURATED FATS

HOW TO DO IT: Saturated fats are found in all foods that come from animals. Cut back on high-fat cuts of meat, fried foods, and full-fat milk products like whole milk, cream, cheese, ice cream, and butter. A good first step is to eat small portions of meat rather than making it the main item on your plate. Make meat a special treat. Use turkey breast for burgers and chili or occasionally have a small filet mignon instead of eating meat every day. Take a cue from Asian cuisines and make stir-fried vegetables your meal's centerpiece, adding a small amount of high-quality cut-up meat if you like.

HYDROGENATED FATS/TRANS FATS

HOW TO DO IT: Trans fatty acids, or trans fats for short, also appear on food labels as partially hydrogenated fats and as hydrogenated fats. They're liquid oils that have been processed so they're solid at room temperature, which increases the shelf life of many products. Hydrogenated means just what it sounds like. Bubbling hydrogen gas through a liquid oil turns it into a solid, so that something like corn oil can then be sold as margarine. These are the trans fats, and they're not good for you in any way. They clog your arteries, increasing your bad LDL cholesterol and decreasing the good HDL. In this way they're just like the saturated fats found in animal products.

Avoid trans fats wherever you find them, and you'll find them everywhere once you start reading labels: in cookies, bakery goods, crackers, peanut butter, frozen waffles, and even some breakfast cereals. Also in solid margarines, french fries, donuts, and fried chicken you eat out. Many microwave popcorns have it too. The good news is that manufacturers have started changing their formulations to eliminate trans fats.

SALT SHAKER SALT

HOW TO DO IT: Put away your salt shaker and retrieve it on rare occasions only. Avoid adding salt when you cook, adding a little sparingly afterward if needed. You can get a better salt taste from a sprinkling just before you eat than you can from teaspoonfuls dumped into the cooking pot.

WHITE-FLOUR PRODUCTS

HOW TO DO IT: Reduce how often you eat foods made from white flour, which is what you get after wheat flour is refined to remove the bran and fiber (the nutritional good guys). White-flour products enter your bloodstream almost as quickly as sugar, spiking your blood sugar instead of taking it on a slow ride upward. The latter is best achieved by eating high-quality carbohydrates (p. 266), which also help your body make serotonin. Again, I'm not asking you to cut out all products made with white flour, but do pretty much reserve for special occasions your intake of bakery goods (donuts, cakes, pies, and white-flour cookies) and non–whole-grain crackers, all of which are also common vehicles for transfats and saturated fat.

Cereals fall into a middle category, many of them high in fiber and good for you, others containing health-damping trans fats and/or highly refined flours and lots of sugar. Read your labels. Even some cereals labeled natural or organic have a lot of added sweeteners—cane sugars and molasses.

Some of our favorite refined-flour products include pasta, freshly baked Italian or French white bread, flour tortillas, and white rice. Enjoy them occasionally, but try to make your mainstay bread a whole-grain version and your regular rice brown or wild. Corn tortillas deliver a lot of flavor. I for one can't abide whole-wheat pasta, though they tell me it's gotten better.

2. INCREASE

One of the easiest ways to focus less on the foods you're reducing is to fill up on the foods you're increasing. If you don't already shop at a market that sells primarily produce, do a little research and try to find one. The diversity of fruit and vegetables is generally broader than at chain groceries, and prices can be better too. Many towns have produce stands or farmers markets in the summer and autumn, when shopping for produce is easiest and eating it most delectable. If vegetables and fruits are new to your diet, start with the ones you enjoy. Then try to incorporate something new each week. Cookbooks and recipes for vegetables abound in bookstores and on the Internet. Even if you're not a cook, you can learn to prepare a vast range of simple veggie dishes. Start by reading the information on vegetable steamers on page 261.

FRUITS: GET FOUR TO SIX SERVINGS A DAY

HOW TO DO IT: Fruit is an easy, nutritious fast food. A skin-on whole fruit like a small apple or pear—or about half a cup of loose fruit like grapes or berries—represents a serving. If you're pressed for time, shop smartly to ensure you've got enough fruit in the house for a week. If it's just you you're shopping for, count out those apples so you've got one for each day of the week and, by the way, shoot for a variety of types, including as many varieties as your store carries (here in the Midwest, our autumn farmers market offers as many as twelve different kinds). To fulfill your daily servings, make sure you've got enough prunes, grapes, citrus, and any other fruit that you like or that's in season. Count out what you'll need for the entire week: 7 apples, a big bunch of grapes, 7 oranges, 7 bananas, and a large bag of pitted prunes (often marketed as pitted dried plums).

Have fruit for breakfast and for at least one of your snacks every day. It's a fine source of the carbohydrates that keep your serotonin elevated (see p. 263).

Variety is the key here, but there are some obvious standbys, including pitted prunes, which are loaded with potassium, iron, and antioxidants. Eat four per day for a serving, either on their own or as a satisfying addition to plain low-fat yogurt. They're also delicious cut up and sprinkled on cereal or oatmeal. Pack an apple and pear and a small chunk of cheese for lunch or a snack at work, or tuck some grapes in with half a sandwich for lunch. You're up to four servings of fruit already and we haven't even covered tossing blueberries or pears into your green salad.

One of my patients has for her breakfast every day a fruit plate that starts with a cup of low-fat plain yogurt topped with a serving each of five different kinds of fruit and a few generous shakes of cinnamon. She says she not only feels energetic when she walks out the door to start her day, but righteously healthy, her daily fruit allotment literally under her belt.

VEGETABLES: GET 5 TO 6 SERVINGS A DAY, MORE IF YOU WANT

HOW TO DO IT: Figure this for a serving: a large handful of loose greens like spinach, kale, or lettuce and a half cup of raw or cooked veggies. Start by being crafty: add nutrient-packed spinach to sandwiches, chop greens and spinach finely and add them to eggs, pastas, soups, and meats. Tuna salad gets a nice boost with finely chopped spinach added to the mix, as does slaw, or add chopped onion or red or green pepper to these salads. Canned diced tomatoes are easy additions to soups, chili, and pastas. Experiment with broccoli and cauliflower using a vegetable steamer (p. 261) and a variety of different toppings. One of my favorite veggies in a jar is roasted red peppers.

Salads are maybe the easiest way to get your veggies, but take a pass on iceberg lettuce as it's just crunchy water. Start with a handful of spinach and a handful of dark romaine lettuce, add a half cup each of four more veggies to meet your day's total. Chop cauliflower and broccoli very fine and add it to other salad ingredients. Toss it all with a salad dressing you love. See page 270 for dressing ideas.

SPICES AND HERBS

HOW TO DO IT: Herbs and spices liven up our foods and many also are helpful in preventing illness and maintaining good health. Do a little research on herbs— fresh or dried—and start sprinkling them liberally into many foods. Used for thousands of years, cinnamon in 2004 was discovered to lower blood sugar and the unhealthy LDL cholesterol. Cinnamon helps insulin move sugar out of the bloodstream and into cells, where it's needed for energy, thus lowering blood sugar. As little as a quarter teaspoon twice a day, sprinkled on your fruit, cereal, or in coffee or tea, is effective and delicious.

Turmeric is another ancient star. This golden orange spice is commonly used in curries, but you can sprinkle a teaspoon into chili, eggs, and soups to gain its beneficial effects, which include acting as an anti-inflammatory, antibacterial, and cholesterol-lowering agent.

Researchers discovered only in 2004 that pungent cilantro appears to be in the antibacterial business in addition to bringing its characteristic flavor to many cuisines. One of the compounds in cilantro (and in its seeds, coriander)— dodecenal—is nearly twice as powerful in killing *Salmonella,* a bacterium that can causes food poisoning, as gentamicin, an antibiotic prescribed by doctors to kill Salmonella bacteria.

LEAN PROTEIN CHOICES, SUCH AS EGGS, FISH, CHICKEN, AND LEAN PORK AND BEEF

HOW TO DO IT: You do need protein (in general and also to generate tryptophan, from which serotonin is made), but you don't need a lot of protein. A good general rule is to eat a palm-sized portion of any red meat or chicken every day, but instead you can combine rice and beans to get a complete protein that has the same value as meat (see What the Heck are Legumes, Anyway?, on page 265). Proteins are made up of amino acids, and when we digest proteins and absorb the amino acids, they're then used throughout our body for our own cell growth and development. You needn't go overboard on protein, but don't skimp, either.

Eggs are an excellent protein and vitamin source—quite good for you—and not the cholesterol villain they were once thought to be. Obviously this means not scrambling them in bacon drippings. You need to make protein choices carefully these days. Various types of meat and chicken may contain hormones. Farmed fish don't have the helpful fats that wild-caught fish do because they're fed a grain-based feed, rather than plankton. In addition, fish are being contaminated with mercury. Doctors aren't sure about the long-term effects, but mercury is definitely a poison—it's toxic to the brain and potentially dangerous to the delicate developing fetal brain. More and more fish are being added to the watch list. I suggest pregnant women avoid tuna and other potentially toxic fish altogether. If you're not pregnant, two or three cans a month probably pose no significant threat. Supplement your omega-3s with fish oil capsules.

WATER AND OTHER LIQUIDS

HOW TO DO IT: You know the drill—eight eight-ounce glasses of water every day. Many of my patients carry water bottles to ensure they're getting enough. Don't listen to anyone who tells you water's not important. It plays an essential role in keeping your digestive system functioning and in moving oxygen-rich red blood cells, which deliver energy, throughout your body, powering your day. Drink sixty-four ounces of water every day, in addition to all the herbal tea and low-sodium vegetable juices you want. Sports drinks are really nothing more than expensive sugar waters and you don't need them.

Yes, coffee is fine. Just don't overdo it—it can cause big swings in your blood sugar (especially sweetened drinks from coffee bars). To keep blood sugar swings to a minimum, drink eight ounces of water after every cup of coffee, and be sure you're eating well, too. Many of my coffee-drinking patients have readily accepted the idea of replacing some of their coffee intake with tea. An iced or warm drink seems to be what many of us are after. Green and black teas deliver real health benefits. They're known to kill cancer cells, lower blood sugar, and reduce your risk of heart disease, in addition to being satisfying.

BENEFICIAL FATS

HOW TO DO IT: As you reduce your intake of butter and other saturated fats, use instead olive oil and other nutritious oils like walnut and flaxseed oils. Healthy fats are also found in avocados, which contain mostly monounsaturated fat, and nuts (an ideal snack), which are loaded with beneficial omega-3s (see Cold-Water Fish, Nuts and Seeds, and Omega-3s on page 261).

HAVE BREAKFAST EVERY DAY

HOW TO DO IT: Breakfast reminds us that we're "breaking the fast," eating for the first time since we went to sleep. It's essential to eat breakfast every day and to eat a breakfast that will sustain your blood sugar at least until a midmorning snack. When researchers took a survey among people who had made it to age one hundred, the single most consistent trait among them was that they never missed breakfast.

Read about fruits (p. 252) for ways to incorporate them into your breakfast. The champion of breakfast foods—oatmeal—is another top choice, and you can add milk, fruit, nuts, or toasted and ground flaxseed to pump up the nutritional value even more. A bowl of oatmeal not only contains soluble fiber that helps maintain blood sugar and lowers bad cholesterol, but also contains phytochemicals called flavonoids, antioxidants that are key to disease prevention. In 2004 researchers found that oats contain flavonoids called avenanthramides that apparently minimize your blood cells' ability to stick to the walls of your arteries. This means they can possibly reduce the accumulation of plaque and also reduce inflammation in your blood vessels, both of which can lead to a heart attack. Oatmeal is a terrific choice for morning, because your body digests it slowly, sending your serotonin upward and keeping your blood sugar even. Plus, it simply keeps us feeling full.

By the way, some people I know like to have oatmeal for lunch or dinner. It's the ultimate comfort food and truly nutritious. It's also a fine afternoon snack at work. Just make sure if you're using an instant oatmeal that it's not loaded with sugar you don't need.

Breaking away from the traditional breakfast food approach, try half a natural peanut butter sandwich on whole-grain bread with a side of fruit (or put sliced banana or chopped prunes on the sandwich) or turkey or chicken on whole-grain bread with spinach. Make the blueberry smoothie recipe on page 269 if you'd rather sip your breakfast.

Eggs remain a fine choice to start your day; add some spinach or other veggies to boost the nutritional value and don't forget to add a slice of whole-grain bread or some fruit as a carbohydrate source.

Q & A: I MISS MY SAUSAGE PIZZA!

Q. I love the way I feel eating the Triple Whammy way, but I long for my weekly sausage pizza with hot peppers and mushrooms. Is there any way it can be part of my eating plan?

A. Absolutely. Remember that your goal is to deposit lots of nutrients into your whole-food savings account (your body). Say you're eating the Triple Whammy way throughout the week, having your fruits and vegetables every day, enjoying lean meats and complex carbohydrates, and restricting or avoiding altogether processed foods. If Friday night is pizza night at your house, don't deprive yourself and feel resentful of everyone around you. Eating the Triple Whammy way most of the time gives you the latitude to enjoy pizza night. It's also worth noting that the cooked tomatoes in the pizza sauce, as well as the mushrooms and peppers, are rich in antioxidants, and real mozzarella cheese is low in fat and very nutritious.

On the other hand, I'm trying but just can't come up with any significant health benefits from sausage. Understand, however, that Chicago-style pizza is a world-famous treat and the sausage contributes mightily to its reputation. So just one word about sausage: moderation.

3. REPLACE

Instead of . . .	*Choose*
Less-than-nutritious midmorning and midafternoon snacks	Soup. A cup of soup can replenish your nutrient stores and fulfill a craving you might think needs to be satisfied by something sweet. Soups that contain beans, potatoes, milk, and/or vegetables will give you a carbo boost to keep your serotonin humming. Take soup to work and heat up a cup when your energy's flagging. You can also try single-serving prepared soups, but please read the ingredient list to be sure there aren't a lot of additives and preservatives.

Popcorn (see p. 267).

Nuts and seeds.

Fruit and a small wedge of cheese.

Quarter or half a natural peanut butter sandwich on whole-grain bread.

Chips made with trans fats (p. 250)	Baked chips (not high in nutrients or complex carbs but nice for an occasional snack).
	Chips that don't list hydrogenated fats as an ingredient. These are low in complex carbs, and high in fat, of course, and you'll want to have them infrequently.
Peanut butters containing hydrogenated fats	Natural peanut butter containing only ground nuts (and sometimes a little salt). Keep it in the fridge and stir the separated layers before using. It's an excellent nutritional choice.
	Other nut butters, which you may have to seek out at your local health food store.
Cookies, including most refined-flour store-bought varieties made with trans fats (p. 250)	Make your own, using oats, oat flour, nuts, and liquid oils.
Butter and hard margarines	Olive oil. Butter's OK in moderation, but try to use it just a couple times a week. Make olive oil your fat of choice for salads, vegetables, and cooking. Or try one of the soft tub spreads that loudly proclaim "no trans fats!" but that do include beneficial flaxseed oil.
Ice cream	Ice cream's a lovely occasional treat, but try replacing it with yogurt—or fruit and yogurt (see Yogurt Blueberry Brain Booster, p. 269).
Most candy	High-quality dark chocolate, which is loaded with antioxidants and also increases serotonin and other feel-good brain chemicals. A small piece makes a great snack a couple times a week with or without a few toasted walnuts (see recipe on page 269).

SPLURGING

What would life be without splurges? If you're following the Triple Whammy Food Plan, congratulations on cutting out most prepared foods, processed foods, and unnecessary sugar. Not only will this do wonders for your good health, it gives you some latitude in the splurge department. Remember that splurges are so named because they occur infrequently, by which I mean not every day but more like once or twice a week. Here are some ideas to satisfy sweet tooths and fat cravings:

– Make a cheese sauce to pour over your vegetables.

– Have half a cup of all-natural ice cream topped with toasted walnuts.

– Savor a small piece of high-quality dark chocolate.

– Sip hot chocolate made with skim or 2 percent milk, real unsweetened dark cocoa, and just enough sugar to satisfy.

TEN WAYS TO EAT THE TRIPLE WHAMMY WAY

1. **EAT DARK LEAFY GREENS THREE TIMES A WEEK AT LEAST.** Purchase kale, spinach, swiss chard, and mustard greens (often available pre-washed in bags) and steam them before adding flavorful additions. Try the dressing recipe on page 270. Or add greens to dishes where they're less noticeable. Chop some raw kale into coleslaw, chop chard finely and toss with hot pasta.

2. **NEVER MISS A MEAL (OR A SNACK, IF YOU'RE A GRAZER).** Skipping meals— or skipping light snacks, if you're a grazer—causes dramatic swings in your blood sugar and brings on a variety of symptoms such as lightheadedness, brain fog, irritability, and tremulousness. Low blood sugar can also send you running for whatever food happens to be closest, like nutritionally empty vending machine snacks or the contents of the donut box sitting out at work. Keep high-quality carbs on hand at home and at work—soups, nuts, fruit, whole-grain bread with a little cheese or natural peanut butter—to eat when you feel yourself approaching a blood sugar "valley." Most important, base your breakfast, lunch, and dinner on the suggestions in this chapter, with plenty of protein and complex carbohydrates (fruits, veggies, and grains), and you'll feel satisfied throughout the day.

3. **HAVE A SALAD FIVE DAYS A WEEK.** Look for the darkest salad greens you can find—they contain the most nutrients. Good choices include dark green romaine and red leaf lettuces, and also one of my favorite fast foods: pre-washed baby spinach. Once your greens are in the bowl, get creative: toasted walnuts, a little intensely favored cheese (such as feta or bleu), and whatever else appeals—

blueberries, sliced pear, or strawberries are lovely for one effect, and so is red onion, sweet pepper, and tomato for another. Make an olive oil and vinegar dressing to pour over. You can get all your veggie servings for the day in one bowl with a little effort, or have your entire meal in a bowl by also adding cooked chicken and half a can of drained kidney beans. Or sauté some ground turkey with onion, oregano, and basil and add it while hot to your greens before tossing in the veggies. Dice a baby eggplant, sauté it in olive oil until soft, and add. Hard-boiled eggs, a mainstay protein addition to salads, are easy to chop and add. Many grocery stores offer salad bars, a boon to your eating plan if you stay away from the potato salad.

4. **ONE NIGHT A WEEK, MAKE IT VEGGIE NIGHT.** Raw or cooked, veggies can in-clude washed and cut raw radishes, carrots, sweet peppers of every color, and a cruciferous vegetable like broccoli or cauliflower. Try baby zucchini or yellow squash raw, sliced lengthwise. Experiment with dips. Make an easy bean dip by putting a can of white beans, red beans, or black beans into the blender with some garlic, fresh lemon juice, and a few drops of olive oil. Add any spices that appeal, such as oregano or basil. Salsas make delicious dips too. Make a creamy salsa dip by adding a tablespoon or two of low-fat sour cream to some red or green salsa. Or steam an assortment of vegetables, drain, and toss with olive oil and some grated intensely flavored cheese (parmesan, feta, bleu, sharp cheddar) and fresh herbs. To have with your veggies, toast whole-grain bread and brush it with a clove of chopped garlic that you've gently sautéed in olive oil. For dessert, enjoy fruit or a little dark chocolate.

5. **MAKE EGGS.** Eggs are a terrific source of protein (remember, you need protein to generate tryptophan, from which serotonin is made), easy to prepare, and don't have the artery-clogging properties of many meats.

6. **ENJOY NUTS.** Great for snacks and adding to salads, nuts are a high-quality car-bohydrate that contain disease-fighting antioxidants and health-giving oils. They're an ideal food to work with for carbo-timing (p. 263) and are especially deli-cious when combined with fruit. Enjoy a third of a cup of any type of nuts every day.

7. **BECOME A SOUP LOVER.** Make a big batch of the Almost-Instant Black Bean Soup (p. 272) and have some for snacks or lunch, or for dinner with a salad and a hunk of whole-grain bread. Soup is enormously satisfying and will give you a carbohydrate/serotonin lift.

8. **RELY ON LEGUMES.** Read "What the Heck Are Legumes, Anyway?" (p. 265) for a primer on this powerful food. Their antioxidant, mineral, and fiber content make them exceptional choices for everyday eating. Plus, you can buy all types of beans and peas already hydrated in cans—this is one prepared food I heartily endorse. Incredibly versatile, legumes are an ideal choice for carbo-timing: half a cup of black beans, for example, contains nineteen grams of carbohydrates. Start looking at your grocery shelf in a new way and experiment with all types of legumes—kidney beans, garbanzo beans (chickpeas), butter beans, and lentils.

Warm them up and add some olive oil and spices. Add meat or not. Chill as a salad and eat for lunch (p. 271).

9. **TIME YOUR CARBOHYDRATES TO KEEP SEROTONIN HIGH THROUGHOUT YOUR DAY.** Learn how on page 263.

10. **STOP DIETING.** Stop dieting and start eating the widest possible range of plant-based foods. Read the healing path "Weight Loss Agonies" on page 188 and enjoy every mouthful of the food you eat.

WHAT ARE THE BENEFITS OF EATING THE TRIPLE WHAMMY WAY?

Boy, am I glad you asked. You will:

- **HAVE MORE ENERGY** as you provide your body with exactly the nutrition it needs to function efficiently.

- **EASE PMS AND PERIMENOPAUSE SYMPTOMS** by eliminating the junk from your diet.

- **INCREASE THE SEROTONIN** in your brain with carbohydrate timing. Once your serotonin levels are higher, you should notice that you're able to tolerate stress better and you should also see improvement in any Triple Whammy disorder you have.

- **BE SMARTER.** With elevated serotonin, B vitamins, fish oil, and protein, your brain will function more efficiently. You may notice your memory is improving.

- **NOTICE DIGESTION IMPROVING** with all the fruits, vegetables, complex carbs, and water.

- **START LOOKING MORE VIBRANT** as your skin, hair, nails, muscles, and eyes benefit richly from the essential fatty acids, amino acids, vitamins, and antioxidants.

- **REDUCE YOUR CHANCES OF DEVELOPING DEGENERATIVE DISEASES,** such as heart disease, Parkinson's disease, macular degeneration, high blood pressure, diabetes, and arthritis.

- **FEEL YOUNGER LONGER** as you slow the rate you age because of antioxidant-rich food choices.

- **HAVE THE TOOLS TO STOP WORRYING ABOUT YOUR WEIGHT,** but only if you also maintain good portion control. Remember, this food plan eliminates calorie-rich, nutrition-poor junk and processed foods from your diet. You'll do even better if you combine the food plan with the brisk daily walk from the Three-Week Cure.

VEGETABLE STEAMER, QUEEN OF THE KITCHEN

Here's a key kitchen implement for Triple Whammy eating: a vegetable steamer. Nothing fancy—just get yourself one of those round stainless steel collapsible devices with holes that sits inside a pot. Put an inch or two of water in the bottom of the pot, drop in your steamer (which opens to accommodate pans of varying sizes), bring the water to a boil, drop in your veggies, and cover. Steaming leaves more nutrients in the food than boiling—which leaves lots in the leftover water—meaning more nutrients reach your cells. Experiment with steaming times. Some highly nutritious vegetables, such as greens (kale, mustard, collards), are quite fragile, requiring just a couple of minutes in the steamer. Others, like green beans and broccoli, need longer to make them tender and palatable. Once you've steamed your veggies, add a flavorful topping, such as the olive oil, fresh lemon, caper, and cheese dressing on page 270, or simply toss the vegetables with a little intensely flavored cheese.

COLD-WATER FISH, NUTS AND SEEDS, AND OMEGA-3s

The oils in cold-water fish and some nuts and seeds contain high concentrations of polyunsaturated fats called omega-3 fatty acids (omega-3s, for short), which your body can't produce on its own. This is the same oil you're taking in the form of fish oil capsules as part of the Three-Week Cure, but it doesn't hurt to get more. The omega-3 called DHA (docosahexanoic acid) increases the amount of serotonin in your brain, which improves your mood and memory in addition to decreasing inflammation and making you less vulnerable to heart disease and cancer.

- **FISH** Here's an idea of roughly how much omega-3s some of the top cold-water fish contain, per four-ounce portion of fish: mackerel (canned), 2.2 grams; salmon (canned), 2.2 grams; sardines, 1.8 grams; and fresh salmon, 1.7 grams. A patient of mine doesn't like fish unless it's exquisitely fresh, and she told me she runs from the room any time her partner opens a can of sardines. If you're among this group, consider your fish oil supplements a true convenience food. They contain the high-quality omega-3s your body needs.

- **WALNUTS AND FLAXSEED AND THEIR OILS** Walnuts are a terrific source of omega-3s, containing 2.6 grams of omega-3 fatty acids per ounce (about 14 halves without shells). Flaxseed is another excellent source of omega-3s (and omega-6 and omega-9) and it's also loaded with lignans, powerful cancer-fighting antioxidants that are also called phytoestrogens because they behave similarly to your own estrogen (see "Adding Soy, Phytoestrogens" on page 263).

To use flax seeds, buy raw whole seeds, grind them in a coffee grinder, and add the flax flour to your oatmeal, muffins, pancakes, cold cereal, cookies, chili (trust me, no one will ever know), and smoothies. Or use them whole by adding a tablespoon to brown or wild rice as it cooks. Flaxseed can also be toasted to enhance its nutty flavor before grinding or using whole. They have about 1.8 grams of omegas-3s per ounce (about 3 tablespoons whole). If you like the flavor of flaxseed oil, a tablespoon contains a whopping 6.9 grams. Walnut oil is a great choice for salads, with just a tablespoon containing 1.4 grams of omega-3s.

ANTIOXIDANT TOP TWENTY: COLOR YOU HEALTHY

Antioxidants are naturally occurring substances found in whole foods that block damage from free radicals to our cells' DNA. Free radicals speed up the aging process and contribute significantly to diseases such as diabetes, cancer, heart disease, and degenerative diseases of the brain. Be guided by the color spectrum in boosting your antioxidant intake: brightly colored plant foods seem to contain the most antioxidants, including the blues of berries and plums, the reds of watermelon, apples, and tomatoes (even more effective after cooking), and the deep purple of eggplant. Scientists at the U.S. Department of Agriculture in 2004 released the following list of the top twenty most antioxidant-rich foods. Include these gems every day in your eating plan, but don't be bound by this list—vegetables like spinach, Brussels sprouts, kale, eggplant, and squash are also loaded with antioxidants.

1. Red beans, small dried
2. Wild blueberries
3. Kidney beans, red
4. Pinto beans
5. Cultivated blueberries
6. Cranberries
7. Artichokes
8. Blackberries
9. Prunes
10. Raspberries
11. Strawberries
12. Red delicious apples
13. Granny Smith apples
14. Pecans
15. Sweet cherries
16. Black plums
17. Russet potatoes
18. Black beans
19. Plums
20. Gala apples

ADDING SOY, PHYTOESTROGENS

Soybean products include tofu, soy milk, many vegetarian meat replacements, and tempeh—a soy cake made by fermenting cooked soybeans. Soybean foods contain isoflavones, powerful natural components of the soy plant that are chemically similar to your own estrogen. Because of their estrogen-like effects, isoflavones are also called phytoestrogens (phyto means "plant-based"). Soy contains many different isoflavones, but two that researchers know about—genistein and daidzein—appear to be the most powerful. And while soy has the most isoflavones of any food, close behind is flaxseed (p. 261), which contains phytoestrogens called lignans.

Phytoestrogens attach themselves to the estrogen receptor sites on your cells, acting like your natural estrogen and reducing hot flashes and other symptoms caused by falling estrogen. If, on the other hand, you have too much estrogen, like during your PMS days, phytoestrogens appear to block the negative effects. Phytoestrogens also help keep your bones strong by increasing their density, again because of their estrogen-like effects.

Researchers aren't yet certain whether the soy isoflavones that are available in pill form equal the effects of soy eaten in its natural state. After all, isoflavones are just one component of soy. For perimenopause/menopause symptoms, try to get 50 to 100 mg of soy once or twice a day. Soy-based protein powders are widely available and easily added to smoothies, soups, and cereal. Soy is also protein-rich with none of the saturated fat of meats. The big coffee chains make excellent soy lattes, which you can easily make at home by adding soy milk (available without added sugar, by the way) to coffee.

STEP TWO: BOOST SEROTONIN NATURALLY WITH CARBOHYDRATE TIMING

Carbohydrate timing might sound complicated, but it's simple once you understand how it works to keep your feel-good serotonin high—and you happy throughout the day. The payoff of timing your carb intake is a nice steady production of serotonin, keeping mood up and the stress protection of serotonin working for you.

Eating a small amount of high-quality carbohydrates periodically through-out the day helps your body make serotonin. Serotonin comes from tryptophan, one of a group of molecules known as amino acids, best envisioned as the building blocks of proteins. But oddly enough, just eating tryptophan-rich foods (like dairy, soy, meats, and fish) isn't enough. In order to transport tryptophan into your brain, you need insulin. And in order to get sufficient insulin to carry the tryptophan, you need to eat carbohydrates.

Here's what happens: when you eat carbohydrates, your digestive system breaks them down into different forms of sugar. As sugar (glucose) is absorbed into your bloodstream, the sugar alerts your pancreas, a gland tucked into the back wall of your abdomen, to release insulin, which ushers glucose into your cells, to be used as energy. Along with its glucose role, insulin also transports tryptophan into your brain, where it's converted to serotonin. You've actually

COST OF THE TRIPLE WHAMMY FOOD PLAN

I hear it all the time from my patients: fresh produce costs a lot, not to mention organic! Let's do some comparison shopping. At my local chain grocery, potato chips (a completely empty food in terms of nutrients it supplies to your body, though lots of fun to eat) cost between $4 and $4.50 per pound. One type of crunchy cinnamon breakfast cereal (another virtually empty food whose ingredient list includes highly refined rice flour and three types of sugar: white sugar, fructose, and dextrose) costs $5.00 per pound. Even a so-called 100% natural cereal made by one of the food giants contains partially hydrogenated cottonseed oil (nothing natural or good for you about trans fats—see p. 250) and comes in at just under $5.00 per pound.

Contrast this to washed baby spinach at $4.96 per pound, but with nutrients galore. Popcorn, at 50 to 75 cents per pound, is the original snack food you make yourself. Natural peanut butters are excellent protein sources and also a fine carbo-timing snack on whole wheat bread or tucked into celery. They run about $4 per pound.

At the low end of the expense scale (and the high end of the nutrient scale) is all manner of fresh produce. A 2004 U.S. Department of Agriculture (USDA) study found that three servings of fresh fruit and four servings of fresh vegetables cost about 64 cents. It's true that some out-of-season fruits and veggies run more, and that's why shopping in season is the way to go. In the summer, fresh corn, tomatoes, and squash cost pennies and themselves make a meal. But even if we double the USDA figure to accommodate your higher servings of vegetables and fruits, your total daily expense sits at about $1.25.

WHAT THE HECK ARE LEGUMES, ANYWAY?

Most of us are familiar with legumes even if we don't call them by their proper name. Legumes are plants that produce pods containing a row of seeds inside, a food group that includes lentils, peas, peanuts, and beans. Researchers have identified more than 13,000 varieties of beans alone—but what's most important here is that legumes are tiny powerhouses of complex carbohydrates that also deliver fiber, protein, B vitamins, antioxidants, and just a trace of fat, while sending your brain the components it needs to produce the all-important serotonin. And they do all this nice and slowly, keeping you feeling full longer and slowly raising your serotonin.

By the way, while legumes are a good source of protein, it's an incomplete protein. Your vegetarian friends will remind you that you need to eat legumes with some sort of grain (including seeds) to get all the amino acids you'd obtain from a complete protein like meat. Here are some combinations that make beans a complete protein source: beans and rice, peanut butter on whole grain bread, hummus made from chickpeas mixed with tahini (sesame paste), and the bean salad on page 271 with a slice of whole-grain bread. Try replacing meat, which has saturated fat, with one of the many legume and grain combinations that provide the same complete protein . . . and complex carbs.

known this all along if you love to eat comfort foods, which are mostly carbohydrates. During periods when serotonin levels are very low, you may crave them. Common during PMS days, your declining estrogen level drags down your feel-good serotonin, and a nice plate of mashed potatoes or chocolate (or some of each) can act like an antidepressant. Mood food.

By the way, studies have shown that when healthy people are deliberately placed on a tryptophan-free diet, their serotonin levels fall and they develop psychological symptoms, including depression. These symptoms reverse when they start eating foods containing tryptophan, which converts to serotonin.

And now you can see why I'm not a proponent of the low-carbohydrate programs. You need the carbs to make adequate serotonin. Without them, you can fall prey to an emotional snarkiness nutritionists call Atkins Attitude. However, on the subject of good-quality carbohydrates, I can't fault the low-carb programs; they've increased everybody's awareness of how different kinds of carbs are handled by the body—the highly refined carbs of foods such as bakery goods and white bread versus what we call high-quality carbs, those found in fruits, vegetables, legumes, and whole-grain pastas, breads, and cereals.

This is all less of an issue for men because we have more available serotonin to begin with. Have you ever met a man who craved chocolate or was calmed down by a big plate of macaroni and cheese?

But back to your brain and serotonin. Once in your brain, tryptophan changes to 5-hydroxytryptophan (5HTP for short) and then to serotonin. Along the way, these reactions need B vitamins, especially Vitamin B_6 (pyridoxine) and certain types of healthy fats, namely the omega-3 oils found in fish. B vitamins and fish oil are an integral part of the Three-Week Cure (p. 45). With these nutritional components in place, your brain itself becomes an efficient serotonin-manufacturing enterprise.

CARBO TIMING

We've established that in order for tryptophan to reach your brain and convert to serotonin, you need to eat carbohydrates. In other words, carbohydrates determine how much serotonin reaches your brain. To increase serotonin and keep it high, each meal of your day (and especially breakfast) should contain some high-quality carbohydrates. I don't mean sugar or sugary foods, like cookies, candy, or refined-carb foods like white bread or chips. Instead, eat periodically from the high-quality carbohydrates suggested below, including whole grain breads, vegetables, nuts, and legumes such as beans (canned is fine), in addition to fruits and dairy products.

Just make sure there's a serving of carbs at each meal. You can achieve this effect if you're following a low-carb diet by spacing out your carb allotment throughout the day. And if you're a grazer, just include some carbs every time you eat.

Timing your carb intake can be as easy as having a cup of skim milk, which has 12 grams of carbohydrate or a half cup of the bean salad recipe on page 271, for about 19 grams of carbohydrates.

HIGH-QUALITY CARBOHYDRATES

High-quality carbohydrates deliver a lot of nutrients per serving. Here we need to briefly address the question of complex carbs vs. simple carbs. The fundamental difference between the two is their chemical structure, but we're most interested in the fact that complex carbs require a longer time to digest, sending

MICROWAVE POPCORN, HOLD THE TRANS FATS

Popcorn is a high-fiber, high-quality carbohydrate that's fun to eat. One of the problems with microwave popcorn, though, is that most of the brands contain partially hydrogenated fats (p. 250), also called trans fats. Some brands of microwave popcorn boast no trans fats, and they're a better option. However, the best choice may still be to make your own with an air popper, adding some fat in the form of spray-on olive oil or even butter for a splurge. Before topping, air-popped corn is about 30 calories per cup. If you pop it with oil, it's got about 55 calories. Some people like to add herbs or grated cheese. It's a quality carbohydrate snack.

your blood sugar and serotonin on a nice slow ride upward and keeping you feeling fuller longer. Complex carbs also contain vitamins, minerals, and other nutrients that support your health. All complex carbs are good for carbo timing; some simple carbs are, too. Let's list some excellent food choices from both categories that you can use in timing your carb intake:

- **COMPLEX CARBS:** Vegetables, potatoes with their skins, legumes (p. 265), brown rice, nuts, popcorn, seeds, whole grains, and whole-grain foods. The package may not specifically use the phrase "whole grains," so look for breads that are heavier by weight and have a coarser texture than cotton-like white bread.

- **SIMPLE CARBS:** Fruit, milk, and milk products such as cheese and yogurt (try plain low-fat yogurt with cinnamon and a little honey if needed).

Other simple carbs—candy bars, donuts, cookies, chips—have virtually no nutrition and because they contain simple sugars they send your blood sugar skyrocketing and then crashing down within thirty to sixty minutes or so.

Q & A: ORGANIC FOODS

Q. Is it worth spending the extra money to buy organic fruit, vegetables, and meat?

A. Nutritionally speaking, this depends on who we believe, with some saying definitely and others maintaining that it makes little difference. To me it makes a lot of sense to go with the organic if you can afford it, and there are four compelling reasons. First, you really don't know for sure what chemicals might have been sprayed on produce that's not organic. Fruits and veggies are shipped from all over the world, from countries using chemicals we banned in the United States years ago. Second, although the U.S. government promises that the pesticides and herbicides our farmers use are safe, the long-term effect of many chemicals on the human body is simply not known. Third, we definitely don't know what effect these chemicals have on the body when you combine two or more of them together. And fourth, let's consider the question from a holistic point of view. Would the entire planet and all its inhabitants be better off if the world were pesticide-free and herbicide-free, and organic produce was everywhere? To me, the answer is an unqualified yes, and we may as well start by supporting our organic farmers.

If you can't afford organic fruits and veggies, get a good dishwashing brush (use it only for produce), immerse your fruits and veggies in soapy water, give them a thorough scrubbing (or in the case of lettuce and other leafy greens, dunking) and rinse before eating them.

You're probably better off with organically raised meat and poultry as well. Although the hormones and antibiotics fed to livestock are recognized as safe by the Food and Drug Administration, I generally recommend that people try to reduce their intake of these as much as possible. The secret here is to do what you can and don't get too anxious about it. If you have an organic grocer near you, try to use chemical-free meat products. If not, you don't want to be driving thirty miles to an organic grocery store to buy chemical-free meats while adding more exhaust fumes to the atmosphere. Many groceries now carry eggs laid by grain-fed chickens that have lived a free-range, additive-free life, and eggs in general are a terrific source of protein.

RECIPES

Yogurt Blueberry Brain Booster

This smoothie is loaded with goodies: the yogurt kicks up your serotonin and makes your belly hum along happily because of the probiotics (helpful bacteria) in the yogurt. Blueberries have a powerful antioxidant effect and you'll get a good shot of iron and calcium from the molasses. The cinnamon slows the rate at which the sugars are taken up by your body and provides a flavorful zing. Buy blueberries fresh in season and then wash and dry them before freezing in a freezer bag. Or buy a bag of ready-to-use frozen blueberries at your grocery.

2 CUPS PLAIN LOW-FAT YOGURT WITH ACTIVE CULTURES (CHECK THE LABEL)

2 CUPS FROZEN BLUEBERRIES (OR ANY FROZEN FRUIT)

2 TABLESPOONS CINNAMON

3–4 TABLESPOONS UNSULFURED MOLASSES

Put everything in a blender or food processor and blend until it's the smoothness you like. Some people like to keep it chunky and eat it with a spoon; others blend until it's drinkable. If you need to thin it, use a little soy milk or skim milk. Add a shake of dry ginger or allspice, some soy powder, some ground flaxseed (p. 261), a cut-up banana, or anything that you like.

Toasted Nuts

Toasting nuts enhances their flavor. Nuts have some of the best fats you can eat and are perfect for raising serotonin because they contain a nice amount of carbohydrates—about 3 grams per quarter cup for pecans; 4 grams for walnuts; and 8 grams for pistachios. We like toasted walnuts especially, but you can toast any kind of nut. Toss them into a green or bean salad, eat them with fruit and yogurt for breakfast, or take them to work for a snack. For toasting, choose raw, unsalted nuts. Make a big batch so you can freeze the extras.

Preheat oven to 350 degrees and put the nuts on a baking sheet that will hold them in a single layer.

Put the pan in the oven and don't walk too far without setting a timer —nuts burn easily. Set your timer for 4 minutes.

After 4 minutes, stir the nuts and shake them back into a single layer. Put back in the oven for another 4 minutes (set the timer), or until you can smell the luscious roasted nut scent. Stir again when your timer goes off. The nuts should be about done, but you can continue roasting for 4 minutes at a time until they're the color you like. (Smaller nuts take less time.)

Cool completely. Store in a covered container.

Dressings for Salads and Hot Vegetables

1. MY FAVORITE THINGS VEGETABLE DRESSING (LEMON, CAPERS, OLIVE OIL, CHEESE)

In a big bowl, put a tablespoon or two of extra virgin olive oil. Add a squeeze of lemon or lime and a tablespoon of capers. When your vegetables are done steaming, drain them and heap them in the bowl. Toss gently to coat and then add a sprinkling of cheese—parmesan, bleu, sharp cheddar, or goat—and toss again. Devour.

2. SALSA AND SOUR CREAM DRESSING

Pour a half cup of good-quality red or green salsa into a small bowl. Add 2 tablespoons low-fat sour cream and whisk or stir until nicely mixed. You can toss this dressing into a cold salad or drape it over steamed vegetables. By adjusting the proportions (one quarter cup salsa to two tablespoons sour cream) you'll have a nice dip for a plate of cold veggies.

Blue Cheese, Pear, and Toasted Walnut Quesadillas

Yum. Have these with Almost-Instant Black Bean Soup (p. 272). Or cocktails.

2 MEDIUM CORN TORTILLAS

¼ CUP CRUMBLED BLUE CHEESE

3 TABLESPOONS TOASTED CHOPPED WALNUTS (SEE P. 269)

THINLY SLICED PEAR, SKIN ON

Chop the toasted walnuts (you have some in the freezer, right?). Place one tortilla in a frying pan coated with a little olive oil over medium heat. Sprinkle on the cheese and the walnuts, and then lay the pear slices on in a star-like pattern. Put another tortilla on top and press down gently. Cover with a lid and turn heat to medium high. Peek after about 3 minutes to see if the cheese is melting. When it starts to melt, use a spatula to flip the quesadilla over. Cook for another 2 minutes, lid on. Cut into wedges and serve. You can use two frying pans to make two quesadillas simultaneously.

TWC Mini Bean Salad

Here's a fast food that gives you a great carbo boost. Take it to work or make it the start of an easy and nutritious dinner. Using the beans and oil as a base, endless substitutions are possible: cooked chopped cold chicken; chopped hard-boiled eggs; onions; raisins; roasted red peppers from a jar; chopped spinach or bok choy; tomato; raw sweet peppers. Sprinkle on some toasted chopped nuts just before eating (so they don't get soggy). Substitute any canned bean and try adding herbs and a squeeze of lime.

1 CAN KIDNEY BEANS

1 APPLE, SKIN ON, CHOPPED

¼ CUP CUBED SWISS CHEESE

1 TABLESPOON OLIVE OIL

Rinse and drain the beans. Put into a bowl, add olive oil, and toss. Add the apple and cheese and toss again. Chill. Or eat it right away if you're hungry.

Almost-Instant Black Bean Soup

This is one of our favorite recipes. Black beans are a high-quality Triple Whammy carbohydrate and incredibly satisfying. You can make this soup in about 14 minutes and then let it simmer to thicken while you get the extras ready, help your daughter with her homework, or have a glass of wine. Serve it with Blue Cheese, Pear, and Toasted Walnut Quesadillas (p. 271). It also freezes well, so make double or triple the amount and freeze in containers you can take to work and microwave for lunch. You can rehydrate dried black beans for this recipe, but large cans of black beans, which cost about a dollar, make this soup easy and economical. Get creative with spices, adding a couple shakes of hot sauce and a teaspoon or two of chili powder, oregano, basil, and/or turmeric as the soup simmers.

1 TABLESPOON OLIVE OIL

1 LARGE ONION, CHOPPED

1 CLOVE GARLIC (OR MORE), CHOPPED, OR A FEW SHAKES OF GARLIC POWDER

1 14.5-OZ. CAN BLACK BEANS, WITH LIQUID

1 14.5-OZ. CAN DICED TOMATOES (LOOK FOR TOMATOES WITH NO SUGAR IN
    ANY FORM, ESPECIALLY THE UBIQUITOUS HIGH FRUCTOSE CORN SYRUP),
    WITH LIQUID

1 BUNCH CILANTRO

½ CUP RED SALSA

⅓ CUP RED OR WHITE WINE OR A QUARTER CUP SHERRY OR BOURBON
(OPTIONAL)

Put olive oil, chopped onion, and chopped garlic in a pot over medium high heat. Cook the onion and garlic, stirring as you inhale the aromas. Open the beans and tomatoes while you stir occasionally.

After about 5 minutes, pour in the black beans and tomatoes with their liquids; add the alcohol now too, if you're using it, and stir to mix.

Cover your pot and turn up the heat to high until it boils. Then remove the lid and reduce the heat to medium, so the liquid simmers briskly and releases its steam, which will thicken the soup. If you'll be eating the soup soon, set your timer for 15 minutes.

While the soup simmers, twist off the tough stem end of the cilantro bunch and wash it well under running water, rinsing and squeezing to get any sand out. Squeeze dry in a paper towel and then chop it.

When your timer goes off, add the salsa, taste the soup, and then ladle into bowls. Add a dollop of low-fat sour cream, which creates a satisfying creamy soup when stirred in, and sprinkle some cilantro on top. Add any of the toppings below.

TOPPINGS:

CHOPPED GREEN OLIVES

CHILES—BOTH HOT AND MILD ARE AVAILABLE IN CANS, OR DE-SEED AND DE-RIB A JALAPEÑO, DICE IT, AND SAUTÉ WITH THE ONION AND GARLIC.

GRATED CHEESE

CHOPPED AVOCADO

GROUND TURKEY OR BEEF THAT YOU'VE BROWNED AND CRUMBLED (THIS CREATES A NICE CHILI WHEN STIRRED IN)

SQUEEZE A SLICE OF LEMON OR LIME INTO THE SOUP AND STIR.

TO GET MORE VEGETABLES INTO THIS SOUP:

Add a chopped green or red pepper at the onion/garlic sauté stage.

Add diced eggplant (skin and all) at the sauté stage. You'll need to cook the soup a bit longer to be sure the eggplant is tender.

Chop a few handfuls of spinach and add to the pot during the cover-off cooking stage. If not everyone in your family appreciates spinach, add some to individual bowls before adding the soup.

Chop some washed parsley and add with the onions/garlic sauté.

22.

USING ALTERNATIVE MEDICINE TO HEAL YOUR WHAMMIES

A woman with a Triple Whammy disorder who schedules an appointment with me does so knowing that I'll likely be recommending some form of alternative medicine as part of her treatment plan. After all, she probably already has an internist, and doesn't need another (though I'm one too), and may have already worked on her condition with her doc, as well as with a specialist or two. She's not looking for a third specialist to order diagnostic tests or prescribe medicine she's already had.

Alternative medicine often dramatically helps women with Triple Whammy problems. Understand, though, that the term "alternative" can be misleading. Today it's widely used to describe treatments like reflexology or aromatherapy that aren't routinely offered by mainstream physicians, though some do offer or recommend them as complementary therapies together with their mainstream treatments. No form of alternative medicine is meant to replace conventional care. Most physicians agree that the strong suits of conventional medicine are surgical intervention and emergency care and also grudgingly acknowledge that medicine does less well with chronic conditions and those whose diagnosis is unclear, like pain and fatigue.

In this section, we discuss the four largest alternative medicine disciplines in the United States, Canada, Europe, and the UK. British and European physicians are far more open to alternative medicine than their American and Canadian counterparts. Herbal medicine, homeopathy, and acupuncture are really rather routine recommendations, encouraged by European doctors and taught to physicians in postgraduate medical school courses. Because chiropractic medicine developed here in the United States, we do have more chiropractors than Europe, but their numbers there are on the rise.

Alternative medicine works best for chronic problems. There is no shortage of good clinical research showing the effectiveness of alternative medicine, whose therapies are regularly described as "safe" and "gentle." The problem has always been that American physicians simply will not read professional journals devoted to chiropractic or homeopathic research. The odds of being injured during a chiropractic treatment, massage, or with an acupuncture needle are about the same as being struck by lightning. And when you add to safe, gentle, and effective the fact that alternative practitioners spend far more time with patients than conventional doctors do, you have a combination that's very hard to ignore.

Will alternative medicine always work for your Triple Whammy disorder? No. Will it help relieve your symptoms, improve your overall well-being, guide you on a path to healthy living, and give you new insights into why you became ill in the first place? Definitely. Is your conventional doctor making a significant error in judgment if she dismisses your idea of trying something alternative? Sadly, yes.

The main challenge you face with alternative medicine is knowing exactly where to begin. Read this chapter and see what appeals to you. Your selection may be limited by what's available in your city. A good alternative practitioner will be aware of her limitations and let you know if she thinks her therapy isn't working. The hallmark of a bad alternative practitioner is one who thinks she can do it alone and encourages you to give up your conventional physician or stop your current medication. If you hear any advice along those lines, do not schedule a return appointment.

CHIROPRACTIC

Chiropractic physicians believe that many health problems are due to imbalances in the musculoskeletal system. Chiropractors check for the presence of imbalances and, using a variety of manual techniques, attempt to get you back into alignment. Philosophically, chiropractic, an American-born and -bred form of alternative medicine, has more in common with traditional Chinese medicine (p. 285) than even most chiropractors realize. It references the body's inner wisdom, a self-healing energy that can be blocked by spinal misalignment. Realigning the spine and clearing blockages called subluxations allow this inner wisdom energy to flow freely and initiate drug-free healing from within.

For many years the American Medical Association (AMA) just wanted chiropractors to disappear. In one of the darker chapters of AMA history, the organization deliberately spread misinformation to the public about the dangers of chiropractic. They blocked chiropractors from admitting patients to hospitals, forbade physician members from making referrals to chiropractors, and blocked chiropractic access to Medicare billing. Then, in 1976, after reading some AMA internal memos about an organized plan to eliminate chiropractic altogether, the chiropractors went on the offensive. A feisty Chicago chiropractor and three colleagues sued the AMA on antitrust violations. In 1990, the AMA lost when the Supreme Court rejected without comment an AMA appeal of a Circuit Court decision finding against the AMA.

Today the relationship between conventional physicians and chiropractors, if not exactly chummy, is cool, and chiropractors acknowledge that they probably brought some of the wrath on themselves. "Straight" chiropractors, a generally declining breed, were convinced that chiropractic was the answer to virtually all medical problems, and that spinal manipulation could cure everything. Up until the 1950s, people asked for and received chiropractic treatment for cancer, heart disease, and infections. We can assume they did badly. Fortunately, the majority of chiropractors are "mixers," meaning they'll combine other therapies, like physical therapy and nutritional guidance, and limit their treatment to conditions associated with the musculoskeletal system.

With almost 40,000 practitioners around the country, chiropractic is extremely popular today. A holistically oriented chiropractic office can be a real resource for a variety of alternative therapies. Many chiropractors are certified in acupuncture, and can help in those communities that have no access to a practitioner of traditional Chinese medicine. Some chiropractors have massage therapists, nutritional counselors, and Reiki practitioners (p. 239) on staff or can help you locate qualified practitioners.

A TYPICAL VISIT TO A CHIROPRACTOR

Your first visit to a chiropractor will last about forty-five minutes. She'll ask detailed questions about your health history, inquiring in depth about your symptoms and how they've affected your life. You'll be asked about your sleeping, eating, and relaxation habits, as well as your response to previous therapies.

A thorough chiropractic physical examination is quite different from one performed by a conventional physician. I've watched my office associate, Dr. Paul Rubin, perform his examination many times, and have marveled about the amount of information he uncovers as he palpates muscles, joints, and bones, both when his patient is perfectly still and then as he moves each joint through its range of motion. Sometimes Dr. R orders X-rays of the spine (and rarely an MRI) to look for disc problems.

Treatment is completely individualized and generally depends on whether the problem has come on suddenly or is more long-standing. It usually begins with soft tissue work, like localized massage, followed by an adjustment of one or more bones of the spine. Each adjustment takes only a second to complete, and you may hear a harmless cracking noise caused by bursting gas bubbles in the fluid surrounding your joints.

In addition to your treatment, a chiropractor will offer advice on posture, stretching, diet, and exercise. You might feel a little sore after your first treatments, and some people like to go home for a short nap. Others feel liberated from the chronic stiffness in their bodies and leave their chiropractor's office bursting with energy.

Just like locating anyone in health care, finding a chiropractor is easy, but finding a really excellent chiropractor may take some effort. Word of mouth is your best bet, so ask your friends: someone probably has a miracle story about a certain chiropractor who "saved her from the knife." Younger conventional doctors are loosening up a bit, so you might ask your doctor for a referral, but don't be discouraged if she says something dumb like "you could be paralyzed," which is what many doctors used to say before chiropractic's name was cleared by the courts.

HOMEOPATHY (HOMEOPATHIC MEDICINE)

If you can envision dogs on opposite sides of a cyclone fence furiously and incessantly barking at each other, you've got a picture, at least in America, of the two-hundred-year-old animosity between conventional physicians and homeopaths. The hostility is so intense that the original by-laws of the American Medical Association included a goal to eliminate homeopathy from the land. Just knowing this, you might sensibly be asking yourself, "Do I really want to get into this?"

From my perspective, the answer is a firm "maybe." Although I've read a lot about the subject, and regularly refer patients to homeopaths, I am not one myself. It takes years of study to be a good homeopath: the books are huge and the language very complex.

Interestingly, it's easier to explain homeopathy to a nonmedical person than to a fellow physician or a medical student. The reason for this, I believe, is that too much scientific thinking narrows a doctor's perspective. Just as acupuncture asks you to accept the existence of *chi* (the vital energy running through your body), homeopathy insists that your knowledge of chemistry and biology may actually be wrong, and that another scientific reality might be possible. Because doctors have years of intensive education invested in mastering their skills, to give in just a little is difficult for them.

LIKE CURES LIKE

Homeopathy teaches that "like cures like." If the fundamentals ever seem confusing, repeat this simple mantra and you'll have it right. A substance that causes the symptoms of a condition when taken in large amounts will cure the condition and its symptoms when taken in small amounts. That's what Samuel Hahnemann, a practicing physician in Germany and the founder of homeopathic medicine, figured out over two hundred years ago. Quick example: If you've got what seems like a bad sore throat and sniffles, find a substance that gives a well person those symptoms, dilute it in the extreme, and you have a remedy. "So what's the big deal?" you might ask. "This is the basic principle of allergy shots and immunizations."

The answer is that most conventional doctors are very (very!) uncomfortable with two additional aspects of homeopathy.

First, Hahnemann proposed that the chosen substance, called a remedy, triggered a change in a person's vital force, an invisible energy (like *chi*) coursing through the body that had temporarily gone awry and was causing the symptoms to appear. Hahnemann's remedies would trigger a self-healing, a concept unacceptable to conventional physicians. In "regular" medicine, when you take a pill, it produces a change in your body. Antibiotics kill germs, anti-inflammatories suppress inflammation and pain, hormones act like chemicals you already have in your body. But nothing triggers your body to get well on its own.

But it's a second issue that really causes near-visible steam to pour forth from conventional doctors' ears. Hahnemann added the concept of *dilution potentization,* which basically means the more you keep diluting your remedy, the stronger and more potent it becomes. (Read that sentence twice before proceeding.) Now, if you keep diluting something, eventually you'll reach a point where no existing molecule of the original substance is left. And that's fine in homeopathy, because now your remedy has reached the level of high potency and is suitable for long-standing chronic symptoms. (Low-potency remedies are best for acute conditions, like colds and sprains.)

This, of course, flies in the face of the laws of physical chemistry, but to Hahnemann, it was all quite logical. With each dilution, the "energy" of the substance was increased and also transferred into the diluting solution, accounting for its increased healing powers.

Today, in the twenty-first century, even after two hundred years of continuous use and even though homeopathy is practiced worldwide, American physicians continue to define the essence of homeopathy as either a placebo effect or outright fraud. Given that statistical data has actually proven homeopathic therapies useful in certain conditions, you'd think they'd lighten up. But they won't give an inch.

THREE REASONS TO CONSIDER HOMEOPATHY

Here are three reasons you might consider homeopathy. If you answer yes to one or more of the following, read on for information on how to locate a homeopath:

– Throughout *The Triple Whammy Cure,* I've addressed both your hormones and neurotransmitters such as serotonin, and how you can normalize their levels to get relief from your symptoms. Along with natural supplements, I do occasionally recommend medications—substances that actually change your body. You personally may not want choose this route, "natural" or not. Instead, you'd like to see if your body can be triggered to self-heal. If this is the case, consider homeopathy.

– The whole concept of energy medicine appeals to you. Intuitively, you are comfortable with terms like *chi.* You believe that if your energy systems could be balanced, good health could be restored. Homeopathy is energy medicine, and you may want to try it.

– You feel a bit squeamish about acupuncture needles and Chinese herbs and would rather be working with an MD, DO (osteopath), DC (chiropractor), or ND (naturopath) who also practices homeopathy.

CHOOSING A PRACTITIONER

Since homeopathy is not taught in U.S. medical schools (U.S. medical schools would rather self-destruct than teach a course in homeopathy), physicians wishing to study it must learn it on their own. Interestingly, homeopathy is one of the most popular postgraduate courses among family doctors in the United Kingdom Physicians take lengthy courses, either by traveling to homeopathic colleges or by correspondence. After passing examinations, they achieve certification.

A mere three states (Arizona, Nevada, and Connecticut) actually license homeopaths; others do not, and the field is largely unregulated. A layperson can become a homeopath, and some are actually quite good, but I would stick with a physician (including osteopaths), a chiropractor, or a naturopath who practices homeopathy simply because they're better trained in understanding disease and the function of the body. In addition, they can turn to more conventional options in case the remedy fails to work effectively.

To find a homeopath, ask friends, check with your local health food store, or use the Internet. The National Center for Homeopathy (http://homeopathic.org/index.html) has a link called "How To Find a Homeopath" that's worth investigating.

WHAT HAPPENS WHEN I VISIT A HOMEOPATH?

A homeopath will begin by taking an extraordinarily detailed health history, asking not only about your current problems and how they developed, but also about seemingly irrelevant details concerning food preferences, sleeping habits, and how your body reacts to various weather conditions. Her goal is to determine the precise remedies for your problem. There are about two thousand homeopathic remedies from which to choose, each made from natural substances (plant, mineral, animal) that, if taken by a totally healthy person in large amounts, would duplicate the very symptoms you are experiencing.

Your remedy will consist of a tiny pellet that melts in your mouth or liquid drops placed under your tongue. During follow-up visits, your homeopath will ask if you notice any changes in your symptoms, and may change or add new remedies along the way. She will likely suggest dietary changes and steps in self-care such as exercise, stress reduction, bodywork (p. 236), or counseling.

Homeopathic remedies are completely harmless; they can be used by children and during pregnancy.

NATUROPATHY (NATUROPATHIC MEDICINE)

Even if you're unfamiliar with the terms naturopathy and naturopathic medicine, you can correctly guess it involves both "nature" and "natural medicine." There are only five schools and barely two thousand practitioners in the United States, and they're licensed in only fourteen states. If you're fortunate enough to live in a state that allows naturopathic medicine, you'll be able to work with a physician who can provide a variety of drugless therapies that have a real possibility of helping you.

Naturopathy has its roots in Europe, where so-called nature cure physicians were immensely popular in the eighteenth and nineteenth centuries. Naturopathy arrived in the United States more than one hundred years ago and spread quickly, with dozens of naturopathic medical colleges and thousands of practitioners. Unfortunately, the quality of both the schools and the practitioners varied widely, and when medicine began to regulate itself by licensing doctors, these numbers went into a steep decline. As "scientific medicine" soared in popularity during the first half of the twentieth century, interest in natural therapies waned, so that by the 1950s the profession of naturopathy was all but extinct. But things do change, and as the public's desire for natural alternatives grew from the 1960s onward, so did the fortunes of naturopathic medicine.

BASICS OF NATUROPATHIC MEDICINE

The fundamentals of naturopathic medicine are actually rather likable and have a commonsense ring to them. The first guiding principle took me a while to pronounce correctly: *vis medicatrix naturae,* or "the healing power of nature." This means that within your body lies the power to heal itself through the energy naturopaths call the "life force." The role of the doctor is to help you remove your personal obstacles to wellness and facilitate your own self-healing process.

The second principle is also that of holistic medicine: treat the whole person. Keep in mind that each of us is a complex interaction of mind and body and that we create and live in an environment that endlessly affects our health. Sadly, this holistic philosophy is rarely practiced in conventional medicine, which most often limits itself to the physical, focuses on disease alone, and employs doctors who specialize in specific parts of the body.

The third notion is shared by practitioners of conventional medicine: *primum nocere,* or "first, do no harm." Of course, since naturopaths don't write prescriptions for drugs and don't perform surgery, they've got a better chance of fulfilling this than their conventional counterparts.

Fourth: identify and treat the cause. This principle resonates well with patients who don't feel comfortable taking medicines that simply suppress symptoms. Many people really would rather find out exactly why they're experiencing a symptom, or why they became ill, and make an attempt to deal with the root cause.

Conventional physicians are in complete agreement with the fifth principle: prevention is the best cure. Doctors of every ilk and breed endlessly wring their hands in despair as patients self-destruct through poor food selections, inactivity, tobacco and alcohol use, and a variety of other unhealthy lifestyle choices.

And finally, naturopaths remind us that the word "doctor" actually means "teacher" (*docere)* and that a physician's role is really to teach the steps you can take toward a long and healthy life.

ECLECTIC HEALERS, AND THE STORY OF AMY

From the dictionary, eclectic means "combining a variety of sources" and if this sounds appropriate for naturopathic medicine, its practitioners would agree with you. In fact, during the nineteenth century, physicians we now call naturopaths were called eclectic healers.

Let me share with you my treatment selections for a recent patient, because they represent a good example of naturopathic eclecticism. I'm kind of glad MDs rarely read books like the one you're holding, written by alternative doctors for an educated public. I certainly would receive some criticism from my professional colleagues for the following:

Amy had just turned thirty, and arrived in my office to learn about alternative therapies for her overactive thyroid gland. She had been feeling generally crummy for the previous ten years (!), either when her thyroid gland was overactive (causing palpitations, fatigue, feeling constantly hot, "wired," and shaky) or when she was on thyroid medicine (which produced acne, hair loss, and more fatigue—almost like she had the flu).

During the previous year, Amy's overactive gland had quieted down with no medication, but after some significant job stress, it started to flare up again. Her doctor wanted to restart medication, but, remembering how ill she had felt while taking it, Amy was opposed. She was also against getting her thyroid destroyed completely using radiation, another option her doctor had presented. When she told her doctor that she wanted to consider alternative medicine, Amy's physician told her to find another doctor and that she was no longer responsible for Amy's care.

In the *Textbook of Natural Medicine,* Pizzorno and Murray devote a whole chapter to managing an overactive thyroid, not one iota of which I was taught in medical school or during my residency in internal medicine. And talk about a combination of therapies! They advise dietary changes (add cabbages, rutabagas, turnips), vitamins (A, C, E), herbs (lycopus, melissa), acupuncture, and stress reduction.

Within eight weeks of starting the program Amy and I agreed she'd try, she was feeling fine and her thyroid tests were completely normal. Would this work for everyone? Probably not. Is it worth a try before radiation or surgery? Ask Amy.

Most conventional physicians who practice alternative medicine are simply incorporating many of the principles and therapies of naturopathic medicine. Much of my own basic training in vitamins, minerals, and herbs for therapeutic purposes came from their schools' textbooks. I had never heard of "functional medicine" in medical school, and it's naturopaths who refined the tests for food sensitivities, digestive and liver function, and measuring hormones using samples of saliva.

Probably more than any group of alternative practitioners, naturopaths want to be regarded as scientists and researchers. The naturopathic schools have been very active in setting up research studies with the National Institutes of Health; naturopathic medical journals publish studies that are as rigorous as any in conventional medicine; and at annual meetings, naturopaths present research papers to fellow members.

CHOOSING A PRACTITIONER

In order to be a naturopathic physician (ND), the candidate must complete four years of training in a naturopathic medical school and pass state licensing exams. During those four years, naturopaths receive a broad education in alternative medicine. By the time they complete their training, they're well versed in herbal medicine and are trained in acupuncture, manipulative therapies (similar to chiropractic and osteopathy), homeopathy, nutritional medicine, physical therapy, and water therapies. Most can also perform minor surgery and deliver babies.

Unfortunately, in those states that don't license naturopathy, anyone can call herself a naturopath and many obtain degrees from one of several mail-order schools. (As a rule of thumb, it's probably best not to turn your health care over to someone learning medicine from a correspondence school.)

In 2005, NDs were licensed in Alaska, Arizona, California, Connecticut, Hawaii, Kansas, Maine, Montana, New Hampshire, Oregon, Utah, Vermont, Idaho, and Washington. They have a legal right to practice in the District of Columbia, Puerto Rico, and the Virgin Islands.

Since the premises of naturopathic medicine include prevention and education, a naturopath is an excellent choice as your primary care doctor. In Illinois, where I live, they're unlicensed but often possess a second "licensable" degree, like chiropractic or acupuncture, and—this is important—work under the supervision of an MD or DO (osteopath). If you decide you'd like to see a naturopathic physician, the primary consideration is education. Make certain they've graduated from one of the accredited four-year in-residence schools. If they have, they'll be rightfully proud to show you their hard-earned degree.

To locate a doctor of naturopathy, contact the American Association of Naturopathic Physicians (AANP), located in Washington, D. C. You can contact the organization online (www.naturopathic.org) or by calling 1-866-538-2267 to verify a practitioner's certification.

YOUR FIRST APPOINTMENT WITH A NATUROPATH

If you're fortunate enough to live in a state that allows naturopaths to practice, here's what will happen during your first appointment. You'll be with the doctor for at least an hour, and you'll be asked lots of questions that go well beyond your medical problem, probing the story of your life and your lifestyle choices.

You'll likely have some diagnostic tests taken—not only the standard blood tests found in every primary care doctor's office, but one or more of the "functional" tests that identify food sensitivities and assess digestive and liver function. You'll learn a lot about healthful eating and you may be prescribed nutritional supplements, herbs, or homeopathic remedies. Your doctor may recommend a course of acupuncture or a bodywork therapy such as Reiki (p. 239), chiropractic (p. 275), or therapeutic touch (p. 242).

Follow-up visits are usually about thirty minutes long. If your doctor believes your condition requires some conventional medicine, such as a prescription drug, she will likely refer you to a physician who either has some knowledge of naturopathic medicine or is sympathetic to alternative therapies.

TRADITIONAL CHINESE MEDICINE (INCLUDING ACUPUNCTURE)

Although the system of traditional Chinese medicine (TCM) began over 2,500 years ago, it took until 1971 for most U.S. citizens to become aware of it as a possible treatment for a variety of ailments. That was the year President Nixon opened up relations with China, and the *New York Times* reporter James Reston was stricken with appendicitis in Beijing during his visit. His post-operative pain was managed by acupuncture, and his story on the front page of the *Times* headlined, "I've seen the past, and it works!"

Among themselves, acupuncturists now divide the history of the world into "Before Reston" and "After Reston," because indeed, their fortunes did change quickly.

As an internist, I must confess an incredible amount of skepticism when the first photos appeared of Chinese patients undergoing major surgery, fully awake and bristling with acupuncture needles, yet apparently pain-free. Years later, when I became interested in alternative medicine and acupuncture, I had the good fortune of tumbling from my bicycle and breaking my wrist.

"Oh, boy!" I thought, "Now I'll get to try some acupuncture."

At the time, this was not the first choice of therapy among physicians, and indeed, I was the first doctor this particular practitioner had ever treated. Lying on a comfortable cot, chatting about nothing in particular, he first asked a few questions, then felt my pulse for what I thought was a unnecessarily long time, examined my tongue with an interest I felt it didn't deserve, and finally inserted three fine needles painlessly into my throbbing arm. In a minute the pain vanished. Gone.

"Wow!" I said, as professionally as possible.

He then suggested I take a nap. I remarked that falling asleep in the afternoon was a problem for me. "Here, this should help," he said, inserting a needle into my scalp. And thirty minutes later, I woke up.

Obviously, an experience such as this can be life-changing. Shortly thereafter, when I made the decision to open the first center in Chicago that would blend conventional and alternative medicine, I discovered I had to rethink my whole concept of the human body in TCM terms if I wanted to understand what had happened during that session.

CORE CONCEPTS

The core concept of TCM says that disease is the result of imbalances in the flow of the body's vital energy, *chi*. Although virtually all fields of alternative medicine have their own word for this energy (homeopathy's vital force, chiropractic's inner wisdom), conventional medicine refuses to acknowledge the existence of *chi*. TCM includes other forms of treatment in addition to acupuncture, such as herbal remedies, dietary therapies, therapeutic exercise and body movement (t'ai chi), and a mind-body therapy called chi-gong.

A TCM practitioner looks for imbalances in your body's energy. So if you hear a phrase like "liver stagnation," it does not mean you have hepatitis, but rather that your *chi* is not flowing smoothly through your body. A head cold may be expressed in the far more poetic "wind-heat invading the lungs." The practitioner may then use the tiny needles to correct the flow of *chi,* or suggest herbs, diet, massage, or daily t'ai chi exercises, all with the goal of restoring your body's energy balance.

Keep in mind that your goal with any form of therapy, conventional or alternative, is positive results. It's reasonable for you to ask how many sessions will be needed before good results can be expected. And if your condition is worsening, you will want to return to your primary care doctor.

The concept that good health can be attained by restoring balance permeates virtually all of alternative medicine. Conventional medicine relies on action (take a pill, have surgery); alternative medicine (including TCM) says something like, "Wait a minute . . . your body has powerful self-healing tools that have been thrown temporarily out of whack. Let's see if we can gently nudge everything back along a path so the body can heal itself."

I've now worked every day for many years with Mari Stecker, an acupuncturist who maintains her own practice adjacent to my examining rooms. If I had a choice of giving up my stethoscope or being without an acupuncturist, the 'scope would be out the window.

We've treated thousands of patients together, and I am still awed in much the same way as when those three needles halted the pain of my broken wrist. I've seen her end an asthma attack that would otherwise have required an emergency room visit, and also a migraine headache that would normally need morphine to quell. I've even seen acupuncture used to rotate a baby in the uterus that otherwise would have been endangered by being born feet first.

A TYPICAL TCM EVALUATION INCLUDES THREE COMPONENTS:

- The first assesses the balance between yin and yang—complementary but opposing qualities that represent the natural dualities of the world, such as male/female, day/night, and hot/cold.

- The second considers the correspondence of the ailment to the five Chinese elements—wood, fire, earth, metal, and water. It is believed that each internal organ and body system is related to an elemental quality and that the body reflects the natural world in this way.

- The third determines which organ or metabolic system requires the most support from therapy.

CHOOSING A PRACTITIONER

Even in China, the initial diagnostic evaluation of a chronic condition or a newer problem is generally done by a conventionally trained physician before acupuncture is considered, and you should do the same. It's really best if you coordinate your care between your doctor and your acupuncturist. If you can't find a pair that will work together, see Locating an Integrative or Holistic Doctor and Alternative Therapists (p. 295) for information on how to find those that will.

The licensing of TCM varies widely from state to state. Most reasonable states license certified practitioners as OMDs (Doctors of Oriental Medicine) or LicAc (licensed acupuncturist). Some states restrict their use of herbs. The education of an OMD is a challenging one: usually three years, with academic and clinic work, an internship, and passing a national board exam. Their numbers are increasing, and virtually every medium-to-large city now usually has at least one acupuncturist.

Chiropractors and naturopaths can take elective courses in acupuncture during their education, but their knowledge is nowhere near the depth of the full course. The University of California offers an extensive course in Chinese medicine for physicians (MDs and DOs—Doctors of Osteopathy). Graduates of this program have an education comparable to that of an OMD, with the additional skills of conventional medicine.

A CAUTION

Chinese herbs are not regulated by the Food and Drug Administration. Your practitioner will be able to tell you of anticipated side effects or any possible interactions with prescription drugs. Usually, American practitioners of Chinese medicine use products from long-established American manufacturers that are well thought of, companies with a history of good, effective combinations of herbs. They stay away from imports from unknown companies.

Q & A: ACUPUNCTURE

Q. I've read my teenage daughter the riot act about not getting a tattoo or piercing because I've heard that unclean needles can carry HIV, hepatitis C, and other serious diseases. Now I want to try acupuncture for my irritable bowel. How can I be sure that the needles will be sterile and safe?

A. Acupuncture needles are never recycled. Instead, your acupuncturist opens a brand new, completely sterile set of needles for you and for each of her patients. In addition, she'll use a new package of needles for each of your visits. Read about how to locate a qualified practitioner on page 295.

APPENDIX

COMPOUNDING PHARMACIES

It may surprise you to learn that at one time, all pharmacies were compounding pharmacies. I myself was raised in one. As a small boy, I well remember my father deciphering what I considered a totally illegible prescription, mixing some powders with a mortar and pestle (proud symbol of the pharmacist), and then painstakingly inserting the powder into empty gelatin capsules. Today, 99 percent of pharmacists dispense already compounded drugs, a shame, really, because the compounding skills they learned at pharmacy school are going to waste.

None of the huge national drugstore chains do any compounding. It's very time-consuming and requires special equipment in a closed space like any good laboratory. But the tiny 1 percent of pharmacies that do compound play an essential role for many physicians and they may be equally important for you. Here's why.

The pharmaceutical industry limits its production to medications from which it will make the greatest profit. These are the drugs the company itself has developed and can sell exclusively—with no competition—and they sell a single version of the medicine, usually in tablet or capsule form, with one or more sizes reflecting different doses.

But many other medications exist, especially older ones and also drugs that can't be patented and owned by a single company. These drugs are sold only in bulk quantities, and you need a compounding pharmacist to measure out carefully a certain amount from the bulk quantity and put it into a capsule, make it into a suppository, or mix it into a palatable liquid. As a physician, I use compounding pharmacies to customize medications so they fulfill precisely the special needs of my patients.

These days, bioidentical hormones for women represent the largest amount of work done by compounding pharmacies, and in the process the pharmacists have become genuine experts in hormone replacement therapy. If you're going to try bioidentical hormones, ask your doctor when she gives you your prescription for the location of a nearby compounding pharmacy. You can also do an Internet search, including the words "compounding pharmacy" and your state or city.

If you need a physician who prescribes bioidentical hormones, visit the website of the Women's International Pharmacy in Madison, Wisconsin (www .womensinternational.com). By clicking on "Resources" and then on "Request a Practitioner Referral," you can request a listing of physicians in your state who have asked to be listed on this referral service.

My patients often ask if medications from compounding pharmacies cost more than other medications; the answer really depends on the medication itself. However, there may be a considerable difference in price between one compounding pharmacy and another, so it definitely pays to shop around.

As for insurance coverage, you need a doctor's prescription to get your medicines (just like any pharmacy), so if you have prescription coverage on your health insurance you're entitled to reimbursement. A few compounding pharmacies will bill your insurance company directly. Most of my patients simply submit the paid receipt for reimbursement. Recently, one health insurance company established a formal contract with a compounding pharmacy and let the enrollees know they could mail their prescription directly to that pharmacy. I looked on this as a big step in the right direction.

CANDIDA (YEAST) OVERGROWTH SYNDROME

There is no disorder that has generated more controversy between conventional and alternative medicine than the one attributed to the microorganism *Candida albicans*—"candida" for short. It's a fungus, and therefore a cousin to the organisms that cause athlete's foot and chronic toenail infections, and the direct cause of vaginal yeast infections. Candida is indeed often referred to as yeast, but is not at all the same as the yeast that makes your bread rise in the oven.

Many years ago, when I was setting up my first integrative medicine clinic in

Chicago, I was called into the office of the chief of medicine of the hospital on which I was a staff member. He had heard rumors of my plan to combine conventional doctors with alternative practitioners and wanted more details. After all, the reputation of "our" hospital was at stake. (The fact that "our" hospital later closed and is now being turned into condominiums has, I hope, nothing to do with my clinic.) The main purpose of this meeting was to inquire if I was going to become "one of those damned candida quacks" whose medical licenses should be taken away because of their professional irresponsibility. Since I was totally clueless about what he was referring to, I replied that I wasn't, but decided on the spot that candida was something worth exploring.

Now, after years of reading more books on candida than I think were necessary, and listening to hundreds of women tell me their tales of woe with candida, I can tell you unequivocally that what follows is a necessary section of this book. By the time you finish, I think you'll agree with me.

Candida albicans normally, and usually quite harmlessly, inhabits our intestinal tracts, and a small amount exists in your vagina as well. Although the population of candida is kept in check by the other microorganisms dwelling in these places, sometimes this internal balance is thrown out of whack, and candida proliferates unchecked, resulting in mild (repeat, mild) mischief. By far the most common trigger for candida overgrowth is taking antibiotics. A single dose of one of the so-called broad-spectrum antibiotics is like an ecological catastrophe to the delicate balance of internal microorganisms. When you take an antibiotic, the candida in your intestines and vagina start to multiply rapidly because, while everything else around it is being killed en masse, your candida is utterly unscathed. In the vagina this is called vaginitis or a yeast infection, and it produces vaginal itching and a whitish discharge.

Candida overgrowing in your mouth can discolor your tongue, a condition called oral thrush. You can also have problems with candida if you have diabetes or take corticosteroid medicines for several weeks, or if you have a condition that destroys your immune system, like HIV/AIDS.

Conventional doctors don't have any argument with these candida infections, but some years ago a pediatrician from Tennessee, William Crook, MD, wrote an immensely influential book about candida called *The Yeast Connection*. He had observed a correlation between women reporting chronic ill health and their previous use of antibiotics, especially when they had used antibiotics for months at a time, like for acne. He proposed that the basis of their symptoms was an overgrowth of candida in the intestines, and honestly, there is some sense to this. Why should problems with excess candida simply be confined to mouths and vaginas? Once an overgrowth of candida had established itself, you could imagine some intestinal symptoms like gas, bloating, changes in bowels, maybe some cramping.

But what Dr. Crook proposed went significantly beyond this. He believed that once the candida was intestinal, it would burrow deeply into the intestinal walls, damage the intestines, and release substances that were responsible for a long list of symptoms. Candida, he proposed, was the main culprit behind previously undiagnosed chronic fatigue, muscle aches, headaches, brain fog, depression, irritability, sugar cravings, chemical sensitivities, increased susceptibility to the side effects of medications, premenstrual syndrome, and decreased libido, especially when all your other diagnostic tests were negative. If this list of symptoms sounds suspiciously like the Triple Whammy symptoms you've been encountering throughout this book, then you'll understand where this is heading.

Getting little response to his theories from the conventional medical community, Dr. Crook took them directly to the public, in his best-selling book and several subsequent titles. The most likely victims of candida overgrowth, he felt, were women suffering most of the symptoms listed, who had also previously taken antibiotics and/or birth control pills. His book attributed both physical and psychological symptoms to candida and, anticipating that a typical reader would get little help from her personal physician, taught you how to treat your candida without a physician, mainly by following an incredibly restrictive diet for months.

Thousands of women identified themselves with the cases Dr. Crook described, and indeed headed off to their family doctors for help. If you were one of these women, you likely were in for a shock. Dr. Crook had anticipated correctly. Not only had your doctor never heard of candida causing these problems, but she also had virtually no interest in reading anything about a condition she felt she'd learned about in medical school. On some misguided principle, conventional physicians almost never touch medical self-help books, and unfortunately close their minds to information that arrives this way.

So there you were. Even though you had been feeling ill for months, your tests normal and your ill health undiagnosed, now you had an explanation for your symptoms. What did you get from your doctor for all your efforts? "There's no such illness," even though the book described your problems to a T. And then your doctor, who probably was seeing other women with the same book, rolled her eyes, took a deep breath, and launched into her version of candida "facts."

Listening, you thought her rather unsympathetic. You'd read that book so thoroughly. You started wondering what to do next.

So then you went back to the book and simply took matters into your own hands. You'd get rid of that blasted candida yourself! Here the nutritional supplement industry stepped in, creating hundreds of confusing products to kill your candida, heal your damaged intestinal lining, restore your good bacteria, and shore up your immune system. Ill-trained alternative practitioners began diagnosing every symptom as candida, prescribing more supplements, more dietary restrictions, and inculcating the idea that the return of any symptom was somehow your fault ("You really ate fudge? With your candida?! Now we have to start all over . . ."). Having a bad day meant a surge of candida "raging" within, and "overwhelming" your immune defenses. Makes you anxious just reading this, doesn't it?

In the meantime, conventional physicians were getting annoyed at what they saw as a form of mass hysteria. Instead of exploring exactly what was going on, giving Crook the hearing he justly deserved, and debating whether or not the syndrome existed, medical societies were actually proposing to remove the medical license of any conventional physician who had the nerve to diagnose or treat a patient with candida overgrowth syndrome. They seriously planned "candida watch" hotlines for patients to report "candida quack" doctors, as my former chief of medicine had described.

Now, years later, I can report that, sadly, the situation has not improved significantly. Each week, I get two or three new patients convinced they have candida overgrowth syndrome as part of their troubles. They learned of it through reading a book or an article in a self-help health magazine or through a well-meaning but misguided alternative practitioner. By the time I see them, I have a pretty good idea what they've been through. Dismissed outright by their family doctor, they're half-starved and depressed from Dr. Crook's extremely strict anti-candida diet, and nauseated from downing dozens of pills a day. They're feeling no better, and even more anxious and more depressed than before they ever heard of candida.

SO WHAT'S GOING ON?

Remember, if you will, the sentence you always hear from your doctor after you've been evaluated with symptoms of the Triple Whammy: "Your tests are normal." You walk out of her office thinking, "There must be an explanation to why I feel so bad. I'm not nuts. I feel tired, achy, bloated, foggy. There must be something happening inside me." You read about candida and think "Aha. It was candida all along."

But it's almost never candida. It's you, understandably wanting an explanation for your chronic ill health. Is it ever candida? Yes, and that's why Dr. Crook's findings deserve serious consideration from the conventional medical community. Some women have indeed taken an extraordinary amount of antibiotics over the years, or tell me that as soon as one vaginal infection clears, another follows in its wake. Women who believe they have a candida problem deserve a serious diagnostic evaluation, not the arrogant dismissal they all too often hear. To diagnose candida overgrowth syndrome, I order a culture of the patient's vaginal discharge and of a stool sample. If a patient has candida growing in her stools and vagina, and her immune system has high levels of candida antibodies, she has candida overgrowth syndrome. If the immune system is busy fighting a candida infection, it reveals itself in the immune antibodies in the blood, so I also measure those, even though the candida itself does not (repeat, does not!) get into your bloodstream unless you have a serious illness that is compromising your immune system, such as cancer or AIDS.

If tests suggest candida, the condition is easy to treat and doesn't require the dietary efforts suggested by Dr. Crook years before medication became available. Prescription medications like Diflucan and Sporanox kill virtually any form of fungus growing in the body, from the chronic toenail variety to vaginal yeast infections. The drugs are really quite safe, but you need to take them for about a month to see an appreciable drop in your antibody levels. If after taking antifungal medications these cultures test negative for candida, the patient's antibody levels fall, and she feels better, this to me stops in its tracks any judgment of placebo effect.

However, the majority of people I see who are convinced that candida is the source of their troubles don't have any evidence of infection anywhere in their bodies. And it's with these patients that I'll discuss the Triple Whammy as the basis for symptoms and previously normal tests, helping them see that a big part of the stress (Whammy #1) that was making everything worse was anxiety about the mysterious candida. With copies of the negative candida tests in front of us, we can move on and begin the real healing by tackling the Triple Whammy.

LOCATING AN INTEGRATIVE OR HOLISTIC DOCTOR AND ALTERNATIVE THERAPISTS

Ten years ago, you would have had a real challenge finding an integrative or holistic doctor or alternative medicine practitioner. Endlessly pressured by medical societies to conform to conventional therapies, physicians interested in holistic medicine or trying to incorporate some alternative therapies into their practices kept a low profile and didn't publicize themselves. Your best bet to locate one was the recommendation of a friend.

Word-of-mouth referrals from satisfied friends remains a reliable source in locating alternative medicine practitioners and holistic doctors, as does asking your chiropractor, acupuncturist, or massage therapist. Health food stores and co-op groceries are places where holistic doctors and alternative practitioners often post their cards.

You can also use the Internet to locate holistically oriented physicians. Search for physician members of the American Holistic Medical Association at its website (www.holisticmedicine.org). These doctors practice the philosophy of dealing with the whole person. When you work with a holistic physician, she'll spend a lot of time exploring how the various factors in your life contributed to your current health condition. What you've been reading throughout *The Triple Whammy Cure* is my own holistic approach to a challenge many of my patients faced.

Members of the American College for the Advancement of Medicine (www.acam.org) may not be any less holistic in their practice philosophies, but are very oriented toward the latest advances in nutritional medicine and innovative therapies on subjects such as antiaging, natural hormone replacement, and memory enhancement.

MOOD DISORDER QUESTIONNAIRE

If you answer "yes" to seven or more in the first section, "yes" to the second question, and "moderate or serious" to the third, share this quiz with your doctor, who will want to evaluate you for bipolar disorder.

                                                        YES   NO

1. Has there ever been a period of time when you were not
your usual self and . . .

YES   NO

... you felt so good or so hyper that other people thought you were not your normal self or you were so hyper that you got into trouble?

... you were so irritable that you shouted at people or started fights or arguments?

... you felt much more self-confident than usual?

... you got much less sleep than usual and found you didn't really miss it?

... you were much more talkative or spoke much faster than usual?

... thoughts raced through your head or you couldn't slow your mind down?

... you were so easily distracted by things around you that you had trouble concentrating or staying on track?

... you had much more energy than usual?

... you were much more active or did many more things than usual?

... you were much more social or outgoing than usual—for example, you telephoned friends in the middle of the night?

... you were much more interested in sex than usual?

... you did things that were unusual for you or that other people might have thought were excessive, foolish, or risky?

... spending money got you or your family into trouble?

2. If you checked "Yes" to more than one of the above, have several of these ever happened during the same period of time?

3. How much of a problem did any of these cause you—like being unable to work; having family, money or legal troubles; getting into arguments or fights? *Please circle one response only.*

No problem   Minor problem   Moderate problem   Serious problem

4. Have any of your blood relatives (i.e., children, siblings, parents, grandparents, aunts, uncles) had manic-depressive illness or bipolar disorder?

5. Has a health professional ever told you that you have manic-depressive illness or bipolar disorder?

NOTES

A WORD ABOUT CLINICAL STUDIES

Almost every day, a patient hands me some new information about the effectiveness, or lack thereof, of a nutritional supplement. Sometimes this is a clinical study, in which a seemingly unbiased researcher wants to publish what she feels is important data. Other times, it's really only somebody's opinion, like "Dr. Jones' Monthly Health Newsletter" reporting that the Chinese herb she happens to be selling is "the new Viagra."

I'd like to think that clinical studies are less biased than Dr. Jones' newsletter, performed with the underlying idea that the results of the study will make absolutely no difference to the researcher. Alas, even conventional medicine is haunted by the fact that often this is not the case. A physician-researcher receiving several million dollars from a drug company knows in her heart that the outcome of the project will affect the renewal of her grant.

Not surprisingly (to me, anyway), most clinical studies performed in the United States to evaluate nutritional products seem to report a large number of "negative" outcomes—mainly "no more effective than placebo." When I examine many of these, I find flaws in the study itself. This may include poor selection of patients, low dosing of a questionable product, and conflicts of interest (should a study on St. John's wort for depression really be funded by the maker of a pharmaceutical antidepressant?)

Finding objective studies in herbal medicine is not that difficult. American physicians should regularly read reports from Europe, especially those performed under the auspices of Germany's Commission E, an institution comparable to our Food and Drug Administration (FDA). For myself, I take with a large grain of salt most U.S. studies that disprove the effectiveness of an herb that has been used abroad with good results for years. To this, of course, I'll add my own clinical experience with thousands of patients over many years.

A critic of the studies listed here might reasonably argue that I've weighted my selection toward positive results rather than negative ones. I wouldn't argue. For every positive study, somewhere you can usually find another that disproves it. My point in listing these studies at all is that there's plenty of evidence in medical literature for the recommendations I make throughout *The Triple Whammy Cure.*

3   *Women are poorly protected against the ravages of stress on their bodies because they have less available serotonin:* Bignall, J., "Serotonin synthesis is depressed in women," *The Lancet,* 24 May 1997, 349:1525.

20   *Because nutritional supplements are generally safe:* The main source for a phrase like "nutritional supplements are safe" comes from the fact that they're all classified as foods rather than "drugs" by the FDA. Regarding every herb mentioned . . . these have been individually evaluated by Germany's Commission E, an institution comparable to our FDA. The vitamins have been available for decades.

20   *A February, 2005, study in the* British Medical Journal: "St. John's wort is effective for moderate to severe depression," *British Medical Journal,* 5 March 2005, 330:503; and doi:10.1136/bmj.38356.655266.82 (published 11 February 2005).

Acute treatment of moderate to severe depression with hypericum extract WS 5570 (St. John's wort): randomised controlled double blind noninferiority trial versus paroxetine. Szegedi, A., managing senior physician, Kohnen, R., head of scientific affairs, Dienel, A., head of clinical trials department, Kieser, M., head of biometry department.

21   *A study published a year and a half ago proved that stubborn hot flashes:* Loprinzi, C.L., et al., "Phase III evaluation of fluoxetine for treatment of hot flashes." *Journal of Clinical Oncology,* March 2002, 20(6):1578–1583.

50   *Although the exact mechanism of production isn't known:* Edwards, R., et al., "Omega-3 polyunsaturated fatty acid levels in the diet and in red blood cell membranes of depressed patients." *Journal of Affective Disorders,* 1 March 1998, 48(2-3):149–155.

54   *In a concentration of at least 400 mg per ounce:* The dose itself is not 400 mg. It's 400 mg per ounce. However, the dosing of progesterone is very confusing, mainly because of the variety of forms it's available in. I recommend conservative doses. The main side effects are skin irritation (obviously from the cream) and drowsiness (from the capsule). Some good studies are: Key, W., Jr., "Medical treatment of PMS," in *Canadian Journal of Psychiatry,* 1985, 30:483–487; Martorano, J., "Differentiating between natural progesterone and synthetic progesterone: clinical implications for PMS." *Comprehensive Therapeutics,* 1993, 19(3):96–98.

An interesting but decidedly biased and not particularly objective (in favor) summary of the clinical uses of natural progesterone. The late Dr. Lee also wrote the extremely popular "What Your Doctor Won't Tell You About Menopause": Lee, J., in *Natural Progesterone: The Multiple Roles of a Remarkable Hormone,* Sebastopol, CA: Bill Publishing, 1995.

The safety of natural progesterone: Hargrove, J.T., "An alternative method of hormone replacement therapy using natural sex steroids." *Infertility and Reproductive Clinics of North America*, 1995, 6:653–674

56 *SAMe as an antidepressant:* Bressa, G.M., "S-adenosyl methionine (SAMe) as antidepressant: meta-analysis of clinical studies." *Acta Neurologica Scandinavia*, 1994, 154 (supp.):714.

56 *Combining serotonin boosters:* There are no studies that I am aware of on 5HTP, St. John's wort, and SAMe interactions. Nutrition-oriented doctors have been using them together for years.

64 *There are no known interaction problems between chasteberry:* I doubt if anyone has ever run a formal study on this. The reason I say "no known interaction" is that they affect different body systems and are metabolized differently.

65 *Valerian:* Leatherwood, P.D., "Aqueous extract of valerian root improves sleep quality in man." *Planta Med*, 1985, 51:144–48;

Lindahl, O., "Double blind study of valerian preparation." *Pharmacol Biochem Behav*, 1989, 32:1065–1066

82 *The exercise will raise your serotonin:* Dunn, A.L., et al., "Exercise Treatment for Depression Efficacy and Dose Response," *American Journal of Preventive Medicine*, 2005, 28(1):1–8.

123 *Take, for example:* There are different opinions and interpretations of the WHI data. This was really the first study that showed increased breast cancer. Most of the previous studies had no such risk (except for one Swedish study a decade earlier). In addition, the risk for an individual woman to develop cancer while taking HRT is still exceedingly small. Current debate now centers around the idea that the synthetic progesterone may have increased the risk. An arm of the study that is testing estrogen only for woman who have had hysterectomies is still underway.

126 *Finally taking a serious look at herbal remedies:* More articles are appearing in the conventional literature. Some are showing effectiveness. "St. John's wort is effective for moderate to severe depression," *British Medical Journal*, 5 March 2005, 330:503; doi:10.1136/bmj.38356.655266.82 (published 11 February 2005)—and others less so. In the latter category, a recent and highly publicized article in the *New England Journal of Medicine* disproved the usefulness of Echinacea when treating the common cold. But even this study has been criticized by herbalists because doses used were below those of World Health Organization's recommendations: Turner, R.B., et al., "An Evaluation of Echinacea angustifolia in Experimental Rhinovirus Infections," *New England Journal of Medicine*, July 28, 2005; 353:341-348

126 *Solid clinical research studies have shown that this herb:* Osmers, R., et al., "Efficacy and safety of isopropanolic black cohosh extract for climacteric symptoms," *Obstetrics & Gynecology*, May 2005, 105:1074–1083 © 2005 by The American College of Obstetricians and Gynecologists.

130 *But we who work with bioidentical hormones:* There are formal studies using estriol, with very good results: Tzingounis, V., "Estriol in the management of
menopause," *JAMA*, 1978, 239: 1638–1641; Wren B., "Oestriol in the control of
postmenopausal symptoms," *Med J Australia* 1982; 1: 176–77.

One researcher has shown that the combination of estriol with estradiol (the
standard blend in (bioidentical hormones) reduces breast cancer risks:

Lemon, H., "Pathophysiologic considerations in the treatment of menopausal
patients with estrogens: the role of estriol in the prevention of mammary carci-
noma," *Acta Endocrinologica,* 1980, 233:217–227.

The micronized oral progesterone is added to natural HRT as the standard protection to prevent overstimulation of the uterus and risk of uterine cancer (like the
'Pro" of "Prempro").

157 *Chasteberry is by far the single most important:* Lauritzen, C., "Treatment of premenstrual tension syndrome with Vitex agnus-castus. Controlled, double blind
study versus pyridoxine." *Phytomed,* 1997, 4(3):183–189 Sliutz G., "Agnus castus
extracts inhibit prolactin secretion in rat pituitary cells," *Horm Metab Res,* 1993,
25:253-255

157 *Nothing in all of conventional medicine has been found to work as well:* This is from
an impressive German study surveyed 1,542 women treated for up to 16 years. 92
percent reported either very good, good, or satisfactory. 1.1 percent discontinued
from side effects. Nothing in conventional medicine matches this.

Chasteberry: Dittmar, F., "Premenstrual Syndrome," *Jiatros Gynakologie,*
1989, 5(6):4–7

174 *Valerian. More than two hundred scientific studies attest to its value:* Valerian.
Leatherwood, P.D., "Aqueous extract of valerian root improves sleep quality in
man." *Planta Med,* 1985, 51:144–48; Lindahl, O., "Double blind study of valerian
preparation." *Pharmacol Biochem Behav,* 1989, 32:1065–1066

279 *Given that statistical data has actually proven homeopathic therapies useful in certain:* Overall, homeopathic data are fraught with controversy. Studies have shown,
for example, that a homeopathic nasal spray was as effective as cromolyn for reducing hay fever symptoms. Vertigoheel, a homeopathic blend for vertigo, was
better than placebo. Conventional doctors with an axe to going will find flaws in
positive studies and praise those that show homeopathy is no better than a
placebo. "Are the Clinical Effects of Homeopathy Placebo Effects? A Meta-Analysis of Placebo-Controlled Trials," Linde, Klaus, et al, *The Lancet,* September 20,
1997:350:834-843

INDEX

ABOUT THE AUTHORS

DAVID EDELBERG, MD, has a long-standing interest in chronic illnesses that have eluded conventional treatment and has been a practicing physician for more than thirty years. From the mid-1970s to the early 1990s, Dr. Edelberg was medical director of Health First, Chicago's largest privately held group of primary care clinics. In 1993, he founded American WholeHealth (AWH), a network of health care centers specializing in integrative care, an approach that combines the best of conventional and alternative medicine. Dr. Edelberg is senior staff clinician at one of six such centers, WholeHealthChicago Lincoln Park.

Dr. Edelberg was chief medical adviser of WholeHealthMD.com, AWH's website. He has written extensively on complementary and alternative medicine in books and articles for the general public and also for physicians considering career changes into integrative medicine. He teaches alternative and integrative medicine to medical students and residents from the University of Chicago, usually providing their first exposure to alternative medicine. He is also assistant professor of medicine at Rush Medical College.

Dr. Edelberg is on the Rodale Medical Advisory Board, has served on the board of the American Holistic Association, and is president of the board of Facets Multimedia, a not-for-profit center of art and foreign film in Chicago, where he lives with his wife and two sons. Be sure to visit Dr. Edelberg's website: www.triplewhammycure.com.

HEIDI HOUGH was editorial director of the American Medical Association Consumer Publishing Division for twelve years, where she directed the development of thirty consumer books, including the best-selling *AMA Family Medical Guide*, the *AMA Encyclopedia of Medicine*, the James Beard Award–winning *AMA Family Cookbook*, and the nineteen-volume *AMA Home Medical Library*.

In conjunction with the Stonesong Press, Simon & Schuster, and the physicians at the Harvard Medical School, she helped to conceive, write, and edit the *Harvard Medical School Family Health Guide*. She has also worked with Reader's Digest Books and the Web-based www.wired.MD, which produces digital health care information. Ms. Hough, who has a deep interest in alternative therapies, lives in Chicago.